Understanding Pregnancy and Childbirth

Understanding Pregnancy and Childbirth

FOURTH EDITION

Sheldon H. Cherry, M.D.
Douglas G. Moss, M.D.

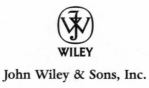

WILEY

John Wiley & Sons, Inc.

Published by John Wiley & Sons, Inc., Hoboken, New Jersey
Published simultaneously in Canada

For general information about our other products and services, please contact our Customer Care Department within the United States at (800) 762-2974, outside the United States at (317) 572-3993 or fax (317) 572-4002.

Wiley also publishes its books in a variety of electronic formats. Some content that appears in print may not be available in electronic books. For more information about Wiley products, visit our web site at www.wiley.com.

Library of Congress Cataloging-in-Publication Data:

Cherry, Sheldon H.
    Understanding pregnancy and childbirth / Sheldon H. Cherry,
    Douglas G. Moss—4th ed.
        p.   cm.
    Includes bibliographical references and index.
    ISBN 0-471-47120-8 (paper)
    1. Pregnancy. 2. Childbirth. I. Moss, Douglas G. II. Title.
RG525.C615   2004
618.2—dc22
                                                     2004040905

Printed in the United States of America
10 9 8 7 6 5 4 3 2

To our wives

Contents

Foreword to First Edition

IN SIMPLER TIMES, an aura of security and even sanctity surrounded the physician and instilled in patients great confidence in the doctor's authority, optimism about treatment, and a bond of mutual respect born of having lived through moments of stress together. This era encouraged the physician to be authoritative and even paternalistic in relations with patients, for all too often the doctor saw this demeanor as a critical means of psychoemotional support when the treatment offered had only pragmatic evidence of value, without substantial scientific support.

In the sophisticated urban and suburban society that is now the environment in which most of our population lives and works, this security about health matters is needed more than ever, but it can no longer be derived solely from the physician's image as a healer. Even obstetricians, who were more frequently the objects of their patients' devotion and love, because they shared with patients and supported them in one of the most profound emotional experiences of their lives—the dramatic, romantic moment of childbirth—have found themselves cast more often now in the role of teacher than that of medicine man. And this is appropriate in an era when the explosion in biological knowledge has been translated into a new understanding of intrauterine fetal life, complex clinical techniques, and electronic instruments that have vastly improved the comfort and the safety of pregnancy and childbirth.

With this new, more scientific approach to the health of mother and infant has come a concomitant rise in the expectation that the obstetrician and associated health workers will inform and translate, simplify, and explain pregnancy and childbirth and other reproductive phenomena in a manner suitable to a more educated generation that derives its security from knowledge, rather than from mystique. With every issue of the public press suggesting new medical advances, the patient demands that her physician, and most especially her obstetrician, concerned now with two patients, act not only as confidant but also as guide through the maze of genuine and spurious discoveries so that wise choices can be made between the scientific and the cultist.

Dr. Cherry's updated *Understanding Pregnancy and Childbirth* is a superb presentation of modern obstetrical knowledge, in a style that is a model of comprehension and clarity. He chooses to refrain from adhering to a single school of obstetrical management with the thought that childbirth is best served by an informed partnership between the patient and her obstetrician. This movement to ask people to take some responsibility for their own health can only result in better care for the public and better education for the physician. Information will replace ignorance, skill will replace magic, and the bond of commitment between the patient and her physician will be strengthened. This volume will surely attain the wide readership that its substance deserves and will make a real contribution to the well-being of those readers who wish a clear understanding of the modern obstetrical era.

S. B. GUSBERG, M.D., D.SCI.,
Distinguished Service Professor,
Department of Obstetrics and Gynecology,
Mount Sinai School of Medicine,
New York, N.Y.

Preface to Fourth Edition

THE FIRST EDITION OF *Understanding Pregnancy and Childbirth* was published in 1973. Since then, a whole generation of women has completed healthy pregnancies by proactively participating in their health care and learning about the glorious and wondrous process of childbearing. In keeping with this tradition, the fourth edition of our book is dedicated to the offspring of the readers of the early editions, who will now be educating themselves on the miraculous process of childbirth. As it did with their parents, this knowledge can help dispel the myths, eliminate fear and confusion, and aid them in having a successful and enjoyable pregnancy.

Since the third edition of *Understanding Pregnancy and Childbirth*, published ten years ago, many major changes have occurred in the management of pregnancy and childbirth. In addition, there have been revolutionary developments in infertility management and treatment. Most couples can now achieve successful fertility by the use of assisted-reproduction techniques. These changes have been incorporated into the fourth edition.

We have expanded on the concept of the fetus as a second patient, both diagnostically and therapeutically. In addition, we are more able to prepare women for pregnancy and have enhanced their comfort, health, and social well-being. There are major revisions of some chapters. A few of the highlights are as follows:

1. An update on preconception care, including genetic testing and vaccination programs
2. The new guidelines for exercise in pregnancy
3. The treatment of infertility, including sex selection, ovum donation, preimplantation genetic studies, and ovum donation IVF
4. A new section on male infertility, including sperm-ovum injection (intracytoplasmic sperm injection)

5. The nonsurgical management of ectopic pregnancy with methotrexate
6. A prenatal testing update, including AFP testing and first trimester sonogram screening
7. Advancements in the induction of labor
8. A new section on depression and the psychosocial aspects of pregnancy
9. Advancements in the management of pregnancy conditions, such as intrauterine growth retardation, prematurity, postdate pregnancy, premature rupture of membranes, and herpes infections
10. New advances in contraception, such as the morning-after pill
11. Abortion update, including medical abortion
12. An update on the management of multiple births, medications during pregnancy, diet and nutrition, and the walking epidural

For this edition I was assisted by Dr. Douglas Moss, a sensitive, bright obstetrician who represents the new generation of physicians in women's health care and who is my colleague in private practice. We welcome you to the amazing process of pregnancy. Your nine-month journey to parenthood should be one of excitement, awe, knowledge, and fulfillment. We hope to help you achieve these goals.

Introduction

CHILDBIRTH, that most natural yet most awesome experience, has in the past been cloaked in superstition and cultural mystique. These beliefs arose over the years to fill the vacuum created by a great deal of scientific ignorance about human reproduction. They have added a supernatural and almost fatalistic aura to the regeneration of the human species, a process that is so much more than a biological occurrence.

Expectant parents of past generations accepted the folktales of childbirth that were passed on from generation to generation, modifying them slightly as new facts about human reproduction have become known. They accepted the perfunctory explanations given in answer to their questions by doctors who doubted their patients' ability to understand.

In the recent past, however, obstetrical care has been changing. The amount of new medical information about childbirth has revolutionized obstetrical practice. While doctors still do not know all the answers to such questions as how two basic cell lines from each parent combine and form skin, blood, hair, muscles, and so many different human systems, they have learned how to tell the sex of the unborn child, how to detect certain development problems during gestation, and, in some cases, how to treat these problems. Young educated adults, who are learning about some of these medical developments in their college science courses, are beginning to demand of their doctors more information about the basic biological aspects of pregnancy.

This book is designed to accommodate these two forces—a great deal of new knowledge and an increasing demand for information—which have come together at this point in time. It includes material never before published in a handbook for parents, in addition to routine and important information about pregnancy, such as diagnosis, hygiene, diet, and physical annoyances.

This book will give you specific information about how the fetus develops. The labor and delivery chapter describes much more

1

than signs of labor: It discusses the whole process of labor as an adaptation between mother and baby; it describes the stages of labor, which many women have never heard of before; and it details the popular Lamaze method of natural childbirth.

Chapter 6 discusses the conditions of pregnancy and attempts to explain such occurrences as miscarriage and tubal pregnancies, so that mothers-to-be can intelligently understand the basic pregnancy process, its alterations, and the risks involved in the common "danger signs of pregnancy." It explains amniocentesis and the analysis of amniotic fluid for abnormalities in pregnant women over thirty-five, since birth defects increase as women approach the end of their childbearing years.

We have included a chapter on chemical and environmental effects on pregnancy, which explains, in part, the effect on the fetus of drugs taken during gestation.

There is also a complete review of contraceptive practice—a subject that may not be of interest to you now but will be after the birth of the baby—as well as a discussion of abortion and the changing laws in this country.

All this information is presented for one purpose: to make childbirth a less mysterious and frightening occurrence, through education. The book holds to no particular dogma. All the current trends in childbirth are discussed, such as breast-feeding and natural birth, complete with appended instructions. But all information is given in the context of every option available to the mother and should be used in conjunction with advice from your physician.

Many women shy away from the explicit approach we have used in this complete handbook to modern pregnancy. They do so on the misconception that knowledge detracts from the intuitive beauty of childbirth. This need not be the case. Our patients tell us over and over how much easier and more enjoyable birth is when they know what to expect. Just the difference between thinking of labor as one continuous pain and knowing that a single contraction cannot last longer than ninety seconds means the difference between approaching labor as an unbearable, frightening experience and seeing it as a manageable, exciting one. Such knowledge makes the mother a participant in, rather than a victim of, reproduction.

Part I

PLANNING FOR PREGNANCY

Chapter 1
Planning for Pregnancy

——⚮——

SOMETHING AS NATURAL as being able to have a baby cannot be taken for granted. Planning ahead for childbirth is important. The body cannot be expected to perform on demand without preparation. In the same way that an athlete strengthens her body to run a grueling marathon with a plan of gradual physical training, a woman can ready her body so that pregnancy will be as comfortable and healthy as possible. Women are starting to recognize that planning ahead and preserving fertility are important. Older women facing a first pregnancy often ask us about the possible effects of a long-ago abortion or an infection. Concern and even fear are common.

Women are having children later in life. The number of births in general is going up, rising 3 percent in the year 2000. Fertility rates have increased by 1 to 2 percent, and there has been an increase in the number of twin pregnancies, reflecting the new reproductive technologies. There has been a rise in the birthrate among thirty- to forty-five-year-old women—women who were once thought to be beyond childbearing years. Births to women in their forties to early fifties were up again in the year 2000. The reason for this is twofold: Women are marrying later and waiting to have children until their educations are completed and their careers established; in addition, 37 million of the postwar babies, the so-called baby boomers, are now older women, whose sheer numbers add clout to any changes that they as a group decide upon. Also, affluence affords many older women access to the advances of reproductive technologies, giving them an opportunity to bear children later in life. In the past, this was not possible.

In these times of women having children later, it has become even more important for you to take care of yourself at an early age. Active participation in your health and well-being is important to maintain fertility later in your life. In our complex society, many factors may affect your future childbearing. They include environmental hazards such as X rays; chemical pollutants in air, water, and food; smoking; and exposure to prescription and nonprescription drugs. Exposure to various illnesses such as rubella and toxoplasmosis can harm a developing fetus. By being informed, you can avoid many potential threats and minimize the impact of possible dangers.

The information in this chapter is intended to give you the best possible chance of having a healthy baby. We will discuss such diverse important areas as genetics, medical history, work environment, medications, eating, and exercises. Planning ahead for a healthy child will help you protect your fertility until the time is right for childbearing and will help you prepare your body and mind once you are ready for pregnancy. Planning ahead will help you get pregnant and help get your baby off to a healthy head start. Years ago not many women thought of having a baby after age thirty-five, but twenty years ago women didn't run twenty-six-mile marathons either. With the right knowledge, the right game plan, and the right care and training, both marathons and healthy pregnancies have become a reality for more women today than ever before.

PRECONCEPTIONAL CARE

Before you become pregnant or stop using birth control, you can begin to maintain a healthy lifestyle, which will help you have a healthier baby and a healthier pregnancy. This includes eating right, exercising, and avoiding alcohol, cigarettes, and exposure to harmful drugs and chemicals. Early medical care and a checkup are also important. All this is part of preconceptional, or prepregnancy, care, ensuring your good health before you become pregnant. Many women do not know they are pregnant until five, six, or even eight weeks after they have conceived. Those early weeks may be some of the most important for the baby because during that time the organs form. Certain substances, such as alcohol, tobacco, chemicals, and some medications, can interfere with that growth. Likewise, medical conditions such as diabetes or high blood pressure should be under special supervision before a woman becomes pregnant.

You should discuss your plans for pregnancy with your doctor. This provides a chance for you to get advice on any questions or concerns you might have. A doctor may also offer suggestions based on your special needs. Women with diagnosed medical problems such as diabetes and anemia have an even greater need for accurate medical advice prior to pregnancy. Find out exactly what the risks are to you and your unborn child, what you can do to reduce them, and what choices you face for risks that can't be entirely predicted or controlled.

Components of Preconceptional Care

The main components of preconceptional care are the same as those of prenatal care: assessing risk factors, promoting good health, and obtaining any necessary medical and psychosocial treatment. The anchor of all other preconceptional care activities is a comprehensive assessment of the risk you and your family carry for a poor pregnancy. You and your doctor can conduct such a comprehensive risk assessment during a special preconceptional visit or as part of a visit for other purposes. It consists of a complete history, a physical exam, and some laboratory tests. You and your physician will both review your health status, identifying any risks for a poor pregnancy outcome, and produce a plan to reduce those risks, revising it later if necessary.

In addition, you should undertake activities designed to promote good health in general. Table 1.1 lists the factors the Expert Panel on the Content of Prenatal Care identified as being important in evaluating preconceptional health. Table 1.2 lists the laboratory tests that may be valuable.

Your doctor evaluates preconceptional care and recommends tests based on their potential to improve not only your health but that of your future child as well. Some tests are of little value to you before pregnancy but are important after conception. (They will be discussed in chapter 7.) Others are valuable during the early first trimester of pregnancy, but since many women do not have prenatal care until the second trimester, those should be performed at the preconception visit. For example, such risks as susceptibility to rubella should be identified prior to pregnancy. Your physician can guide you as to which laboratory tests are important for you.

Infectious Risks

When an infection occurs, for the most part, pregnant women have a normal immune system. While some infectious conditions may have only minor or no effects on a pregnant woman, the effects on the fetus can be devastating. Conversely, potentially serious infections may have little or no effect on the fetus.

HIV/AIDS

Frequency of HIV—human immunodeficiency virus—infection among women varies greatly among different population groups. Heterosexual women represent the fastest-growing group of newly diagnosed HIV-positive cases. Although recent studies have shown a decline in the incidence of HIV in high-risk populations, such as those who use IV drugs, identification of HIV-positive pregnant women has become

TABLE 1.1
Preconceptional Risk Assessment:
History and Physical Examination

Medical Factors
  Sociodemographic data
  Menstrual history
  Past obstetric history
  Contraceptive history
  Sexual history
  Medical/surgical history
  Infection history
  Family and genetic history
  Nutrition

Physical Examination
  General physical examination
  Blood pressure/pulse
  Height
  Weight
  Height/weight profile
  Pelvic examination and
    gynecologic examination
  Breast examination

Psychosocial Factors
  Smoking
  Alcohol
  Drugs
  Social support
  Stress levels
  Physical abuse
  Mental illness status
  Pregnancy readiness
  Exposure to teratogens
    (drugs producing fetal
    abnormalities)
  Housing, finances, and so on
  Extremes of physical work,
    exercise, and other activities

SOURCE: *Caring for Our Future: The Content of Prenatal Care,* a report of the Public Health Service Expert Panel on the Content of Prenatal Care (Department of Health and Human Services, 1989).

extremely important. In 2001 the U.S. Public Health Service updated the 1995 guidelines for routine AIDS counseling and voluntary testing of all pregnant women. It is now customary at your first prenatal visit for your obstetrician to request a test for the AIDS virus. The reason for this is twofold. First, HIV-positive women are at risk for many different infections, which could put their lives and the lives of their unborn children at risk, and there are now treatments that can minimize the risk of developing such infections. Second, medicines, such as zidovudine (ZDV), have been developed that can fight the AIDS virus. ZDV can be administered to women before and during labor and can be given to babies after birth to prevent children from developing this disease. In recent studies, HIV-positive women were treated with ZDV before delivery, and the babies were given ZDV after birth. As a result, the chance of a baby developing AIDS was reduced to less than 3 percent. Having a C-section, instead of a vaginal delivery, may also reduce the risk of transmitting the virus to the baby. Given this

TABLE 1.2
Preconceptional Risk Assessment:
Laboratory Tests

Hemoglobin or hematocrit	Hepatitis B
Rh factor	Toxoplasmosis
Rubella titer	CMV (Cytomegalovirus)
Urine: protein, sugar	Herpes simplex
Pap smear	Varicella
Tuberculosis screen	AIDS (HIV) test
Gonococcal culture	Genetic tests: Tay-Sachs, sickle cell,
Chlamydia culture	parental karyotype
Syphilis test	Illicit-drug screen

SOURCE: *Caring for Our Future: The Content of Prenatal Care*, a report of the Public Health Service Expert Panel on the Content of Prenatal Care (Department of Health and Human Services, 1989).

new therapy, pregnancies may be safer in this expanding population of patients with AIDS.

Hepatitis B (HB) and Hepatitis C (HC)

About 0.3 percent of all adults in the United States are chronic hepatitis B carriers. Approximately 300,000 new cases of HB occur annually. Acute HB occurs in 1 to 2 per 1,000 pregnancies, and chronic HB occurs in 5 to 15 of every 1,000 pregnancies. An estimated 18,500 births occur among these women annually. Without the HB vaccine, approximately 4,300 newborns would acquire HB infection from these women each year. Unless treated, about 1 percent of infected infants will develop a fatal infection, and 85 percent to 90 percent will become chronic HB carriers.

To prevent newborn HB infection, doctors must first recognize the mother's infection. Then they can immunize and administer HB immune globulin promptly after delivery. Screening during pregnancy can identify positive cases.

Women at substantial risk of having or acquiring the HB virus include those who have had sexual contact with HB-infected partners, users of illicit injectable drugs, prostitutes, institutionalized women, those with tattoos, and certain immigrant groups, including Southeast Asians. Those with an ongoing risk of acquiring HB infection should have a preventive vaccination.

HB screening is now legally required of all pregnant women in many states. It makes sense to obtain a screening prior to pregnancy.

Hepatitis C (HC) appears to affect as much as 0.6 percent of the pregnant population, and the risk factors are similar to those for HB. Unlike HB, there is no vaccine to prevent infection and no treatment to offer pregnant women to reduce the risk of transmission to the baby. Pregnant women with HC should not breast-feed because there is a 2 to 3 percent risk that the virus can be transmitted this way. Approximately 7 to 8 percent of pregnant women with HC will produce offspring with HC infection.

Rubella (German Measles)

A pregnant woman infected with German measles, particularly during the first sixteen weeks, risks spontaneous abortion, stillbirth, or a baby with congenital rubella syndrome. The incidence of congenital rubella has declined by more than 99 percent since 1969, the year the rubella vaccine was licensed.

All women should be tested for rubella immunity. If you had rubella as a child, you are not necessarily immune as an adult, so routine susceptibility testing should be conducted. Most studies carried out during the early 1980s found that 10 to 20 percent of women of childbearing age had no immunity to rubella. Women considered susceptible to rubella should receive the vaccination prior to conception and then avoid pregnancy for three months. Should conception occur soon after vaccination, however, there is not a great risk of infection from the vaccination.

Toxoplasmosis

Toxoplasmosis is an infection caused by a one-cell parasite named *toxoplasma gondii*. It can be found in the feces of infected cats and in raw or uncooked meats. Foods that are in contact with these contaminated meats can also be infected. It is not found in raw fish, so fear not, sushi lovers!

About one-third of adult women in the United States have antibodies to toxoplasmosis; the remainder may be at risk for a primary infection during pregnancy, which can result in fetal infection. If a pregnant woman is infected during the first or the second trimester, chances are greater that the fetus will be severely affected than if the woman is infected during the third trimester. Although earlier exposure in the pregnancy has more severe consequences, the actual risk of fetal infection is much less in the earlier trimesters.

If preconceptional testing shows that you lack immunity, you should be advised about the proper cooking of meat and during pregnancy avoid close contact with cats, cat litter, or soil that may contain cat feces.

Acute infection in an adult is often subtle. Symptoms, when present, generally are nonspecific and include fatigue, swollen glands, and fever.

If symptoms develop during pregnancy, prior testing can help your physician identify whether an acute infection is due to toxoplasmosis. If repeated testing during pregnancy shows the presence of toxoplasmosis antibodies in a woman who previously had negative antibodies, then acute infection is indicated. In the absence of such prior information, the interpretation of tests obtained during pregnancy may be confusing. Labs in the United States can now pinpoint the time of exposure to the parasite quite accurately, so that women can be adequately advised. Screening of those women who own or have regular contact with cats, especially outdoor cats, is very important. Probably all women considering pregnancy should be screened.

Fifth Disease

Fifth disease is usually a childhood illness caused by a virus named parvovirus B19. Children who get infected have a rather mild illness, characterized by very red cheeks (slapped cheeks), and they completely recover. Adults who get exposed to this virus often have no symptoms at all. Most adults already are immune to this virus (over 60 percent) and therefore need not worry. When outbreaks of this virus occur (usually in the spring), around 50 percent of people who are exposed and not immune will catch this virus. Typically, the virus can be transmitted five to ten days before the appearance of the rash. If pregnant women were to seroconvert (become infected with parvovirus B19), up to one-third of them would infect the fetus, according to some studies. If fetal infection occurs, there is a small risk of fetal loss (2 to 9 percent), and it may cause a condition known as hydrops fetalis. Long-term development appears to be normal in the fetuses with congenital parvovirus when the fetus does survive. Your doctor has blood tests available that can check your immunity to this virus, should you be exposed, and can test to see if you have become infected.

Varicella Zoster Virus (Chicken Pox)

Most women of childbearing age are immune to chicken pox. Infection during pregnancy is quite rare (0.4 to 0.7 per 1,000 women). If a nonimmune pregnant woman develops chicken pox within the first half of her pregnancy, there is a small risk of major birth defects (around 2 percent). However, if a pregnant woman develops chicken pox from five days before delivery to two days after delivery, there is a very high risk of neonatal death due to neonatal infection. Therefore, women who are not immune to chicken pox should strongly consider receiving the vaccination prior to pregnancy. (This is a live virus vaccine and cannot be given to pregnant women.) If a pregnant woman is not immune, she should avoid contact with those who may be infectious.

Herpes Simplex

There are two types of herpes infections, type 1 and type 2. Although both types can occur along the birth canal, type 2 is more commonly found there. About 45 million adult Americans have been infected with genital herpes, and 1,500 to 2,000 newborns contract a herpes infection each year. Newborns who develop a herpes infection usually get infected while traveling through an infected birth canal. The newborns can get a localized infection of the skin, the eyes, and the mouth; an infection of the central nervous system; or an infection throughout the entire body. With a localized infection, there is no risk to the baby, but if the nervous system is infected, 15 percent of babies can die. If there is a generalized infection, 57 percent can die. The biggest risk to the baby occurs when the mother develops her very first outbreak (primary herpes) at the time of delivery. Some studies show that the baby can then get infected 50 percent of the time. For recurrent infections, the risk is substantially less, at around 0 to 3 percent. Because the risk to the baby is so high, it is generally recommended that if a woman has a clear infection at the time of labor, whether primary or a recurrence, she should have a cesarean section so that the baby avoids contact with the birth canal. Many doctors are now using antiviral agents, such as acyclovir, during the later weeks of pregnancy to reduce herpes recurrences and decrease the risk of needing a cesarean section.

Although uncommon, first-time outbreaks early in the pregnancy may lead to an increase in miscarriages and birth defects.

Other Infectious Diseases

Screening for syphilis, gonorrhea, and chlamydia should be performed as part of general preventive health care. These infections may affect your ability to conceive and may increase the risk for ectopic pregnancy. The routine testing for cytomegalovirus, varicella, and herpes simplex has not yet been recommended by the Expert Panel on the Content of Prenatal Care, but your own physician may want to test for these.

Maternal Medical Disease

Advances in the effectiveness of medical treatment and the greater number of pregnancies in women in their late thirties have resulted in more women with various types of chronic diseases deciding to conceive. It is reported that 15 percent of women may have medical problems at their first prenatal visit. In women over forty years old, 25 percent are often found to have medical conditions that predate the pregnancy.

If you have a preexisting chronic medical condition, preconceptional care should include an assessment of your disease status and an evaluation of the likelihood that pregnancy will affect your health and the medical condition will affect your pregnancy. Your therapy may have to be modified to optimize the pregnancy outcome. For women with certain conditions, this may include advice regarding the timing or the avoidance of pregnancy.

Modifying and identifying a drug treatment before pregnancy can be very important. Harmful drugs should be eliminated whenever possible; some medications may be replaced with alternatives that are safer in pregnancy; and the goals of therapy may be reevaluated in relationship to a pregnancy. These issues must be considered before the pregnancy.

It is impossible to list all the medical conditions of importance to a pregnancy, but some of the more common ones are:

High blood pressure
Chronic kidney disease
AIDS
Diabetes
Alcoholism
Thyroid disease
Anemia
Tuberculosis
Cardiac diseases
Chronic infections
Liver disease
Breast cancer history

Cardiovascular diseases, including chronic hypertension, are the most common chronic conditions among women of childbearing age. Many women have heart murmurs that have not been evaluated. A medical or a cardiological workup in such conditions may be helpful in counseling women regarding the potential impact of a pregnancy upon their health. For some women, corrective surgery may even be advisable before conception. Women who are found to have a congenital cardiac defect may also benefit from genetic counseling.

Depending on the age group, 0.5 to 1.5 percent of women who become pregnant have preexisting *diabetes mellitus.* The children of these women are twice as likely as those of healthy women to have congenital defects. Most of the common congenital malformations in infants of diabetic mothers arise before the seventh week of gestation, so steps to reduce the rate of malformations must be taken before most women seek prenatal care or even recognize they are pregnant. Rigorous control of sugar levels at conception and during the first trimester may reduce such defects.

Special care and counseling diabetics who are planning pregnancy have resulted in significantly lower rates of congenital malformation and of affected newborns. Chronic diabetic women who receive adequate education, counseling, and preparation prior to conception are more likely to participate in controlling their diabetes and achieve a more successful outcome.

Other Medical Conditions

A woman may have a history of a successfully treated medical disease that nonetheless can seriously jeopardize her pregnancy. Special testing and care prior to conception may identify her need to arrange for high-risk care during pregnancy. These diseases include thyroid disease, a history of immune thrombocytopenia, lupus erythematosus, kidney disease, and many others.

Other medical conditions may be screened for and treated as a part of routine health maintenance. For instance, identification and treatment of iron deficiency anemia can be done prior to pregnancy. Screening for tuberculosis may be of benefit in some high-risk groups. A Pap smear and treatment of chronic gynecologic infections are all important health maintenance measures, which will benefit a future pregnancy. The diagnosis of fibroid tumors of the uterus, ovarian cysts, or endometriosis may have potential reproductive effects.

EXERCISE BEFORE PREGNANCY

A strong, fit, healthy body is an essential element in a happy, secure, and psychologically healthy pregnancy. The time to get your fitness level up and your eating habits in line is well before you start trying to get pregnant. A strong body adapts to the physical challenge of pregnancy more easily. A well-nourished body has the nutrient reserves for the developing fetus to draw on: calcium for building bones, iron to manufacture red blood cells, and so on. Once you are pregnant, some of these basic rules will change. Later in the book we will discuss diet and exercise guidelines to follow during pregnancy, but your goal prior to pregnancy should be to get or stay in shape for your own health and the health of your future child.

There are many components of physical fitness, each important in its own right. The three most important are body composition, that is, how much of the body is fat and how much is lean muscle, bone, and water; flexibility, or the degree to which muscles and joints let us bend, stretch, and twist; and cardiovascular or aerobic efficiency, which measures the body's ability to extract oxygen from the air we breathe and speed it via the blood to every cell in the body. Although each aspect of fitness is important to health, you should balance your exercise program to meet your own particular goals.

Getting in Shape

Exercise is appropriate for every woman at every age. It is particularly important for you when contemplating pregnancy. Being overweight at any age takes a health and a psychological toll, but for a woman planning a new pregnancy, it poses additional problems. For one thing, obesity increases the risk of toxemia and diabetes. For another, dieting is not wise during pregnancy since it would deprive the fetus of necessary nutrients. The best plan, then, is to get to a normal weight before pregnancy.

It is difficult to lose weight and keep it off by diet alone. The body seems to sense when you are dieting and lowers its metabolic rate. In other words, when you suddenly start to eat less, the body prepares to wait out a possible famine by slowing down in order to conserve fuel. If, instead of cutting calories to tip the fuel and energy balance in favor of weight loss, you increase the body's need for calories through exercise, the metabolic rate will remain stable and even increase. Therefore, the combination of reducing food intake and increasing activity will produce slow and steady weight loss. The best types of exercise to add to your routine for weight loss are those that expend large amounts of calories. They include cycling, jogging, skiing, swimming, and aerobic dancing—activities that keep a large percentage of the body's muscles working over an extended period of time.

It is difficult to be patient when setting off on a weight-loss plan, but it is important to start up slowly. Joining a health club or an exercise class is an excellent way to get through the critical early stage of an exercise plan. During the first six months, as many as 50 percent of women lose their resolve and drop out. It takes a long time to lose 20 pounds, perhaps six months or even a year, but keep in mind that it is only one year to shed weight that may have accumulated over a period of many years.

Flexibility

Joints and muscles can lose flexibility with age and lack of use, leaving the body stiff and injury prone. Proper stretching can correct and enhance your mobility. Increase flexibility by moving each joint gently, without bouncing, and then stretching it a bit beyond the current limit. This tension should not become painful. Stretching to increase flexibility in any joint can loosen stiff muscles. Tightness in the back, the trunk, and the back of the thigh muscles is associated with back problems, which often worsen during pregnancy due to the added weight of the fetus. To test your flexibility in this area, sit on the floor and slowly reach for your toes, keeping your feet flexed so that the toes point to the ceiling. If there is a gap of more than 2 to 3 inches between your fingertips and your toes, your back muscles need to be stretched. Use this test as an exercise, holding the reach for ten to twenty seconds until you feel the tightness in your back and hamstrings ease.

Aerobic Capacity

The rate at which you can keep steadily running, walking, or bicycling depends on your aerobic fitness. Aerobic fitness is the body's ability to take in, transport, and use oxygen. If exercise is too intense, your body can't supply the oxygen fast enough. It makes up the difference with less efficient anaerobic (without oxygen) metabolism. This produces a substance called lactic acid in the muscles. A large amount of this acid interferes with your muscles' smooth and efficient functioning and may cause cramping pain. The idea is to reach a balance and push the body only to the point at which lactic acid can be whisked away in the blood as quickly as it is produced. Then you can continue to exercise for long periods of time.

Of all the measures of fitness, aerobic capacity is probably the most important. Unlike flexibility or muscle strength itself, the ability to endure an exercise—that is, to jog 2 miles or bike 10—is linked to some of the most important qualities of overall good health. Aerobic exercise can change your cardiovascular system and decrease your risk of heart disease. Regular exercise may cause healthier patterns in your lipoproteins, which are the carriers of fat and cholesterols in the blood. Levels of low-density lipoproteins (LDL) tend to be lower in active people. Lowering LDL has been shown to reduce the risk of heart attacks.

High-density lipoproteins (HDL) protect against coronary artery disease. They seem to remove cholesterol from the tissue, including the inner walls of the blood vessels. Cholesterol left on blood vessels can form plaques that narrow vessels and eventually block the blood supply to the heart. This may cause a heart attack or, if the blood vessel goes to the brain, a stroke. Very active women, such as runners, have been shown to have much higher HDL levels.

Aerobic workouts must be reasonably vigorous, equivalent, say, to at least 10 miles of running per week for at least six months, to have an effect on your cardiovascular system. With aerobic fitness, your blood pressure tends to go down; your heart learns to do more work more efficiently, and your heartbeat slows down. One way of getting to know more about your fitness is to measure your resting pulse rate before you get out of bed. Eighty beats per minute or higher is common for unfit women, whereas sixty beats or lower may occur for a highly trained athlete.

How can you tell if you are aerobically fit right now? One test is to measure how long it takes you to walk or run a mile and a half on level ground. For a young woman, eleven minutes is excellent, fourteen minutes is average, and seventeen minutes is poor. To improve your score, you must train your body to improve its ability to use oxygen.

The "sing-talk method," although not very precise, can also be used to measure how hard you are working out. If you cannot talk without gasping for breath while exercising, you have probably exceeded the target zone. If you can sing while exercising, you are probably not pushing hard enough. In order to achieve a training effect, an aerobic workout should last twenty to thirty minutes and be done at least three times a week. Starting out slowly will minimize the risk of injury as your body adapts to the increased activity.

The intensity, the duration, and the frequency of aerobic exercise should be increased gradually, one component at a time. A day off between workouts is sensible, to minimize stress on the joints and the ligaments. By gradually increasing your capacity, you may be able to exercise daily. Varying your type of workout will relieve parts of the body from continual stress and will create a welcome change of pace for your mind as well. Exercise should feel pleasurably tiring. If it is just pleasant, you are probably not working hard enough. If it is only tiring, you are working too hard. An hour after finishing your workout you should feel good and rested but not exhausted.

A well-rounded exercise program should aim at improving strength and flexibility, as well as aerobic capacity. Muscle building, calisthenics, or weight lifting can be added to strengthen parts of the body neglected by your choice of aerobic exercise. This may include the abdominal and the upper-body muscles. You might alternate days of aerobic workouts with days of strength training. Whether done alone or as part of a longer workout, the aerobic segment should begin with a warm-up and be followed by a cool down.

There is an additional advantage to regular exercise, besides enhancing cardiovascular health and making weight control easier. Getting in shape can improve your psychological well-being. Regular exercisers feel better about themselves in general, and many report finding relief from tension, anxiety, and depression. These good feelings of mental and physical health often encourage us to improve other habits as well—eating better, sleeping more regularly, and cutting down on smoking and on alcohol and drug use. The goal of complete fitness is to strengthen your muscles and increase your endurance so that your body, on command, can walk to the store, play three sets of tennis, or carry a baby with grace and energy to spare.

Pregnancy is quite a bit like a marathon. It is physically demanding, takes a long time to complete, and requires that you have a last burst of energy in reserve for getting over the finish line. Fortunately, you don't have to be in marathon form for pregnancy, but being in shape and having strength, stamina, and a feel for your body's responses to physical demands can be a big advantage.

NUTRITION BEFORE PREGNANCY

All of an unborn baby's nutrients come from you, the mother. How well nourished you are at the time of conception seems to play a role in the health of your developing fetus. Studies have shown that if you are well nourished and have a balanced diet when you conceive, you are more likely to give birth to a healthy baby.

A balanced diet is basic for good health at all times in your life, but especially before and during pregnancy. Eating wisely means choosing your meals from four basic food groups. In general, you will be well nourished if you eat plenty of fresh fruit, vegetables, and whole grain products, as well as two servings a day of meat, fish, poultry, or other protein food. Calcium, found mostly in milk, cheese, and other dairy products, is also important during pregnancy.

Women who are underweight and subsequently gain little weight during pregnancy are at high risk for fetal and neonatal morbidity and mortality. One recent study found that more than half the infants born to women with a prepregnancy weight of 80 percent or less than standard weight and who gained less than 23 pounds during pregnancy were of low birth weight. At the other extreme, marked obesity is associated with gestational diabetes, hypertension, large infant size, and resultant prolonged and difficult labor. A study done in 2002 demonstrated that women who were obese prior to pregnancy were more likely to gain excessive weight during pregnancy and were, on average, 18 pounds heavier than their prepregnancy weight 6 months after delivery. The optimal weight gain for very obese women during pregnancy is not definitely known. Thus, for both significantly underweight and very obese women, preconception nutritional intervention is highly desirable.

A proper medical assessment of your nutritional status should include an individual and a family history, height and weight measurement, and a discussion of your optimal weight. The history will elicit special diets, food allergies you may have, your habits and attitudes, and your knowledge of proper nutrition. Lactose intolerance may be identified and the adequacy of your dietary calcium intake assessed; lactose enzyme or calcium supplementation may be prescribed if indicated. Women on vegetarian or other special diets should receive nutrition counseling to assure the adequacy of their diet prior to and during pregnancy. Women with preexisting medical conditions, including diabetes, anemia, liver disease, and gastrointestinal disease, may require special diets. Fad diets or unusual dietary practices should be identified and discussed.

A nutritionist may be of help in evaluating and counseling you on the adequacy of your diet for pregnancy. If bulimia, anorexia nervosa, or other emotional problems affecting nutrition are identified, psychiatric counseling as well is important, particularly for women contemplating pregnancy.

Some women may benefit from special nutrition counseling due to their life situation. These include adolescents contemplating repeat pregnancy, women with a low income or a limited food budget, or those without budgeting or cooking skills.

Neural tube defects (NTDs) such as spina bifida may be prevented by early vitamin supplementation, especially with preparations containing folic acid. NTDs are more common among women of lower socioeconomic status and those with dietary histories demonstrating vitamin deficiencies. One recent study demonstrated a rate of NTDs of 3.5 per 1,000 among infants of women who never used multivitamins before or after conception. In contrast, the rate for those who used multivitamins containing folic acid during the first six weeks of pregnancy was 0.9 per 1,000. Note that the neural tube is formed soon after conception, so it is very important to begin taking folic acid while you are trying to conceive. By the time you discover that you're pregnant, the neural tube has mostly formed and it is too late. To date, many studies have proved that folic acid can reduce the risk of this birth defect. How much folic acid should be taken? The average prenatal vitamin has 0.4 mg of folic acid. According to a large study, 0.4 mg of folate will reduce NTDs by 36 percent, whereas 5 mg will reduce the risk by 85 percent. Therefore, either through diet or supplementation, a woman should try to get at least this amount. For those who used multivitamins without folic acid during the first six weeks of pregnancy and those who began using multivitamins with folic acid at seven weeks of pregnancy, the prevalence of NTDs was similar to that among nonusers.

Energy Balance

If you want to gain weight, you have to take in more calories and burn up fewer. If you want to lose weight, you have to take in fewer calories and burn up more. This is easy to say but difficult to translate into everyday practice. Since we eat to satisfy much more than our body's simple need for nutrients, cutting down on eating is in itself no simple task. It is also difficult to determine exactly how many calories your body needs. There is a certain baseline requirement just in being alive. Added to this basic rate is your caloric need to support movement, whether walking up a flight of stairs or running a marathon. But even that doesn't describe the complexity of the calorie in–calorie out balance.

Table 1.3 shows how many calories walking or running uses up, but these numbers are just approximations. Your exact need may vary, depending on many factors: the shape you are in, for instance; what your body's proportion of fat is; how old you are; or how hot it is outside. The only way to know what will work for your body right now is to cut back a bit on calories and see what happens.

What you eat is also critical to your health and well-being. Try to eat a little bit less to lose weight; a mouthful here and there can make an astonishing difference over a month. Of course, if your diet is too high in fats or simple carbohydrates, you should try to bring them into healthier balance as well. As far as weight loss goes, it's the total number of calories that counts. A healthy weight loss is usually no greater than 2 pounds a week. More than that and you are probably

TABLE 1.3
Comparative Table of Calories In/Calories Out

| FOOD | CALORIES | Minutes of Activity Required to Burn Up Calories | | |
		IN WALKING	IN BICYCLING	IN RUNNING
Apple	100	19	12	5
Beer (1 glass)	115	22	14	6
Raw carrot	42	8	5	2
Cottage cheese (1 tbsp.)	27	5	3	1
Ice cream (1/6 pint)	193	37	24	10
Pizza (1 slice)	180	35	22	9
Hamburger	350	67	42	18
Orange	68	13	8	4

SOURCE: Modified from *Complications of Pregnancy,* ed. S. H. Cherry, M.D., and I. Merkatz, M.D. Baltimore, Md.: Williams & Wilkins Co., 1991.

disturbing the body's water balance and excreting water, rather than burning fat. You won't be able to sustain that rate of loss anyway. If you were to eat 500 fewer calories per day and increase the amount of exercise to burn another 500 calories, you would be reducing your total calories by 1,000 a day, or 7,000 a week. That is exactly 2 pounds' worth of calories per week.

As soon as you start to think about getting pregnant, you should plan to first get your body in shape. If you are not sure what a healthy weight is, ask your doctor. Then you can work backward from your planned conception time, following the 2-pounds-a-week rule. Give yourself some leeway so the process can be as relaxed, gradual, and enjoyable as possible. By the time you are ready to get pregnant, you may just be in better shape than ever before.

HAZARDS TO PREGNANCY

Certain hazards to a healthy pregnancy can crop up and affect reproduction. The damage can be done long before you get pregnant. Environmental hazards can damage your eggs, for example; render men sterile; or cause them to produce mutant sperm incapable of fertilization. Such hazards can crop up in what we normally think of as the environment—air, water, and soil—or from things like drugs and X rays that become part of our environment when we get sick. They may arise from things you choose to do, such as smoking, consuming alcohol, drinking excessive amounts of coffee, or using various recreational drugs. They may also come from things you are not aware of or have no direct control over, such as toxic substances in food, water, or air; pesticides; food additives; industrial pollution; and contaminants.

When exposure occurs during pregnancy, the harmful effects vary, depending on the stage of fetal development. Different kinds of damage may occur during the preimplantation period, during the third to twelfth weeks, and after twelve weeks of gestation. Sometimes there may be long-term disabilities in our offspring, such as development of behavioral disorders or cancer, that do not become apparent until later in life. Knowledge of these potential hazards is important in preparing for pregnancy, for some of them will affect your body prior to pregnancy, while others may be hazardous during the early weeks when you may not even know yet that you are pregnant.

Medications That Endanger Pregnancy

Between 1957 and 1962, thousands of people took a drug called thalidomide as a tranquilizer. Since it was available without a prescription, people assumed it was a safe drug. Inevitably, it was taken by some pregnant women, many of whom did not even know they were pregnant at the time. The problem was that this drug, if taken between the twentieth and twenty-fifth days after conception—only about two to three weeks after a missed period—interfered with the development of the fetal limbs. As soon as the association was confirmed, thalidomide was taken off the market, but not soon enough to undo the damage it had caused. The thalidomide tragedy focused much-needed attention on the effects of drugs on pregnant women and their fetuses. It served as a stimulus to intensify drug safety studies and underscored the extreme caution that must be used in prescribing any drugs during pregnancy or taking any drugs while trying to conceive.

Many studies have shown that most women take one or more drugs during their pregnancies. A Centers for Disease Control report from 1987 questioned 492 pregnant women in New York and found that 90 percent took drugs, either over-the-counter or prescription. Average drug consumption was about four medications, and this probably underreports actual maternal use.

The drugs pregnant women reported taking were from many different classes, including analgesics, antibiotics, and tranquilizers. More recently, drugs with known teratogenic effects contain very specific warning labels in both graphic and text form. Unfortunately, in

2001 researchers at the CDC found that of the drugs that harbored teratogenic effects and therefore contained warning labels, only 21 percent of people surveyed had interpreted these labels as meaning that the drugs should not be taken while attempting conception and that pregnant women should not take the medications. If you are trying to conceive, review closely your drug history with your doctor.

There is an increasing general awareness that recreational, prescribed, and over-the-counter medications may contribute to fetal damage. It has been estimated that 1 to 2 percent of congenital anomalies today are caused by drugs, environmental chemicals, or both.

Table 1.4 lists some commonly encountered drugs administered to pregnant women and their relative safety. Consult your physician before you take any medication while trying to conceive or while pregnant.

Toxins in the Workplace and the Environment

The number of chemical and physical agents that pose a potential threat to some aspect of reproduction is enormous. Over 100,000 chemicals are now used in industry, of which only a small portion have been tested for possible effects on men's and women's reproductive capacity or a direct effect on a developing fetus. While most chemicals have been tested for their potential to cause cancer, the standards for reproductive safety in occupational exposure lag far behind. Table 1.5 lists some of the factors that may be hazardous to reproduction.

It is a good idea to identify hazards both you and your partner may be exposed to and to inform your doctor. Consider the environment of your home, your job, and any other places you frequent. To evaluate possible reproductive hazards, your doctor must know the type and the duration of the exposure and the stage of your pregnancy at the time of exposure, along with your history of adverse outcome in previous pregnancies.

Accurately estimating the stage of pregnancy at the time of exposure is essential because there are critical periods when the fetus is most susceptible and the potential harm can be the highest. Also, different organs have varying susceptibility to hazardous agents at different times during pregnancy. It is only during the second to the eighth week after conception (the embryonic period) that most structural defects occur.

When assessing the workplace, consider all potential means of exposure, including inhalation, skin absorption, and ingestion. Pay attention to routine exposures, as well as peak exposures, accidents, and spills.

TABLE 1.4
Drugs in Pregnancy

DRUG	SAFETY
Antibiotics	
Penicillins	Safe
Tetracycline	Unsafe
Cephalozimines	Safe
Erythromycin (Base)	Safe
(Estolate)	Unsafe
Sulfonamides (first and second trimesters)	Safe
(third trimester)	Unsafe
Clindamycin	Safe
Metronidazole	Controversial
Miconazole (topical agents for fungus)	Safe
Acyclovir (for herpes)	Okay for indicated cases
Isotretinoin (Accutane)	Very unsafe
Progesterone (natural)	Safe
(synthetic)	Not approved
Anticoagulants	
Heparin	Safe
Warfarin	Unsafe
Anticonvulsants for epilepsy	None proven totally safe— some used with monitoring
Psychotropic drugs	None safe—some used carefully, if necessary, under doctor's observation
Lithium	Unsafe
Prozac	Acceptable when indicated
Zoloft	Acceptable when indicated
Hormones	Unsafe for the most part— check for specifics
Aspirin (third trimester)	Unsafe
Baby aspirin	May be therapeutic in certain pregnancies
Ibuprofen	Unsafe but can be used temporarily to treat certain conditions
Acetaminophen (Tylenol)	Safe

Since many employees may be exposed to wide varieties of potentially hazardous substances, it is extremely difficult to demonstrate that a specific substance is a reproductive hazard. In such cases, groups of occupational hazards, rather than a specific agent, are evaluated.

TABLE 1.5
Hazardous Occupational and Environmental Exposures

EXPOSURE	POSSIBLE OUTCOME
Anesthetic gases in the operating room	Spontaneous abortion, prematurity, fetal malformation
Lead in paint, glass, pottery, glazing	Spontaneous abortion, low birth weight, abnormal sperm production
Mercury	Cerebral palsy, mental retardation, fetal malformation
Beryllium and selenium	Birth defects
Polychlorinated biphenyls (PCBs) from industrial use, fish contaminants	Low birth weight, intrauterine growth retardation
Herbicides with dioxin	Spontaneous abortion, intrauterine growth retardation
Pesticides	Decreased sperm production
Benzine and other solvents in dry cleaning and other industries	Increased menstrual flow, anemia, bleeding disturbances
Carbon disulfide in the textile industry	Medical disorders of various types, decreased fertility, excessive fetal loss from miscarriage, stillbirth
Chemicals at toxic waste dumps	Spontaneous abortion, intrauterine growth retardation
Arsenic in pesticides, industrial waste, and copper methinemissius	Small infants, fetal malformation
Air pollutants such as carbon monoxide	Increased miscarriages, abnormalities
Cadmium and nickel in the electroplating industry and in cigarette smoke	Fetal malformation, small infants
Hyperthermia (increased body temperature in saunas and hot tubs)	Fetal malformation
Radiation (X-ray technicians, physicians)	Fetal malformation, male infertility, future cancer in offspring
Smoking	Increased miscarriage, prematurity, low birth weight, neonatal death
Formaldehyde and other sterilization media	Increased miscarriage
Vinyl chloride in plastics	Fetal malformation

High-Risk Behaviors

Smoking

From 1965 to 1990, there was a 40 percent decline in the overall prevalence of smoking; subsequently, there has been no change. Approximately one-third of women who become pregnant are smokers, but about 20 percent will quit by their first prenatal visit. Five percent of infant deaths and 14 percent of all premature deliveries in the United States have been attributed to maternal smoking. Still, 15 to 29 percent of pregnant women smoke throughout pregnancy. Smoking has been associated with increased early fetal loss, ectopic pregnancy, ectopic pregnancy, preeclampsia, placental abnormalities, intrauterine growth retardation, and congenital anomalies. Maternal smoking during pregnancy has been estimated to account for 12.8 percent of deaths from sudden infant death syndrome. A 2002 study found that smoking increased pregnancy-related health-care costs over $360 million per year in the United States. A 1985 study showed that approximately one-third of women who smoked were unaware that smoking increased the rate of miscarriage, contributed to stillbirth, caused premature birth, and increased the risk of low birth weight. While up to 20 percent of women will quit smoking after becoming pregnant, the majority relapses during or immediately following pregnancy.

All women who smoke and who are contemplating pregnancy should be offered special counseling or programs designed to help them stop. Since most people try to quit several times before they are successful, preconceptional intervention may be particularly worthwhile. Some women may be motivated by learning about the impact of smoking during pregnancy. Heavy smokers, and those who have tried to stop but failed, may benefit from nicotine gum or a patch, as well as from a referral to a stop-smoking program. Nicotine gum and patches are considered during pregnancy only when counseling has failed. Recently, the FDA has approved Zyban as a drug to curb the craving for smoking. Zyban is actually an antidepressant, also known as Wellbutrin, and its potential effects in pregnancy are unknown.

Alcohol Consumption

About 3 percent of women nationally are estimated to take three or more drinks per week during pregnancy, although much higher rates have been reported in specific populations. While many women reduce their consumption of alcohol once they learn they are pregnant, those least likely to are moderate to heavy drinkers.

The adverse effects of alcohol on the fetus may begin early in pregnancy, often before a woman realizes she is pregnant. A safe level of alcohol consumption during pregnancy has not been established. Women who consume two to four drinks per week during the first trimester are at double the risk of spontaneous abortion. At a level of three drinks a day, the average IQ of offspring in a middle-class white population has been found to be decreased by five points, and the rate of offspring with IQs less than 85 tripled. The working executive who has a drink at lunch, a second while preparing dinner, and a third during dinner is incurring significant risk if she is pregnant.

Fetal alcohol syndrome was described as recently as 1973. It clearly showed a group of newborns' problems as being due to the ingestion of alcohol by pregnant women. We now know that more than 50 percent of infants born to alcoholic women have features of this syndrome—namely, growth retardation, brain and spinal cord abnormalities, and characteristic facial changes. Since the initial report of fetal alcohol syndrome, numerous studies have appeared in the medical journals. Today the two main concerns are: What is the minimal dose of alcohol that will produce adverse effects? When during pregnancy is the fetus most vulnerable? Recent data indicate that the prevalence of this syndrome in the 1980s and 1990s was between 0.5 and 2 cases per 1,000 births.

Severe fetal alcohol syndrome occurs only in children whose mothers were heavy drinkers during pregnancy. While a decrease in alcohol consumption by these heavy drinkers before pregnancy results in less fetal problems than those observed in women who continued to drink heavily, adverse effects of alcohol as measured by psychological testing have still been seen in infants whose mothers quit drinking even early in their pregnancy. Some studies have shown significant drops in birth weight and a greater frequency of malformations in children of alcohol users. The stillbirth rate among women consuming three drinks a day was found to be two and a half times that of women drinking less than this amount. Spontaneous miscarriages are more than twice as common in pregnant women drinking moderately twice a week or more.

All of this poses a dilemma to the obstetrician and to women who are pregnant or contemplating pregnancy: How much drinking, if any, is really safe? It would seem simple to just advise complete abstinence, but such a recommendation is often not followed, especially by women who have, in fact, consumed alcohol in the past and produced normal and even exceptional children. A recommendation for complete abstinence might also cause considerable guilt and anxiety among women who drank before they knew they were pregnant. Perhaps a total alcohol ban might lead women to substitute other drugs, which could be even more risky. Despite these realities, the medical community's official response has been that women should beware of any alcohol at all and even the small amounts of alcohol that are present in some foods and drugs. Some doctors have taken a more moderate approach, advising women of the hazards of excessive drinking and discussing this matter with each pregnant woman on an individual basis. This seems like the logical strategy, since it is not yet possible to form rigid guidelines concerning a safe quantity of alcohol during pregnancy.

Caffeine Use

Caffeine has been shown to produce abnormalities in the offspring of laboratory animals. Some studies in humans have also suggested that excessive use may be bad for the fetus. One study, in which 30 ounces of coffee were consumed a day, showed a high incidence of miscarriage and prematurity among pregnant women. However, a recent study of coffee consumption involving 12,000 women did not reveal any relationship between prematurity or malformations and coffee consumption. Some studies have looked at an association between caffeine consumption and poor fetal growth. A 2002 study found that women who used caffeine and smoked substantially increased their risk for having a small baby, compared to that of women who only smoked. Our advice to patients attempting pregnancy or already pregnant is to cut coffee down to one cup per day; drink weak tea; cut out medications with caffeine, such as Empirin and Anacin; and watch out for excess cola consumption.

Recreational Drug Use and Substance Abuse

The use of cocaine, heroin, and other illegal substances may lead to spontaneous abortion, intrauterine growth retardation, low birth weight, congenital defects, and fetal or neonatal death. An estimated 10 to 15 percent of women use cocaine, heroin, methadone, amphetamines, PCP, marijuana, or any combination of these, during pregnancy. Those with serious addiction problems are unlikely to seek preconceptional care. However, most women using these substances do so only occasionally.

A careful history to identify occasional use of illegal substances is part of a preconceptional evaluation. Users often do not consider occasional recreational use to be a problem, nor may they be aware of its dangers during early pregnancy. Use of cocaine during the first trimester may be associated with subsequent problems or with congenital defects, even if use does not continue later in pregnancy.

Occasional drug users should be encouraged to abstain completely, especially if they are not actively preventing pregnancy. Women who regularly use cocaine or other illicit substances should maintain effective birth control until their substance abuse has been properly treated.

In summary, all mood-altering drugs have adverse effects on the fetus and the newborn baby, although to varying degrees. It is best to refrain from all such substances during pregnancy.

GENETIC COUNSELING

Advances in the science of medical genetics have dramatically increased our understanding of genetic disorders. As researchers uncovered the principles behind the inheritance of genetic abnormalities, they recognized that a small number of diseases followed specific patterns as these were passed from generation to generation, and that the likelihood of their occurrence with any particular couple could be determined. In the last decade, there has been an astonishing increase in the amount of information gleaned from genes and even more so in the number of ways this information can be applied. For example, some genetic defects can be corrected after the baby is born. Some chromosome abnormalities and metabolic disorders can be accurately detected in utero with little risk to mother or fetus.

Approximately 3 percent of newborns are affected by genetic defects. A careful history can identify genetic risk. If you have a specific indication, such as a previous affected pregnancy, a family history of genetic disease, advanced maternal age, toxic exposures in the environment or at work, or a specific ethnic background, you may obtain genetic counseling and screening. Common disorders for which genetic screening is recommended include Tay-Sachs in Ashkenazic Jews, beta-thalassemia in Greeks and Italians, alpha-thalassemia in Southeast Asians and Filipinos, and sickle-cell anemia in Africans and Hispanics. In addition, if either you or your partner is affected by a genetic disease or has an affected relative, you should receive genetic counseling and possibly genetic testing.

The number of individuals and couples seeking genetic services increases each year. The number of centers offering such counseling is also growing. There are now more than 600 hospital-based genetic programs in the United States, with associated laboratory services to do studies. Some major medical centers have developed satellite clinics that reach out into surrounding communities to provide education and improved services. Your local medical school and the March of Dimes program in New York City are good places to call for advice on finding a genetic-counseling program.

The progress of medical genetics has come during a time when attitudes toward abortion and population control are evolving, but ethical, social, religious, and economic issues remain to be resolved. The choices a couple faces are extremely difficult ones. Partners should not hesitate to lean on anyone available—especially each other—for emotional support. And they should dig up every scrap of information they can so that whatever their decision, they feel it is right for them at that time and is based on medical knowledge and careful, honest self-questioning. Then they will know they've done the best they could under the circumstances.

Basic Genetic Principles

Genetic disorders fall into three basic groups: chromosome, single-gene (or Mendelian), and multifactorial.

Chromosome Disorders

These disorders are classified as genetic because they involve genes. They are not necessarily genetic in the way most people think of the word. They can be one-time mutations that spontaneously occur at the time of early cell division and are not inherited or passed on to offspring in succeeding generations. However, most chromosomal disorders *are* inherited.

The cells of all living organisms contain a specific amount of genetic material in their nuclei, which generally stays the same throughout the organism's lifetime. This genetic material is arranged in distinct units called chromosomes. Chromosomes are made up of special proteins called bases. These bases are arranged in a special order to make up genes. Each chromosome is believed to contain hundreds, if not thousands, of genes, and each gene is responsible for a particular characteristic of the organism. Through advances in genomic technologies, the order or the sequence of these bases has nearly been unraveled. Around 3.1 billion bases have been sequenced, and there are around 30,000 genes. In humans, every cell contains forty-six chromosomes arranged in twenty-three pairs—every cell, that is, *except* the reproductive cells. The ova of a woman and the sperm of a man come in halves, each with twenty-three unpaired chromosomes, which will make a new, complete, unique combination of genes when they come together to form a new human being.

Of the twenty-three chromosome pairs in all nonreproductive cells, twenty-two pairs are called *autosomes*. The last pair, the sex—or X and Y—chromosomes determine whether the person is male or female. A normal human female is designated 46XX because she has the correct total chromosome number of forty-six, or twenty-three pairs, one of which is XX, the combination of two X chromosomes that makes her female. A normal male is designated 46XY—he, too, has a total chromosome number of forty-six, that is, twenty-two autosomal pairs plus one pair made up of the single X and single Y chromosome combination that makes him a male.

Chromosome analysis can be done on the white cells in the blood, on cells in the bone marrow, on skin cells, on cells shed from a fetus into the amniotic fluid, or on a small sample of the placenta. The cells are grown in tissue culture so that some can be caught at the precise time in the division process when the individual chromosomes can be seen—in a normal, nondividing cell they're invisible. The chromosomes are counted and arranged in pairs according to the size, the shape, and the dark-and-light patterns they display. Each pair is then carefully numbered according to a uniform identification system.

In 1959 an extra number 21 chromosome was discovered in white blood cells grown from individuals with Down's syndrome. These people are said to have trisomy-21, another name for a type of Down's, which simply means they have three number 21 chromosomes instead of the expected two. This was an amazing genetic breakthrough: It was the first time a specific, visible chromosome abnormality was linked to specific physical defects in a human being. Since then, many other human chromosome abnormalities have been documented—some, like trisomy-21, associated with a structural alteration of the autosomal chromosomes' genetic material, others associated with a change in the sex chromosomes.

It was to be expected that these initial discoveries were made in people with obvious problems—abnormal sex characteristics, physical malformations, mental retardation, or diseases such as leukemia. But it was extremely surprising that, eventually, laboratory studies on cells from people who appeared absolutely normal sometimes showed extreme chromosome deviations. Genetics is clearly an area in which we have much left to learn.

Chromosomal surveys done on infants show that approximately 1 in 200 has a major chromosome variation, which may or may not have a negative impact on the baby's life. The most frequently seen chromosome disorder is trisomy-21, or Down's syndrome, which occurs in approximately 1 in 600 live births.

Single-Gene, or Mendelian, Disorders

Mendelian disorders occur when one member of a pair of genes is abnormal. More than 2,000 genetic variations of this type have been discovered by charting inheritance patterns, although how often most of them occur is unknown. These disorders follow the nonclassic patterns first described by Gregor Mendel in 1865. Remember that genes containing specific biochemical information occur in pairs, which are located at specific places in the chromosomes. Normal individuals receive one gene (half of each gene pair) from each of their parents. Mendelian single-gene disorders are classified according to the way they are inherited: autosomal dominant, autosomal recessive, or X-linked recessive.

Autosomal dominant means the problem, whatever it is, will show up when just one abnormal gene is present. That single gene will "dominate" the other normal one. These problems are thought to arise through spontaneous mutations, which can then be passed directly from one generation to the next. These are different from the one-time mutations discussed previously. It is estimated that a person with a known autosomal dominant condition has a fifty-fifty chance of transmitting the mutant gene to his or her child. There are over 1,200 autosomal dominant disorders known today, and new ones are being discovered all the time. While these disorders are generally not familiar names, one example is neurofibromatosis—the Elephant Man's disease.

Of course, not only genetic *problems* are inherited in the autosomal dominant manner. Brown eyes are dominant over blue: One blue-eyed gene from the mother and one brown-eyed gene from the father produces a brown-eyed child.

Autosomal recessive conditions occur when both members of a particular gene pair are abnormal. A person is said to be a carrier if he or she has only *one* abnormal gene: The single gene isn't strong enough alone (as the dominant genes are) to make the carrier have a disorder, but the gene can be passed on to a child. If two carriers of the same abnormal recessive gene have children, there is a 25 percent (one in four) chance that their offspring will receive a double dose of the harmful gene and actually have symptoms of the disorder. Statistically, a carrier couple has *the same* 25 percent chance with each pregnancy of giving birth to a child with a recessive disorder: The chances don't go up or down, depending on whether one child does or doesn't have the disease. But the couple also has a 50 percent (two in four) chance of having a carrier child and a 25 percent (one in four) chance of having a child with no abnormal genes at all.

Recessive genes are also involved in the inheritance of normal traits. Remember, blue eyes are recessive. If two brown-eyed parents both have a gene for blue eyes, each child has a one-in-four chance of having blue eyes.

There are over 900 known autosomal recessive disorders, including many disorders of metabolism, such as Tay-Sachs disease. Babies born with Tay-Sachs (but *not* carriers) lack a specific enzyme, which results in the buildup of a fatty substance in the cells of the brain and the spinal cord. Symptoms—neurological problems—first appear in infants at about six months; death is inevitable by about four to six years. There is no treatment for this disorder. It occurs primarily in Jews of Eastern European origin, with a frequency of approximately 1 in 3,000 live births. Sensitive, reliable genetic tests can determine whether prospective parents are carriers, and amniocentesis can determine the genetic status of a fetus of carrier parents.

Phenylketonuria (PKU) is another metabolic problem passed by autosomal recessive inheritance. Here, too, an enzyme is lacking that is necessary for normal central nervous system function. In most of the United States, inexpensive, simple, and accurate tests for PKU are required by law for newborns. If affected babies are put on a special diet from birth, a substantial amount of otherwise inevitable mental retardation can be prevented. However, there is no carrier test available for PKU.

X-linked recessive disorders are problems that occur primarily in men but are passed along by women. This occurs because, as was explained earlier, men have one X and one Y sex-determining chromosome, while women have two Xs. So if a woman inherits a single X gene for one of these diseases, she won't *have* the disease—since in recessive disorders the single healthy X will dominate—but she will be a carrier, capable of passing on that one abnormal X to a child. Men, on the other hand, have only a single X gene; if they inherit a faulty X, they will have the disorder. There are approximately 150 X-linked recessive disorders, including hemophilia and Duchenne's muscular dystrophy.

Multifactorial Disorders

These are due to the interaction of many gene pairs with one another and with environmental factors (X rays, drugs, and so forth). Multifactorial disorders result in congenital malformations such as a cleft palate, cleft lip, and defects of the nervous system. The frequency of these disorders is unknown, but the risk of recurrence in subsequent children is low.

Genetic Counseling

Genetic counseling is a very detailed, complex, and time-consuming process. The first thing the genetic counselor does is determine the reason a couple or a person is seeking counseling. Then a complete history, or "pedigree," is obtained, including a review of all past and present medical problems and information about age, nationality, habits, diet, hobbies, education, and vocation. Exposures to various infections and environmental hazards, such as X rays and chemicals, are investigated. If you have had a child with a genetic problem, the counselor may review all information about that child's conception, abortions or stillbirths, and your methods of contraception. The counselor will study all available records, including birth, medical, and autopsy reports, and sometimes even family records and photographs if available. A physical examination will sometimes be done, and consultations with neurologists and ophthalmologists may be set up. Biochemical and chromosome tests may also be run.

The genetic counselor then assembles and reviews the information and makes a diagnosis. If there is a problem, the counselor must first decide if it is genetic or environmental. If it is genetic, the type of inheritance is figured out. The diagnosis and the implications will then be explained in an interview. Mode of inheritance, recurrence risk, and, finally, all possible options are fully explained and considered.

Carriers of Genetic Disorders

The ability to detect carriers of genetic disorders can sometimes seem like a double-edged sword. Screening programs, available to test populations at risk for such disorders as sickle-cell anemia and Tay-Sachs disease, provide valuable genetic information. Genetic disorders—and carriers of them—are no longer viewed as a threat to society's well-being, but rather as an individual or a family problem. Being labeled a carrier is an understandably upsetting experience—so much so, in fact, that some people may avoid genetic studies and all the benefits that can follow good counseling, because they fear they simply can't deal with the knowledge.

Carrier detection may have an enormous impact on mate selection and childbearing decisions. For example, people who find out before marriage that they are carriers of a recessive disorder may, after counseling, decide to restrict their choice of mates in order to prevent the birth of abnormal children. Deciding when to tell this to a potential mate is an extremely difficult task; this is just one small example of the kind of pressure this knowledge can bring. Carrier detection *after* marriage brings its own set of problems, which may lead to discord and even divorce. Parents of a child with a genetic disorder are usually devastated, frightened, and full of grief and guilt. Studies of mothers of hemophiliac children suggest that their severe guilt may come from their perception of themselves as being genetically responsible for their baby's condition.

Much more needs to be learned about the effects of disclosing the carrier state, so that doctors, friends, potential and actual mates, and the carriers themselves can better cope with this extraordinarily difficult situation.

Ashkenazi Jewish patients are now requested to test for a myriad of genetic diseases before attempting pregnancy. Examples include testing for Tay-Sachs disease, Canavan's disease, cystic fibrosis, Gaucher's disease, Nieman-Picks disease, Bloom's syndrome, Fanconi's anemia, mucolipidosis, and familial dysautonomia.

Genetic Prenatal Testing

The use of amniocentesis and the new technique of chorionic villus sampling are prime examples of the way genetic advances in sterile laboratories can benefit women in real-life situations. These techniques (explained in detail in chapter 7) remove fetal cells so that their genetic makeup can be determined. Such prenatal diagnosis usually provides reassuring news. When these tests do reveal a genetic problem in a fetus, couples have the option of terminating the pregnancy.

Unfortunately, while prenatal testing can rule out a number of problems, it can't guarantee a healthy baby. Diagnosis is still not possible for many congenital abnormalities or Mendelian single-gene disorders. For example, prenatal testing can determine the sex of a fetus but *not* whether the fetus actually has an X-linked disorder such as hemophilia. Interestingly, a new technique has been developed to actually test the egg before fertilization for evidence of the abnormal gene. In vitro fertilization (IVF) is used to fertilize a normal egg and then implant it into the mother. This could assure the parents that the baby doesn't have the disease.

All women should have knowledge about prenatal tests and the kinds of information they can and cannot provide. Great advances have been made in current genetic counseling, fetal diagnosis, and screening for carriers of problematic genetic traits. Sometimes, however, a couple caught in the middle of a terribly difficult situation may feel that what is known simply isn't enough. That is true, in many ways, and will continue to be true for the foreseeable future. But sometimes a little bit of knowledge can make a big difference, and in many cases, genetic innovations have reduced human suffering.

THE PREPREGNANCY CHECKLIST

The following list summarizes all the things a health-conscious couple should take care of before trying to become pregnant.

- Get a checkup and discuss with your physician possible effects of existing medical conditions on pregnancy.
- Discuss possible laboratory tests to screen for toxoplasmosis, syphilis, and HIV.
- Check on your immunization to rubella and hepatitis.
- Stop smoking. Ideally, give your body a period of adjustment—say, six months. Short of that, throw away your last pack of cigarettes with your last packet of contraceptive pills or when you tuck away your diaphragm or have your IUD removed.
- Cut down on alcohol. The official word from the surgeon general is that no alcohol should be consumed during pregnancy. Since that period includes the critical time before you'll even know for sure that you are pregnant, you should stop drinking from the time you start trying to conceive. If that seems unreasonable, ask your doctor to suggest more workable guidelines.
- Maximize nutrition. If you have weight to lose, try to drop it. If you have a few pounds to gain, start eating. Remember, these things take time—a two-pound weight change per week in either direction is a safe, healthy maximum. But that's not all: Even normal-weight women often have remarkably irregular eating habits. It's time to change this, too. A body built on a strong nutritional bedrock is likely to have a healthier, easier time supporting pregnancy.
- Get fit. Pregnancy is a physical challenge, and like any other physical challenge it will be faced most comfortably with a strong, fit body. Since it's not a good idea to tackle a fitness plan once you are pregnant, the time for physical conditioning is before conception.
- Have a dental checkup. Although almost any dental work can be done during pregnancy if necessary, why worry about the possibility? Also, your dentist may want to see

you more frequently during pregnancy because of gum changes brought about by pregnancy hormones, so set up a schedule now.
- Have a gynecologic checkup three to four months before conception. It should include:

    A breast, a pelvic, and a general physical examination

    A Pap smear

    Tests for sexually transmitted diseases

    Blood tests as indicated, such as hemoglobin, blood sugar, and liver tests

    A rubella test and, if necessary, immunization

    A toxoplasmosis (rare infection from raw meat, fish, or cats) test if you have or have had a cat

- Have a genetic screening if there's any question of family diseases on either partner's side.
- Avoid drugs, medications (unless prescribed by your physician), X rays, and environmental hazards while trying to conceive.
- Stop birth control. The pill should be stopped three months before you try for a pregnancy. An IUD can be removed a month or two ahead of time. Barrier methods should be used during the intervening months, then stopped with your period when you want to start trying to conceive.
- Record when your last menstrual period occurred to accurately date the onset of pregnancy.

Part II

PREGNANCY

Chapter 2

Becoming Pregnant

NOW THAT YOU HAVE made the decision to have a child, there is much you still need to know about becoming pregnant. Starting a much-wanted pregnancy may not always be as simple as you might think. Knowing a bit about the most common hurdles, as well as about some of the complexities of the process of conception, can go a long way toward easing the stress of waiting for the big event. You have already prepared for pregnancy by getting a thorough gynecologic history and a physical examination, appropriate tests, and genetic counseling, if necessary. Your exercise and nutrition habits are now the healthiest possible.

It may surprise many young couples, especially those who have been careful about birth control, that pregnancy does not always happen as soon as you decide to try for it. It will take the average couple about four to six months to achieve pregnancy, and after a year of trying only four out of five couples will produce a pregnancy. If conception does not occur after one year of intercourse without birth control, it is time to seek medical advice. If you are over thirty or your partner is over fifty, a medical evaluation is in order after six months of trying. It tends to take older couples longer to achieve pregnancy, and at the same time, they have fewer fertile years left in which to evaluate and treat any problems that may be present (see chapter 14).

No matter what your age, it is best to just relax and have fun with sex during the time you are trying to get pregnant. Try not to keep deadlines or adhere to schedules for conception. Taken to the extreme, the stress of trying to get pregnant can even throw off your menstrual cycle and ovulation, just as any stress can make pregnancy more difficult to achieve. This can be a unique and beautiful time for most people. There are no worries about remembering birth-control pills or using diaphragms or condoms. That freedom and the excitement of what's ahead can make this a special time. Remember that becoming pregnant can take time. Relax and enjoy it!

FERTILIZATION

Your knowledge about ovulation and subsequent fertilization can help you achieve a planned pregnancy. Fertilization is defined as the moment when a sperm enters the ovum. From that second, this microscopic bundle of genetic material has all the basic elements it needs to develop from embryo to newborn infant. The female ovary usually releases one egg each month into the reproductive tract to be fertilized. This ovulation process usually occurs ten to fourteen days before the next menstrual period starts, no matter how long a woman's cycle. Therefore, a woman with a twenty-eight-day menstrual cycle will usually ovulate about two weeks before the onset of her period, right smack in the middle of a twenty-eight-day cycle. On the other hand, a woman with a thirty-eight-day cycle will usually ovulate on the twenty-fourth day of her cycle (thirty-eight minus fourteen). A menstrual cycle begins with the first day of bleeding and ends with the first day of the next period. If you keep track of the length of your menstrual cycle over six months, you will soon get a clear idea of when to expect ovulation. The illustration shows the timing of ovulation in relation to the basal body temperature. This is discussed in chapter 14.

Once ovulation has occurred, the ovum is transported into one of the fallopian tubes, where it is moved along by the tube's muscular efforts and by the brushings of the tiny hairlike cilia that line it. In the tube the egg meets the oncoming sperm, one of the millions of sperm from a single ejaculation. Once fertilization happens, the egg takes about three days to travel down the tube into the uterus. The endometrium, or uterine lining, has been built up during the cycle to receive and nourish the fertilized ovum. If the egg is not fertilized, the uterine lining will be discarded as menstruation and the whole cycle begins again. Since sperm can live about two days within the female reproductive tract, intercourse must occur within forty-eight hours of ovulation for conception to occur.

With these facts in mind, you can start to formulate a plan for increasing your chances of fertilization each month. Once you have figured out about when ovulation will occur, and keeping in mind that sperm will live for about forty-eight hours, you might want to try to have intercourse at least three times around your projected time of ovulation. If ovulation is expected on or about day fourteen, as in a twenty-eight-day cycle, if you have intercourse on days ten, twelve,

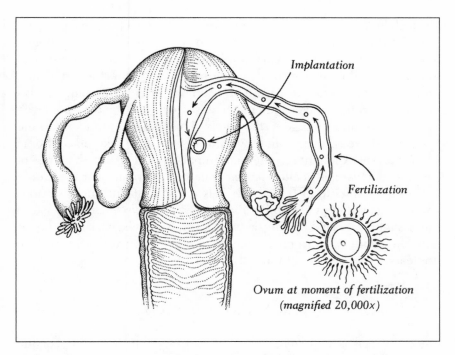

Implantation

Fertilization

Ovum at moment of fertilization
(magnified 20,000x)

FERTILIZATION AND IMPLANTATION

fourteen, and sixteen, live sperm will most likely be present at suitable intervals to achieve fertilization. There are other, more precise methods to determine ovulation. The use of the basal body temperature curve requires measurement of your basal temperature upon awakening each morning. If this is charted on a graph, your temperature will remain below 98°F prior to ovulation and will rise above 98° after ovulation. By doing these temperature curves, you can determine the timing of ovulation and use this information in a subsequent cycle. In addition, intercourse can be continued every forty-eight hours until the basal body temperature rises above 98°F, thus ensuring that in a long cycle the timing is correct. (See chapter 14.)

Chemical methods are also available now for precisely determining ovulation time. These ovulation predictor kits measure the amount of luteinizing hormone (LH) in your urine. LH rises twelve to twenty-four hours prior to ovulation. By measuring the LH peak, you can accurately predict ovulation. These tests are quite accurate, simple to perform, and relatively inexpensive, and they can help you time ovulation and intercourse to achieve fertilization and pregnancy efficiently.

Some women say they can detect their ovulation by feeling a watery discharge in their vagina at this time. (In fact, the amount of cervical mucus increases ten times at ovulation.) The cervical secretion becomes thin and slippery, due to the higher level of estrogen prior to the moment of ovulation. The purpose of this thin cervical mucus is to allow sperm to penetrate more easily into the cervix and move into the uterus. If a woman examines herself internally at this time by inserting a finger in her vagina, she will feel the increased wetness and a distinct change in the cervix. This increased mucus and the open cervix are sure signs that ovulation is about to take place. Some women even experience some abdominal pain at about the time of ovulation. This pain, called *mittelschmerz* (a German word meaning "pain in the middle of the month"), is unpleasant but not dangerous and does not affect your ability to conceive. *Mittelschmerz* may cause some slight vaginal bleeding as well, which can be alarming but is only the result of hormonal changes. Though *mittelschmerz* may be unpleasant, at least it will remind you that you are ovulating.

EARLY PREGNANCY

Once the egg is fertilized, it usually burrows into the lining of the uterus. This process is called *implantation*; it starts two to three days after the fertilized egg reaches the uterus and may be marked by a small amount of vaginal bleeding, which can last a few days. Once implantation occurs, the endometrium nourishes the fertilized egg and allows it to develop. After implantation, menstruation, of course, does not occur. During days twenty-one to twenty-eight of the menstrual cycle, there is rapid growth of the fertilized egg and the placenta begins to develop, even before you miss a period. The placenta is the embryo's life-support system. This interface between mother and fetus provides food and oxygen to the growing fetus and takes away its waste products of urine and carbon dioxide. The placenta grows and continues to do its job right up to the end of pregnancy.

By the end of what is called the first month of pregnancy, the fertilized egg is actually about fourteen days old and is smaller than a pea. At about this time the placenta has begun to produce enough of the hormone human chorionic gonadotropin (HCG) to be measured by a common urine test. This is the main hormone of pregnancy and is one of the stimuli for many of the changes your body undergoes during the course of pregnancy. In actuality, the first traces of this hormone can be detected in your blood by very sensitive tests called immunoassays as early as nine days after fertilization, or five days *before* you've missed your period. The level of this hormone rises rapidly as pregnancy continues, and at about the time you miss your first period, its level can be detected by home pregnancy tests.

THE SEX OF THE FETUS

The sex of the baby is determined at conception. During fertilization, there is an exchange of genetic material that determines the physical characteristics of the baby. Genes are grouped and carried in structures called chromosomes. Every adult, male and female, has forty-six chromosomes in each cell—twenty-two matched pairs and one set of sex chromosomes.

The exceptions to this rule are the sperm and the ovum cells, which each carry twenty-three single chromosomes. Fertilization, then, combines the twenty-three chromosomes in the sperm with the twenty-three in the ovum, restoring the full complement of chromosomes. As explained, the chromosomes that determine sex are labeled X (female) and Y (male). All eggs have X chromosomes exclusively; sperm cells are equally divided between X and Y. If a sperm cell carrying an X chromosome fertilizes the ovum, this XX combination produces a female baby. An XY combination results in the development of a male baby.

Sex Selection

Sex selection is the method for determining the sex of the baby using medical technology. This may be necessary to avoid the risk of serious sex-linked genetic disorders like hemophilia. In these cases, 50 percent of boys born to women who carry the gene for hemophilia will have this condition. In addition, parents who have two boys, for example, may want a third child only if they can have a girl. Clearly, the former requires serious medical attention, while the latter may only provide some psychological comfort. Although doctors now know how sex is determined, predetermining the sex at conception can be quite challenging. To date, the only reliable method of sex selection has to be done postfertilization (after the sperm and the egg have fused). Techniques used for prefertilization sex selection (before the sperm and the egg have fused) have not been shown to be reliable.

Prefertilization

The sperm determines the sex of the baby because it carries either an X or a Y chromosome. The old wives' tale in which one could encourage the "male sperm" or the "female sperm" to fertilize the egg has at best limited success. The concept, however, stems from the fact that male sperm and female sperm move differently because the latter has more genetic material and is technically heavier. This can be exploited in a scientific way by two recognized methods that have been shown to "enrich" X- or Y-bearing sperm. Both of these methods can be done in a human reproductive laboratory, which is usually available to your doctor. One method is called "flow cytometry" and the other is called "12-step Percoll." Recent studies seem to indicate that the flow cytometry method seems to significantly enrich both the male- and the female-carrying sperm, but the 12-step Percoll really can enrich only the female-carrying sperm and not by much. Sperm that was enriched with either male or female could be used for artificial insemination. Despite the advanced technology, success is limited, and a couple must be able to deal with potential failure.

Postfertilization

Sex selection performed after the sperm and the egg fertilize can be extremely reliable. With in vitro fertilization, the egg is fertilized outside the body and is allowed to grow. Before the fertilized egg is put back into the woman's uterus, it can be biopsied, and the potential sex of the embryo can be determined. This has moral and ethical considerations (e.g., one can use only male embryos). This is quite costly and is usually reserved for cases involving sex-linked genetic disorders.

Sex selection can be performed after implantation. In the early stages of the pregnancy (nine to ten weeks), chorionic villus sampling can be used to determine sex, and a decision about terminating the pregnancy can be made.

PREGNANCY TESTING

Measurement of human chorionic gonadotropin (HCG), the hormone produced by the placenta, is the basis of all current pregnancy tests. This hormone was first detected in the urine of pregnant women in 1927 by two researchers named Ascheim and Zondek. At first, HCG could be measured only indirectly, using laboratory animals such as rabbits. This is where the term *rabbit test* came from. These animals were injected with a woman's urine and examined after a period of time for changes in the ovary, which would indicate that HCG was present. The process took days and was not completely reliable.

Pregnancy-testing methods have developed rapidly over the years so that performed directly on a woman's blood or urine, they can produce very rapid and accurate results. The new test, called the radioimmunoassay, or RAI, is so sensitive it can detect the HCG in the blood only one day after implantation or nine days after conception. Most physicians have a urine test available that is sensitive enough to turn positive after you miss your first period. The home versions of these laboratory tests are now also sensitive enough to become positive only a few days after you miss your period.

Recently, urine testing achieved a major breakthrough that puts it close behind blood testing in speed and accuracy while maintaining the advantage of easy sampling. The difference is monoclonal antibodies, substances that react only with HCG and make the test extremely accurate. Home pregnancy tests can be purchased for $10 to $20 in most pharmacies. The tests are easy to use: in a few minutes, a color change can mean pregnancy and no change means no pregnancy.

Pregnancy testing is more than just a way to satisfy a couple's very understandable curiosity about whether or not pregnancy has occurred. The sooner you know, the sooner you can be more careful of your habits: eating healthfully, getting enough sleep and exercise, and cutting out possible harmful habits, such as smoking, drinking, and drug taking, if you haven't already. And home tests allow partners trying for pregnancy the privacy to savor the excitement of a positive result together, if only for a few hours or days before going to the doctor. A negative result can save couples the time and the expense of an unnecessary doctor's visit. However, patients should be cautioned not to rely on a home pregnancy test without having a physician confirm it.

Besides using just the presence of HCG to confirm a pregnancy—a kind of yes/no evaluation—measuring the precise amount of HCG in the blood has also become an important tool in the hands of your physician. Having several checks of the HCG levels through a test called the beta sub unit (BSU) over a period of time during the pregnancy can provide valuable clues as to whether or not a pregnancy is healthy. For example, an impending miscarriage can sometimes be predicted by the failure of BSU levels to rise. Ectopic pregnancies—those that implant outside of the uterus, most often in the fallopian tubes—can also sometimes be diagnosed by low levels of BSU. Many physicians obtain a baseline level of BSU when a woman has had a previous abnormal pregnancy or when there is any suspicion that the current one may present problems. The BSU level in a normal pregnancy should double approximately every three days. The lack of this rise in BSU, coupled with abnormal bleeding, suggests to your physician that a sonogram should be performed to help rule out a possible miscarriage. (See chapter 6.)

DATING A PREGNANCY

Once your physician confirms your pregnancy, your probable delivery date will be calculated. The length of the average pregnancy is approximately 266 days. But since the exact day of ovulation is usually not known, an approximation is made by using the date of the last menstrual period. Since this is usually 14 days before ovulation, 14 days is added to the 266 days for a total of 280 days, or 40 weeks. By convention, we use 40 weeks from the date of the last menstrual period as the estimated date of delivery (or EDC, for estimated date of confinement). If you have long cycles or are irregular, however, this EDC will not be accurate. In those cases, sonograms are used for accurate pregnancy dating.

The customary way physicians estimate the expected date of delivery is to count back three months from the first day of your last menstrual period and add seven days. If, for instance, your last menstrual period began June 10, your expected date of delivery would be March 17 (June 10 minus three months is March 10; add seven days to get March 17).

Less than 5 percent of all pregnant women actually go into labor on the estimated date. About one-third deliver within five days of that date. Most women give birth within two weeks of the due date. Since most calculations are based on the average twenty-eight-day cycle, ask your doctor for a special calculation if you menstruate more or less frequently.

It is wise to think of your due date as an estimation, rather than as the exact day when you can expect to go into labor. If you have conceived after you stopped taking the birth-control pill, your dates may be completely wrong because the first ovulation following the use of birth-control pills can be quite delayed. It sometimes takes several months to establish a normal menstrual cycle after stopping birth-control pills. Therefore, you might be off by even a month in your due date. However, ultrasound can very accurately date a pregnancy. Accurate dating of pregnancy benefits management of a pregnancy, especially for those women who are at risk for complications that might require active intervention. These conditions include diabetes, hypertension, heart and kidney disease, and previous cesarean delivery. Accurate dating improves our ability to diagnose fetal growth retardation and postmaturity and to handle many other problems.

The following criteria can be used to accurately date a pregnancy and are listed in approximate order of accuracy:

1. A basal body temperature (BBT) chart with a record of sexual relations.
2. An ultrasound measurement between seven and ten weeks of pregnancy.
3. Two ultrasound measurements of the fetus prior to twenty-six weeks that are in agreement on fetal size and age.
4. Blood pregnancy hormone levels. (A level of 5,000 units will date a five- to six-week pregnancy.)
5. A urine pregnancy test that turns from negative to positive. (This indicates a four- to five-week pregnancy.)
6. A last menstrual period that is normal, regular, and certain.

You can help date your pregnancy accurately by keeping records of your menstrual periods and seeing your physician within six weeks of pregnancy.

You may experience some early signs of pregnancy, other than missing your period. Breast changes occur during the first few weeks of pregnancy in preparation for lactation. Your breasts may feel tender and heavy quite soon after missing your first period. Later on (past three months), the brownish circles around the nipples, the areolae, become darker and the little bumps on them become prominent. If you are pink-skinned, you may notice that the lacy network of blood vessels in your breasts, as well as the blue veins that run over the breasts, have become more prominent.

Another common sign of early pregnancy is nausea. This can occur at four to five weeks. These waves of sickness can happen early in the morning, but they may also occur in the early evening or at other times in the day. Some women feel sick; others actually vomit. Fatigue contributes to nausea, but so does an empty stomach. Small frequent snacks may relieve the feeling. A few crackers or dry toast immediately upon waking may prevent nausea. If you experience nausea, cut out all greasy, spicy, and fried foods, as well as tobacco and alcohol.

Tiredness occurs because your whole body has to adjust to the process of growing a baby. It is not surprising that you may feel you cannot carry on as before. Enormous metabolic changes are taking place. Many women complain of extreme fatigue in the first eight to ten weeks of pregnancy, but as your body adjusts to the pregnancy the fatigue vanishes. You may find the middle months easier. If you are feeling tired, it is sensible to heed this message and go to bed earlier or perhaps take midday naps. Try to organize your life as well as you can, with at least a short time every day when you are completely free from responsibilities. Women having a second or third pregnancy are often exhausted by the nonstop pace of their older child's daily life.

Another early symptom of pregnancy is increased frequency of urination. Since the growing uterus may press on your bladder, you will probably need to urinate more frequently. This may be an early sign of pregnancy. Some women also state that their vaginal secretions change during pregnancy. They get thicker, whiter, and stickier. This change is noticed very soon after a missed period.

Of course, one of the most important symptoms of pregnancy is the cessation in menstruation. It is reasonably safe to assume that a woman who is menstruating normally is not pregnant and that one who can conceive and suddenly ceases to menstruate is probably pregnant. But certain conditions other than pregnancy can delay menstruation; these are changes in climate and environment, external psychological influences, severe illness, menopause, and lactation, as well as recent cessation of the use of contraceptive pills. Various drugs can inhibit ovulation and menstruation as well. While the absence of a menstrual period is not definite evidence of pregnancy, it is eventually useful at fixing the date of conception and determining the duration of the pregnancy. Be wary, though, for vaginal bleeding, which is indistinguishable from menstruation, can continue following conception. It is not rare for a woman to have one or two periods if she is pregnant, but usually this type of vaginal bleeding is less profuse than that associated with your menstruation.

Ultrasound for the diagnosis of pregnancy is quite valuable as the first definite sign of a live pregnancy. The fetal heartbeat can be visualized through ultrasound as early as six to eight weeks of gestation. Most obstetricians will use vaginal ultrasound within the first three months of the pregnancy. First-trimester ultrasound is done for two reasons. First, after six weeks fetal viability can be confirmed. Ultrasound can also provide accurate dating to help manage late potential obstetrical problems.

The use of ultrasound in pregnancy is one of the major advances of the past twenty years and is discussed fully in chapter 7. However, the early use of real-time ultrasound, especially the vaginal type, has certainly changed our ability to diagnose a live pregnancy, as well as to make a diagnosis of an ectopic pregnancy.

PREGNANCY SIGNS IN THE SECOND TRIMESTER

During the second three months—the second trimester—of pregnancy, new signs appear in a normal pregnancy. Your doctor will watch for these symptoms as an indication that your pregnancy is progressing smoothly and that the baby is continuing to grow. If you are not already aware that you are pregnant by the end of the first trimester (which is highly unlikely), these new signs should prompt you to seek medical advice.

Abdominal size. If it has not happened earlier, by the beginning of the fourth lunar month of pregnancy, the abdomen should begin to protrude. This protrusion may come all of a sudden, following a rapid increase in the volume of amniotic fluid during the fourth month of gestation. You will not mistake the growing abdomen as an ordinary potbelly. The abdomen housing the fetus is low and very firm. It will probably be well hidden under loose-fitting clothes for the first few months of pregnancy but will be very obvious when uncovered.

Quickening. Sometime following the fourth month, you will feel a slight, indescribable sensation in the abdomen. At first, you will just make a mental note of it, but within several weeks, the feeling will be quite pronounced and will resemble the fluttering of tiny birds' wings or the rising of bubbles along the wall of the uterus. These sensations are called "quickening," and they represent the first perceptions of fetal movement. The movement is noticed earlier by women who have felt it before. Quickening is only of presumptive value to diagnosis, since

TABLE 2.1
Main Events in Early Pregnancy

Day 1	Onset of last menstrual period
Day 14	Ovulation
Day 20	Implantation of the early pregnancy
Day 22	Earliest detection of HCB by chemical assay
Day 28	Missing first menstrual period—positive home pregnancy test
5 weeks	Early pregnancy sac detectable in uterus by ultrasound
7 1/2–8 weeks	Positive fetal heartbeat detectable on vaginal ultrasound
16–18 weeks	Quickening, or the perception of fetal movement by the pregnant woman, occurs

intestinal movements or abdominal muscle contractions can give the impression of fetal movement.

Fetal movement. Persistent fetal movement can be observed as early as the sixteenth week. If you look, you will be able to see a slight, momentary bulge of the abdominal wall, or the passage of a limb across your stomach. Sometimes the movements are so vigorous, they are visible through clothing. If you or your partner lays one hand on your abdomen, you may feel a weak knock or a stroke. This is a positive sign of fetal life.

Uterine contractions. Intermittent uterine contractions may be felt any time after the tenth week, and they may continue right up to the time of labor. The uterus is so sensitive to touch that it can harden at the slightest pressure during the doctor's examination and will relax as quickly as the hand is removed. These contractions are a sign of pregnancy and are normal.

Fetal heartbeat. The fetal heart can be heard by a doctor using a Doppler machine usually from about the fourth to the fifth month on. The heart becomes stronger and louder as the child grows, until by the seventh month, your partner might be able to hear it by placing his ear on your abdomen. (Caution: A heavy head will be kicked.) What he will hear is a fast ticktock, which sounds as if it were muffled by a pillow. The rate will change from 120 to 160 beats per minute, almost twice the pulse of the average adult. The fetus has a lot of work to do!

Fetal structure. By the end of the second trimester, the doctor should be able to feel several key parts of the fetus merely by feeling your abdomen. A trained hand can feel the head and the back quite easily.

CHOOSING THE DOCTOR

You will probably have several choices of medical care for your pregnancy. Your family doctor may care for you and deliver your baby, or you may choose to go to one of the many fine hospital clinics available. But chances are, you will choose a doctor who specializes in obstetrics, the branch of medicine concerned with birth. An obstetrician's primary concern is the management of pregnancy, labor, delivery, and postpartum care. In England, midwifery carries the same meaning as obstetrics does in the United States. As a matter of fact, in this country there is a resurgence in the use of nurses trained as midwives, working directly with physicians, to deliver babies. This medical team usually works at a family health center, which is another alternative to the private obstetrician for the management of pregnancy, one that will probably cost less. But if you are planning to use a private physician and have not yet chosen one, you should be aware of certain facts before making your choice.

Before 1930, an average of 60 maternal deaths occurred for every 10,000 live births. Today, only about 1 maternal death occurs per 10,000 births, and most of those are women who enter pregnancy with a previous disease. This overall reduction is a superb testament to the improved quality of obstetrical care. Many factors are responsible for the reduction, including the development of antibiotics to fight infection. But the most important factors are probably better education and training in the field of obstetrics.

The American Board of Obstetrics and Gynecology, which certifies specialists in the field, has very high standards. A doctor seeking certification must be a graduate of an accredited medical school and must thereafter complete one year's internship and three years' residency in an accredited hospital. After that, he or she must practice in the specialty for several years and then pass both written and oral examinations.

It can be as difficult to find a competent obstetrician as it is to find a good gynecologist. With the increasing publicity over the various types of childbirth available and the large number of cesarean sections performed, many women have become more aware, more informed, and more careful about finding competent obstetricians who can fulfill their particular needs and care for them with respect. They also look for physicians who are associated with hospitals they trust. This development in better doctor–patient relationships is a good one.

When you begin your search for an obstetrician in the hospital, you must establish your own standards for care. Do you prefer birthing rooms and rooming-in? Do you prefer a more homelike environment? Also, there is the practical matter of how much you can or are willing to pay for care.

The safest environment for you and your baby during the labor, the delivery, and the immediate postpartum period is the hospital setting, in which a team of professionals, including an anesthesiologist, an obstetrician, and a pediatrician, is available to respond to emergencies. Within the hospital setting, many facilities have a combined waiting-labor-delivery area called a birthing room, where family members or other support people can remain with you as long as possible throughout childbirth. Birthing rooms are intended for uncomplicated vaginal deliveries. If problems occur, delivery then takes place in the traditional delivery room.

It is important for a woman who is pregnant for the first time to see a physician who is informed about the latest trends in obstetrical care and who has time to answer questions. Your obstetrician should offer superior care and technical competence. This is important for obvious reasons, because pregnancy and birth are critical times. But besides possessing skill and experience, you want your obstetrician to be able to fulfill specific emotional and psychological needs. Here you have to evaluate your priorities for yourself. One couple may be so concerned about safety or technical competence that the partners will consider a doctor only if he or she has great experience and outstanding qualifications. Others may value understanding and sympathy above all. They want someone whom they can easily relate to and who makes them feel comfortable and secure. Sometimes obstetrical practices vary from one hospital to another; you should make sure that you are comfortable with the hospital rules and the type of facility that is available.

Many doctors who call themselves specialists in obstetrics are not board-certified obstetricians. They may have conducted hundreds of deliveries and have valuable practical experience, but they may not have taken courses required to qualify for board certification. To be board-certified, a doctor must take an approved four-year residency in ob-gyn and then pass a certifying examination. If they are not board-certified, they are not governed physicians. A specialty board constantly keeps in touch with its members regarding new developments in the field and also requires that all members attend a certain number of postgraduate classes to keep them abreast of new practices.

You can find out an obstetrician's qualifications by going to the library or to your local county medical society and looking up his or her name in the *Directory of Medical Specialists.* The *Directory* will list your doctor's birthday, medical school, hospital affiliations, and board certification. When the term *board certified* does not appear in a doctor's biography, you have to make up your own mind about how important this is to you.

In listing a doctor's hospital affiliation, the *Directory* can often give you an idea of his or her skill, since the most competent physicians are generally affiliated with the best hospitals. In major urban areas the most desirable hospitals are often the ones associated with large medical centers and medical schools. One of the advantages of choosing a larger hospital is that the hospital administration (or specially appointed boards of physicians) closely monitors its physicians' standards.

Another choice to be made is between solo or group practice. Obstetricians often prefer to decrease the stress and the strain of obstetrical practice by joining a group. This option has become very popular and is often the only choice. In a group practice doctors tend to monitor one another and, by sharing responsibilities, have time to attend meetings and classes to expand their knowledge. And, of course, the physical stress of being constantly on call is diminished. If the qualifications and the reputation of the senior partner in a group practice are good, there is a good chance that he or she is very careful before accepting associates into the practice.

Most obstetricians charge a flat fee that includes prenatal care, attendance at delivery, and a schedule of postnatal visits. Some insurance companies pick up only part of the cost for the obstetrician, so you will probably end up paying much of the obstetrical bill yourself. Many insurance companies participate with physicians in what is called a managed-care arrangement. Agreeing to get your prenatal care from a participating physician may decrease your out-of-pocket expense substantially. Unfortunately, many such participating physicians are overburdened due to the need to increase their volume of patients, as the doctors' reimbursements are usually much less than their usual fees. It is important to discuss fees early in your care and to be sure that you and your partner are comfortable with the financial arrangements. Many factors go into the physician's fee, and it's important to know what those are. Remember, a high fee does not necessarily mean quality care.

In some cases a perinatologist, as well as an obstetrician, may be helpful. A perinatologist is a specialist in the management of high-risk pregnancies. In addition to a regular residency, perinatologists have had an additional two years of training, concentrated in the latest research in the management of high-risk pregnancies. The largest medical centers have perinatologists on staff. These perinatologists are available for consultation and evaluation if the pregnancy is complicated by major problems. They are often the ones who perform very extensive ultrasound examinations and do high-risk evaluations (see chapter 7).

THE CHRONOLOGICAL DEVELOPMENT OF THE FETUS

First month. During the first month of pregnancy, rapid growth of the fertilized egg and the development of an early placenta take place. At the end of the month, the fertilized egg is about fourteen days old and is smaller than a BB shot. (Remember, doctors date a pregnancy from the last menstrual cycle before conception, not from the date of conception.)

THE DEVELOPING FETUS

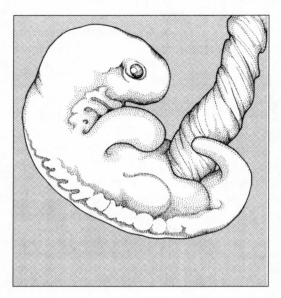

THE FIRST FOUR WEEKS: *The heart is pulsating and pumping blood. The backbone and the spinal canal are forming. No eyes, nose, or external ears are yet visible. The digestive system is beginning to form. Small buds that will eventually become arms and legs are present.*

SECOND MONTH (EIGHT WEEKS): *The fetus is about 1 1/8 inches long and weighs about 1/30 ounce. The face and the features are forming; eyelids are fused. Limbs are beginning to show distinct division into arms, elbows, forearms, hands, thighs, knees, lower legs, and feet. A distinct umbilical cord has formed. Long bones and internal organs are developing.*

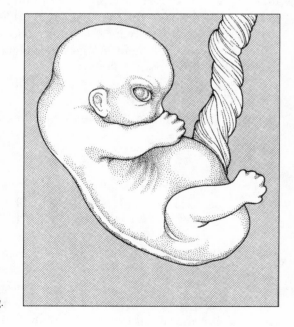

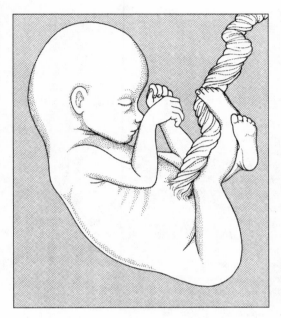

THIRD MONTH (TWELVE WEEKS): *The fetus is now about 3 inches long and weighs about 1 ounce. Arms, hands, fingers, legs, feet, and toes are fully formed. Nails on the digits are beginning to develop. External ears are present. Tooth sockets and buds are forming in the jawbones. The eyes are almost fully developed; the eyelids are still fused.*

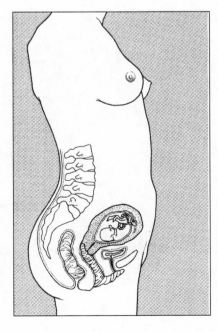

THIRD MONTH (TWELVE WEEKS): *The uterus begins to enlarge with the growing fetus and can be felt extending about halfway up to the umbilicus.*

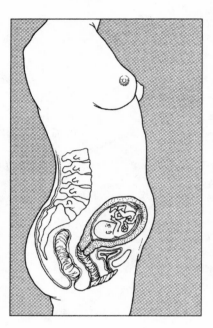

FOURTH MONTH: *The fetus is now 6 1/2 –7 inches long and weighs about 4 ounces. It has a strong heartbeat, fair digestion, and active muscles. Its skin is bright pink, transparent, and covered with fine, downlike hair. Most bones are distinctly indicated throughout the body. The head is disproportionately large at this stage. The eyes, the ears, the nose, and the mouth are nearing their typical appearance. The eyebrows appear.*

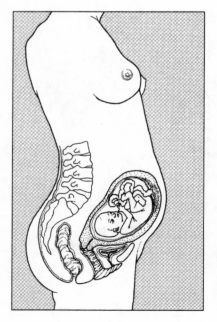

FIFTH MONTH: *The fetus measures about 10 inches long and weighs 1/2 –1 pound. Its skin is still bright red. Its increased size now brings the dome of the uterus to the level of the navel. The internal organs are rapidly maturing, but the lungs are insufficiently developed to cope with conditions outside the uterus. The eyelids are still completely fused at the end of five months. Some hair may be present on the head.*

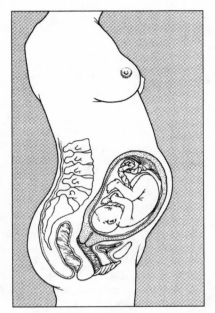

SIXTH MONTH: *At the end of the sixth month, the fetus measures 11–14 inches and may weigh from 1¹/₄ –1¹/₂ pounds. The skin is quite wrinkled, still somewhat red, and covered with a heavy protective creamy coating. The eyelids are finally separated and eyelashes have formed. The fingernails now extend to the end of the fingers.*

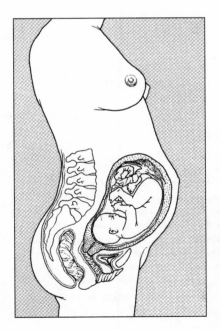

SEVENTH MONTH: *The fetus is about 3 inches longer, and its weight has about doubled since last month. It still looks quite red and is covered with wrinkles that will eventually be erased by fat. The premature baby at seven months has a good chance for survival in nurseries cared for by skilled physicians and nurses.*

EIGHTH MONTH: *The growth and maturation of the fetus in the last two months are extremely important. From 2 1/2 to 3 pounds at the beginning of the eighth month, it will put on some 2 to 2 1/2 more pounds and lengthen to 16 1/2 to 18 inches by the end of the month. The bones of the head are soft and flexible. If born now, it stands a much greater chance for survival than does a seven-month fetus, contrary to a popular fallacy.*

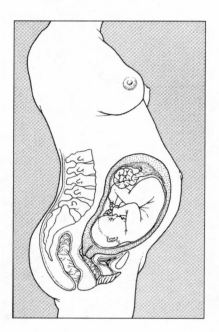

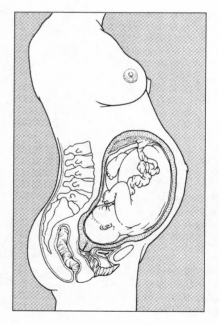

NINTH MONTH: *At birth, or full term, the baby weighs on average about 7 pounds if it is a girl or 7 1/2 pounds if it is a boy. Its length averages about 20 inches. Its skin is paler but still coated with the creamy coating. The fine, downy hair has largely disappeared. Fingernails may protrude beyond the end of the fingers. The size of the soft spot between the bones of the skull varies considerably from one child to another and will close within 12 to 18 months.*

The placenta is producing the hormone HCG, which allows the mother's body to make a multitude of changes to support pregnancy. This hormone will now show up in the mother's blood so that a laboratory test at this time could confirm a suspicion of pregnancy.

Six weeks. The fertilized egg with its nutritive material is about the size of a marble, but the developing baby is only half that size. Yet, in the four weeks of growth since fertilization, it has developed a complete circulatory system and a placenta, its embryonic heart has begun to beat, and it has the beginnings of a real heart, brain, limbs, ears, a nose, and eyes. The uterus is continuing to develop muscles and elastic tissue to support the fetus.

Eight weeks (two lunar months). At eight weeks, the ovum is about the size of a hen's egg; the developing embryo is slightly larger than the yolk. It has developed limbs and external genitalia. The cavity within the placenta is enlarging to accommodate fetal growth and already contains the amniotic fluid in which the fetus floats. The uterus also continues to grow and begins intermittent contractions, called Braxton-Hicks contractions, which continue through pregnancy. The fetal heart can be heard by ultrasound fetoscope and be seen beating by sonogram. The first tiny movements occur.

Twelve weeks (three lunar months). The ovum at twelve weeks is about the size of a tennis ball, while the fetus itself is about two-thirds that size. In this third month of growth, the fetus develops fingers, toes, and nails and continues to mature. The tiny fetus is complete and moving.

Sixteen weeks (four lunar months). The fetus is about seven inches long at sixteen weeks and weighs about one-fifth of a pound. It has breathing movements and swallowing reflexes. The uterus has rounded suddenly because of a large increase in the amount of amniotic fluid.

Between the fourth and fifth months, the fetal movements, known as quickening, can be felt by the mother. At first, the movements are very slight and may resemble mild gas pains. Eventually, there is no mistaking them. Usually by the start of the fourth month, the doctor will be using a small machine called a Doppler that translates movement into sound, which will allow anyone in the room to hear the baby's heartbeat. It is unmistakable and sounds like a galloping horse! Both movement and heartbeat become stronger as pregnancy progresses. Amniocentesis for genetic diagnosis can be performed at this time because of the accumulation of approximately a pint of fluid.

TABLE 2.2

Average Fetal Size through the Weeks of Pregnancy

WEEKS OF GESTATION	WEIGHT (LBS.)	LENGTH (IN.)
8	0	1.6
12	0	3.0
16	0.2	6.3
20	0.6	9.8
24	1.5	11.8
28	2.4	13.8
32	3.11	15.7
36	5.2	17.7
40	7.3	19.7

Twenty weeks (five lunar months). The fetus at twenty weeks is ten inches long and weighs a little more than half a pound. Its body is covered with a cheesy white protective material called *vernix caseosa.* The facial features are fully developed, although the face is wrinkled and shriveled, causing the baby to look like a little old man. Early toenails can be seen. This is an excellent time for the doctor to either perform or order a directed ultrasound, which is a special ultrasound with which the baby can be evaluated closely for many defects. (This will be discussed later in the book.)

Twenty-four weeks (six lunar months). At twenty-four weeks, the fetus is about 13 inches long and weighs about 1$^{1}/_{2}$ pounds. If born at this time, it might possibly survive a few hours, although the lungs are usually too immature to sustain life. Its skin is shiny and red and is covered with a fine hair known as lanugo. Parts of the fetus can be discerned by the doctor by feeling the abdomen.

Twenty-eight weeks (seven lunar months). The fetus is 15 inches long after twenty-eight weeks and weighs about 2$^{1}/_{2}$ pounds. Each day from this point on, its chances of surviving premature birth are better and better. The baby is getting larger and may be moving less because it has less room. The eyes open now, and good hair development occurs.

Thirty-two weeks (eight lunar months). By eight months the fetus is about 16 inches long and weighs approximately 3 pounds. Its chances for survival are increased (despite the popular fallacy that seven-month babies live, but eight-month babies do not). The closer the mother is to term, the better the baby's chance for survival.

Thirty-six weeks (nine lunar months. The baby is fully formed after thirty-six weeks, measures 18 inches, weighs a little more than 5 pounds, and spends all its time maturing and building up fat tissue to provide it with warmth after birth.

Term. The baby is ready and waiting for some unknown signal that will precipitate labor. It measures about 19 inches and weighs an average of 7 pounds.

Chapter 3

Adjusting to Pregnancy

—⊶⊷—

ONCE YOU KNOW that you are pregnant, there are new concerns and adjustments to be made so that you can fulfill your goal of having a happy, healthy baby.

To help you achieve this goal, let's examine some important factors to consider at this time. And quite a few areas do demand attention. For example, if you would like to work throughout your pregnancy, what will the impact of your job be on both your own body and that of your developing fetus? And what about the reverse: Will your pregnancy affect your ability to do your job? Are you exposed to any chemicals at work or at home? Do you take any medications your doctor should know about in helping you plan for a healthy conception? How different is it to have a baby when you're over thirty, thirty-five, or forty? Should you start to eat differently or change the type of exercise you do? As for genetic counseling before pregnancy, how do you or your partner even know whether it's necessary? Some of the facts in this section may surprise you.

If you've been taking good care of your health and any health problems as they arise, you've already done much to increase the chances of your future children being healthy. Your obstetrician will work with you once you become pregnant, perhaps suggesting various tests to monitor the health of your fetus, such as blood tests, ultrasound, and amniocentesis, to help ensure that those good odds continue. (The various tests are discussed in chapter 7.)

ADJUSTING TO PREGNANCY

No matter how much you want a child, you are bound to have some worries and conflicting emotions once you find out you actually are pregnant. Changing the structure of a family—and that's exactly what

64

the birth of a child does—always requires some adjustment. Conflicting emotions may be even greater for a woman having a child at a later age. After investing so much time in building a career, a relationship, an entire life that doesn't contain a child, it's normal to feel torn at the thought of what might have to be given up, and at the changes you will have to make.

Many women are facing similar dilemmas, as more and more professional women in their thirties start families. Interestingly, in recent decades the female labor force has increased substantially in many countries. In the Netherlands, for example, only 25 percent of women ages fifteen to sixty-five worked outside the home in 1960. Today, more than 50 percent of women are working. In the past, it was theorized that combining work and children could potentially damage a woman's health because the increased stress and fatigue could lead to illness. In 2002 a study looking at 1,000 women actually showed that the combination of caring for a child and working led to improved health!

Martha, a thirty-four-year-old physician who was pregnant with her first child, commented, "It's very exciting, and not just a little frightening. I'm used to scheduling my time in a logical and disciplined manner, knowing exactly what's required of me. But I can't yet see exactly how my life will be affected by this new human being. For the first time, I can't plan for every minute. I just have to wait and see."

While you can't plan exactly how a baby will affect your life and your work, that doesn't mean you can't plan at all. You can make some basic decisions that will work with your life and your needs and build in some flexibility so that you can accommodate the unforeseen. Some women plan to work full time after having a child. Others decide to resolve their need for both babies and work by having a part-time job. Still others think they will simply put their careers on hold for a while. But if you survey a few friends who have been in this position, you may realize that even the best-laid plans sometimes take a 180-degree turn: The woman who was convinced that staying home with an infant for six months would drive her batty couldn't drag herself away from her baby for a year. And the mother who thought it would be a nice change to stay out of the office rat race for a while finds herself hungering for the challenges that her years on the job trained her to meet. It's not a bad idea, then, to make a second or even a third backup plan so that whichever one ends up seeming right, some planning will already have gone into it. By being sensitive to, and honest about, your own feelings and the needs of your family, and by talking things over with your partner, you should be able to make decisions that are right for you and your family. And if one decision doesn't work, plans can always be scrapped and a new strategy tried.

"It's incredibly stressful and exhausting," said Emily, a forty-year-old mother of three and a medical news reporter in New York City. "But I knew that if I took a break during this critical time in my career, I would never be successful."

Obviously, your relationship with your partner also undergoes changes when you have a baby. If you've been a couple for a long time, you've probably developed daily routines and leisure activities that are comfortable and satisfying. Change, even longed-for change, can present a difficult challenge for couples. It also can end up, as it does in most cases, adding richness and intensity to your feelings for each other. Pregnancy and childbirth are exciting and immensely rewarding events. Age should not prevent you from being able to have a child safely and happily. Your obstetrician, your partner, and your friends are all there to help. Use them to air your fears, to lean on when you need them, and, finally, to share with you the joys of having a child.

THE WORKING WOMAN AND PREGNANCY

Over the last ten years, the number of women in professional occupations has increased by nearly 60 percent. Approximately 50 percent of the workforce is female today. The number holding managerial positions has more than doubled. The number of women in sales, service, and clerical jobs has also increased. The proportion of women obtaining professional degrees has increased dramatically, especially in such fields as medicine, dentistry, law, optometry, and theology. In some of those areas, the number of women graduates has increased tenfold. And behind those impressive statistics are creative, intelligent, ambitious women who also plan to be mothers.

Today nearly half of all children under the age of six have working mothers. Over 60 percent of kids ages six to seventeen also have mothers who work. Why have women sought employment outside the home in such dramatic proportions? One reason is that two-wage-earner families have become necessary in some parts of the country to maintain even an average standard of living. Sometimes women begin to work for special projects—a child's college education or buying a home—and never stop. One in five American children lives *only* with the mother, who must work to support the child. Still other women need the feelings of achievement and the social contacts they gain from paid employment. Some find the very special responsibilities of child care overwhelming without the balancing factor of work. Finally, many well-educated women possess the abilities for a professional career and, quite simply, want to achieve that status without giving up the option of having a family.

The life of the working woman and mother involves considerable compromise in order to keep the family, the job, and herself going. Sometimes it is very difficult to excel in a career and, at the same time, raise a family well. As one thirty-seven-year-old working mother of three explained it, "I'm always torn. When I'm at the office, I worry about the kids at home. When I'm with them, something left undone at work nags at me. But then I remind myself that all mothers worry about their children, and all professionals feel there's more work to do than time to do it. I'm glad I have the chance to do both."

There are sacrifices involved in juggling work and home responsibilities. Although more women than ever are working and shouldering the same responsibilities as men, most mothers still carry the burden of managing the household and raising the children. A working wife enjoys substantially less leisure time and sleep than her spouse does. Women who work and are married find very little time in the course of the day to just relax and unwind. In addition, the ingrained cultural ideals about the way children are supposed to be raised remain alive, leading to feelings of guilt and inadequacy on the part of some working women.

Eventually, all this can take its toll. Many talented and self-confident women who began climbing the corporate ladder in the 1970s are now dropping out, having decided they couldn't do both and continue to meet the high standards they set for every aspect of their lives. Says one mother of two preschoolers, "I could not be an excellent bank executive *and* an excellent mother. I choose to concentrate on one thing for now: my kids. In a few years, when they're in school full time, I might want to go back to work. For now, I'm happier knowing I'm at least doing one thing to the best of my ability."

Other women try to work it out differently. "Housekeepers and husbands are the key," one mother said. "You can't do it all yourself. And you shouldn't feel guilty for that either."

Another category of working mother today is the single mother. Often divorced or widowed, these women have a tough time because they must make all the decisions and the arrangements alone. Part of this group consists of unmarried women who have chosen to have their children alone. The number of single women giving birth has been steadily rising in the last three decades. While this includes many women who were not planning to become mothers, middle-class, career-conscious, unmarried mothers-by-choice comprise an increasing share of this number.

Between 1993 and 1997, more than 65,000 children born to single women were studied in the United States. Surprisingly, those children were no more likely to seek and obtain health care than were children of two-parent homes. In fact, the level of maternal education was more predictive of obtaining health care than was family structure.

Planning Your Family

There is no such thing as a totally convenient time to have a child. It used to be that couples fresh out of high school or college would have babies immediately. Now many men and women are hesitating, waiting longer to get married and have their children. While this can then make the change from being a couple to becoming a family a bigger step, there are advantages to waiting.

A working couple, by delaying parenting, is usually in a stronger financial position to weather the costs of children and child care. Job advancement usually means larger salaries and greater ability to afford housekeepers and day-care centers. Delayed childbearing also helps ease some psychological strains of balancing this often difficult money situation.

Maturity is a big bonus that can make some of the work-versus-motherhood struggles easier. Once your reputation has been established, the workload may decrease naturally, or it may be easier to do it by choice. It becomes less necessary to prove yourself to your employer or your colleagues. The longer a woman works, the more likely it is that her employer has a vested interest in keeping her. Seniority may even win special concessions, such as maternity leaves, more flexible working hours, and variable vacations.

Delayed parenthood also gives women time to forge a solid professional identity—build up a track record and achieve promotions. Once in this position, even if they take a few years off to have children, women are likely to have an easier time coming back into the professional arena.

Ten years ago, more working couples were scaling down their family size. The birthrate in this country was lower than in the late 1950s, when it reached a record high. In the early 1990s, the American family averaged less than two children; many families stopped at one. But recently, the National Vital Statistics Report of 2002 disclosed an increase in birthrates. In fact, the total fertility rates in the year 2000 were above replacement for the first time in more than thirty years. We are seeing many of our patients adding the third child they never thought they would have. The economic boom of the late 1990s may have something to do with the change.

If you want more than one child, spacing the children two to three years apart seems to be best. This is medically sound, and psychologically it reduces the strain on parents and on the firstborn child.

By age three, a child has become slightly more independent and is less likely to resent the intrusion of the new baby. Also, by this time the older child is usually more manageable, out of diapers, and amenable to reasoning. However, there is no one best spacing time for all families. Many couples I know have children less than two and a half years apart, and, of course, women who have postponed pregnancy until their late thirties may not have the fertile time to wait three years between children.

Working while Pregnant

Millions of women, working in a wide variety of jobs, become pregnant each year. Many will work until just before delivery and return to work within weeks after birth. Because of this trend, we must examine the question: Is it safe for pregnant women to work?

A pregnant working woman should discuss her own particular job situation and conditions with her physician. Basically, if you are a normal, healthy woman with an uncomplicated pregnancy and a normally developing fetus, you can work at no increased risk right up to when labor begins. You can also resume working several weeks after giving birth. But if your job is strenuous and requires a lot of standing or walking, your physician may ask you to cut back on your work hours and, perhaps, to stop working a few weeks before delivery.

Some job situations may expose you to work conditions that could be harmful to you or your baby. In those cases you may have to be transferred to another job or stop working. Women with a history of certain maternal problems—such as miscarriages or premature births—or who are carrying twins may be advised to stop working.

Toxic substances, physical strain, and stress may adversely affect pregnancy. Certain metals, chemicals, or X rays can cause abnormal fetal development, miscarriages, defects at birth, or problems later in your child's life. The following is a partial list of potentially hazardous jobs:

Job	Potential Hazard
X-ray technician	X-ray exposure
Operating room personnel	Anesthetic gasses
Paint, glass, ceramic, and battery manufacturing worker	Heavy metal exposure
Toll booth attendant, road worker	Lead exposure
Laboratory and dental office technician	Mercury vapors

Radiation from microwave ovens, video display terminals, and television sets is safe because this type of radiation is nonionizing.

Heavy physical work, such as lifting heavy objects, strenuous labor, and climbing, can cause discomfort. The dizziness and the fatigue of early pregnancy can also increase the risk of accidents. Balance is often affected, and you may be vulnerable to falling. Of course, if you have any question as to what is safe, ask your physician.

The decision to continue working during pregnancy will depend on your preference, your overall health, the progress of your pregnancy, your age, and any problems you may have had during past pregnancies. The type of work you do, the number of hours you work, and any job-related threats to you or your fetus should also be considered.

If you work while pregnant, take good care of yourself. Have regular checkups. Keep nourishing snacks such as fruits and nuts near your workstation. Try to rest during breaks. Housework and the care of other children at home do not stop during pregnancy and may be equally strenuous. You may need to share more responsibility with your partner or others to ensure adequate rest. Avoid stress and strain by careful planning and sufficient sleep. If you are working, it is even more important to take care of yourself and maintain a healthy pregnancy lifestyle.

Practical Aspects of Working and Pregnancy

The twenty-first-century woman is likely to be working at the time her first pregnancy begins. Being prepared for the many challenges that exist in balancing work and motherhood is prudent.

Announcing Your Pregnancy

You may wish to wait until after your first trimester to tell colleagues that you are expecting—at that point, the greatest risks have passed. By then, of course, an announcement may not even be necessary because people may be able to tell that you're expecting. However, if you are experiencing discomfort that is obvious to others and that prevents you from fulfilling your job responsibilities, or if you need to schedule a lot of doctor visits, it may be best to announce your pregnancy during your first trimester.

Morning Sickness

Don't let morning sickness interfere with your job. Nausea and vomiting are the most common symptoms experienced in early pregnancy, occurring in 70 to 85 percent of women, with about half of those experiencing vomiting. These symptoms typically last until about sixteen weeks. The following suggestions may help:

- Eat some protein and a little natural starch or natural sugar—cheese, fruit, and cereals are good choices—before going to bed.
- Recent studies published in 2002 have shown a reduction in severe nausea with the use of vitamin B6 (pyridoxine).
- The ancient Chinese discovered that acupuncture or acupressure at Neiguan-point, or P6 (a spot located on the wrist), reduced nausea. A recent review of the literature supports this contention in pregnant women. Try to find specialized wrist bands that apply wrist pressure for a safe and effective way to cut down on nausea and vomiting during pregnancy.
- Try brewer's yeast and oral ginger root extract.
- Never let your stomach get empty; small snacks throughout the day help.
- Drink plenty of liquids, but start the morning with dry crackers or toast.
- Greet the morning in slow motion—rushing tends to aggravate nausea.

Sometimes the nausea and the vomiting become so severe that weight loss and dehydration occur. This can be severe enough to lead to electrolyte and fluid imbalances in the blood. When this condition occurs, it is called *hyperemesis gravidarum*. Fortunately, this is a very uncommon occurrence. If this condition persists, there can be serious complications. Be sure to get in touch with your doctor if you notice that you are losing weight. If all else fails, talk to your doctor about the new medications that are now available to prevent nausea, which appear to be perfectly safe in pregnancy.

Maternity Leave

If your company has no maternity leave policy or has a flexible policy, make specific recommendations to your boss. Be prepared to address and negotiate the following:

- How long a leave do you plan to take?
- How will you be compensated?
- Who will cover your job while you're on leave?

- Will you be responsible for training that person and will you need to be available to answer questions while you're on leave?
- Do you plan to return to work?

It's wise to learn about your company's maternity leave policy *before* you become pregnant. A common policy is six weeks' paid leave and up to three months' unpaid leave. Legally, pregnancy is considered a medical disability, which is why many companies won't give paid—or even unpaid—leave to adoptive mothers. Inquire about paternal leave if it makes sense for you and your husband. Many companies are changing their policies on maternity leave, so be sure that you get the most up-to-date information.

Determining the length of your leave is a very personal decision, based on your health, your mental readiness, and your financial circumstances.

Only you and your doctor can decide exactly when you should begin your leave. It might be a full month before your due date or just days before you deliver. Keep your boss and your coworkers posted on your delivery date, and work with them to ensure that a smooth transition is made. Apply all of your work management skills to organize the work you leave behind.

Planning Child Care

It's never too early to think about child care. With more mothers in the workplace than ever before, many options are available today. Whether it's a day-care center, a sitter's or a relative's home, or a nanny, you need to examine your choices carefully. Much will depend on whether you will be returning to a well-scheduled job or one with long, uncertain hours. Economics may play a deciding role as well.

Begin researching child-care options as soon as you know you are pregnant. Contact referral services, and seek out new mothers in the company who are willing to share what they have learned. Invest time and effort to find the best, most affordable care available.

You'll perform better at work if you can trust the child care you've arranged. Your peace of mind is well worth the investment in time.

If you plan to hire a sitter or a nanny, begin researching about the sixth month of your pregnancy, but don't be discouraged if a solution isn't reached until the last two or three weeks. Finding the right person is hard to do. During candidate interviews, identify other commitments or constraints that the person may have. Be sure to discuss transportation, sick days, and vacation time. Check references carefully. Although you are an employer, you want to make a positive connection with your caregiver. Finding someone who shares your values takes time. Once you do, be sensitive to meeting that person's needs so that he or she stays.

Making a Successful Transition to Pregnancy

You may think that you feel self-conscious about being pregnant on the job, but people are not shocked by figure changes as much as by *style* changes. As your body changes, try to keep your present style. If you ordinarily wear tailored suits and muted colors to work, look for maternity clothes designed in that mode. If you have difficulty finding appropriate maternity clothes, look for looser styles in larger sizes than you normally wear.

Many working women find that it's important to maintain a stylish, energetic look at work. They take extra care to treat cosmetic problems like blotchy skin and acne that may develop. Making sure that your shoes are comfortable is also important. Replace four-inch heels with stylish, low-heeled shoes.

Don't let your pregnancy become the constant subject of office conversation; curtail discussions of your physical ailments. When you are pregnant—*and* working—it's more important than ever to eat right, get plenty of rest, and exercise per your doctor's instructions.

Keeping in Touch with the Office

Soon after the baby is born, call the office. Your colleagues have followed your pregnancy with interest and will want to hear about the baby from *you*. Let everyone know you're thinking of them. Remind them of the day that you can take calls at home if they need your help.

After that, be responsible to your job and your coworkers by calling the office regularly to make sure work is progressing smoothly. You keep the connection to your job strong when you demonstrate that you are interested and involved.

Thanks to modern technology, there are many ways to stay involved with the office while you are on leave. Fax machines and computers allow you to stay in close contact, and you may be able to persuade your company to share the costs.

Returning to Work

Just as you planned your departure, you need to plan for your return. Agree on a specific date with your employer, and make sure that you are up-to-date on all projects.

Begin working the kinks out of your child-care plan a month in advance. Arrange to spend some time away from home to make sure your caregiver is capable and responsible.

Check your wardrobe, your hair, and your makeup. You may have returned to your prepregnancy weight but might still discover that your clothes need alterations. The better you look, the better you'll feel, and that will make your return much smoother.

Creating a Child-Care Contingency Plan

Who will help you if your caregiver or your child is sick? Every working mother can use several emergency plans. Relatives, at-home mothers, or a sick-child care center are just a few of the options. Research them in advance. Back-up plans will make your career and your peace of mind possible.

Identifying Part-Time Options

Suppose you promised you'd return within six weeks, but now you're not so sure you want a full-time job. Your new baby commands your full attention and interest, and you decide that you'd prefer to spend more time at home. As soon as you decide to explore the possibility of part-time work, schedule an appointment with your boss.

Don't go empty-handed. Prepare a plan for restructuring your job. You might propose that you work two or three days a week or even five mornings. Create a schedule that will work well for you *and* your company. Some organizations offer a trade-off. You might take just six weeks off and then work three days a week for a year or two years. After that, the arrangement is subject to negotiation. Another option is to consider freelancing on a project basis.

Deciding Not to Return to Work

It's impossible to predict the effect that a newborn will have on you. Even though you intended to return to work, you may discover that you feel strongly about staying home with your baby.

If you make that decision, schedule an appointment with your employer right away. Don't just call and announce that you won't be returning. Flatly announcing your decision leaves your job in a bind and makes you look unprofessional. The way you handle the announcement will affect the references you get.

Striking the Balance

Being a parent and having a career are both dynamic experiences. Each has its constant ups and downs and moments of boredom, frustration, and exhilaration. You *can* strike a balance, but the balance will always be changing.

In attempting to do both to the best of your ability, you will find that you can have it all some of the time, but you can't have it all *all* of the time. It is impossible to focus your full energy in both directions at once.

The key is to learn how to channel your time, your attention, and your emotions so that you can move forward in your career *and* nurture and shape the development of your child. Learn to make choices about what is most important at each point in time. This means always being willing to reevaluate, be flexible, and make changes. What works for you when your child is an infant may not work at the toddler stage.

Above all, be fair to yourself. Accept the fact that there are times when your career takes precedence and times when your child will come first. Be sensitive to the changes, and you will find rich satisfaction in both worlds.

Disability

Your doctor's advice may vary during the course of pregnancy, depending on changes in your condition, your job, or your lifestyle. Your pregnancy may also lead to disabilities that prevent you from performing your usual duties. Such disability usually falls into one of three categories:

1. *Disability due to the pregnancy itself.* Some women have pregnancy-related side effects, such as nausea, vomiting, indigestion, dizziness, or swollen legs and ankles—all of which may cause temporary problems while working. Your doctor will reevaluate these problems at regular intervals, giving you guidelines each time.

2. *Disability from a complication of pregnancy.* Most serious complications—infection, bleeding, rupture of the amniotic sac—may make you physically unable to continue working. Medical conditions you have before becoming pregnant, such as heart disease, diabetes, or high blood pressure, may also make working while pregnant more risky.

3. *Disability related to the job.* Some disabilities may be work-related, such as exposure to toxic substances or strenuous labor.

If your doctor decides that your pregnancy is disabling, he or she can verify to your employer that you are eligible for any disability compensation the company offers. On the other hand, if your doctor says you are able to keep working, your employer may request a letter written by your doctor stating so.

Maternity policies vary from job to job. Only about 40 percent of employed women in the United States are entitled to a paid six-week disability leave for childbirth. Others are forced to use sick leave or vacation time or to take time off without pay. The Pregnancy Discrimination Act passed by Congress in 1978 requires employers who offer medical disability to treat pregnancy-related disabilities in the same manner as all other disabilities. This means that if you are temporarily unable to work because of pregnancy, your employer must give you the same rights as other employees temporarily disabled by illness or accident. If your employer regularly assigns lighter work to other partially disabled workers, the same must be done for you. Unfortunately, many employers offer no disability benefits at all and therefore are not obliged to provide maternity leave. If no disability plan is offered where you work, you may qualify for temporary disability benefits from your state. Your local unemployment office is the best place to find out about state benefits and how you may qualify.

Disability related to job exposure is often hard to establish. There is still much to be learned about the effects on pregnancy of toxic substances, physical strains, stress, and other possible health threats the working woman may encounter. The few studies that have been done have produced conflicting results. Until more is known, common sense on your part and a knowledge of established hazards on your doctor's part are the best ways to minimize risks involved in working during pregnancy.

PREGNANCY AFTER THIRTY-FIVE

Many more women today are having their first child later in life. In the last thirty years the rate of women between ages thirty and forty-four having children rose significantly. In 2000, the total number of births rose about 3 percent. While teenage births have continued to drop, births to women in their forties and fifties have gone up. In 1979, nearly 20 percent of children born to thirty-four-year-old women were first children—double the percentage of just ten years before. And in the next ten years the birthrate among women ages thirty to thirty-four rose by 40 percent. Most of these women were college graduates and professionals who wanted to establish their careers before starting to raise families. In fact, one-third of children born in 1988 had mothers age thirty or older.

Women who are considering having children in their thirties or forties often have many questions and concerns about their ability to conceive, the ability of their bodies to carry and deliver a baby, and the health of a child born to an "older" woman. Worries like these are not entirely unwarranted, but it is important to understand that nothing is magic about age thirty-five. People age bit by bit, not all at once.

We also age unequally. A "young" forty-year-old might have no more problems with a pregnancy than an "old" twenty-five-year-old. The woman of forty might be slim and well muscled, have lots of stamina and energy, eat and sleep healthily, forgo smoking, and drink only an occasional glass of wine. Her younger counterpart might be plump, smoke like a chimney, and pant breathlessly after trudging up one flight of steps. Age is only one factor involved in a healthy pregnancy. Even age-linked problems can be minimized by working closely—right from the start of your planning stage—with your obstetrician.

Age and Fertility

Recently, much attention has been focused on fertility in women approaching age forty. Every day we hear about a famous woman having a baby well into her forties. "I read in *People* magazine how this actress had her first child at age forty-seven," said Molly, a patient in her mid-forties. "I'm forty-four and I'd like to start my family."

What these magazines do not explain is that many of the pregnancies in older women are made possible through egg-donation programs. Unfortunately, infertility rates rise exponentially after age thirty-five, and despite the nuances in reproductive technologies, the success rate for achieving pregnancy in the best reproductive facilities in the country after age forty is less than 10 percent. Many studies have tried to examine the precise relationship between infertility and maternal age. The main reason older women have more difficulty seems to be related to the age of the egg. Due to advancements in reproductive technology, older eggs, or oocytes, have been studied. As women age, they produce more and more abnormal eggs. It becomes more difficult to fertilize these eggs successfully. Another reason has to do with the hormone production of the ovary. As a woman ages, her ovaries are less able to keep up with demands placed on them to achieve normal ovulatory function. In addition, certain areas of the brain—specifically, the pituitary gland and the hypothalamus—are important in ovulation and also suffer the effects of aging.

As you get older, you're more likely to have encountered some of the hazards that can affect fertility, such as pelvic infections from sexually transmitted diseases, endometriosis (growth outside the uterus of the tissue that normally lines it), fibroids (noncancerous tumors in the uterine wall), and the effects of other pregnancies on your body. Finally, aging increases the risk of women developing certain medical conditions, such as high blood pressure and diabetes, which can impair fertility. Many studies looking at age and fertility have been criticized by experts in the field for not "controlling for," or taking into account, enough of the possible variables, such as the health of the father and the number of menstrual cycles covered in the study.

In order to try to eliminate these confounding variables, a now-classic French study looked at the success of artificial insemination (in which donor sperm are deposited at the top of a woman's vagina) in women who had never conceived and in men who had produced no sperm. The results showed a slight but significant decrease in the conception rate starting at age thirty and becoming more marked after age thirty-five. Even this study has been criticized for not accounting for the differences between natural and artificial insemination and between childless women and those who already had children. Still, along with all the other studies, the French report does seem to indicate that there is a slight but constant fall in fertility as women get older. See Table 3.1.

Since your ovaries produce fewer functional eggs as you grow older, you might have to spend several extra months trying to conceive, so be prepared: It may take longer to become pregnant.

As usual, though, that's not the only factor. How often you have sex, your partner's health, and your own gynecologic history all will have an impact.

Since 80 percent of all couples conceive within twelve months of starting to try, about a year's trying is recommended before a couple

TABLE 3.1
Percentage of Women Infertile by Age Group
(Average of Three Studies)

AGE	PERCENTAGE INFERTILE
20–24	5.3
25–29	5.8
30–34	9.8
35–39	20.0

SOURCE: Adapted from *Obs-Gyn Survey*, vol. 45, no. 2, p. 108.

seeks a full-scale infertility investigation. However, if you're over thirty, you might want to seek professional advice after six months, simply because you have a shorter period of fertility ahead. New diagnostic and treatment strategies enable many couples who previously were not able to procreate to have children.

Pregnancy and Delivery after Thirty-Five

Other problems besides difficulty with conception may also increase slightly after age thirty-five. Again, it's difficult to say just how much higher the chances of, for example, a miscarriage after thirty-five really are. For one thing, now that we can diagnose pregnancy so much earlier than ever before, what appears to be a higher miscarriage rate may only be a more accurate counting of miscarriages that were occurring all along. New data are leading experts to suspect that nearly half of all fertilized eggs may abort spontaneously, without the woman's even knowing that she became pregnant. It's the body's way of quickly and easily dealing with a defective pregnancy, without disturbing the rhythm of the menstrual cycle. Nevertheless, as women age, they are more likely to have miscarriages. Just as the "older" eggs are more difficult to fertilize, they are more likely to produce defective pregnancies. Table 3.2 demonstrates this fact.

In women over thirty-five, the proportion of stillbirths (babies born dead) is slightly higher than in women ages twenty to thirty. The proportion of low-birth-weight babies is also slightly higher for women over thirty-five. The proportion of women having cesarean sections for delivery is again slightly higher for women having their first child after thirty-five. A study done between 1995 and 2000 found that women

TABLE 3.2
Risk of Miscarriage with Increased Age

MATERNAL AGE (YEARS)	SPONTANEOUS ABORTION (%)
15–19	9.9
20–24	9.5
25–29	10.0
30–34	11.7
35–39	17.7
40–44	33.8
> 44	53.2

SOURCE: From "Reproductive Potential in Older Women," by P. R. Gindoff and R. Jewelewicz. *Fertility and Sterility* 46 (1986): 989.

over thirty-five were 6.5 times more likely to have a cesarean section than were women between ages twenty and twenty-nine. One reason for the latter may be, of course, that many obstetricians are quicker to opt for surgery over a more wait-and-see approach for an older woman at delivery.

Birth Defects

The possibility of birth defects is a major concern to many older women considering pregnancy. It should be reassuring to know that most children in the United States are born healthy and normal. The cause of birth defects isn't always known, although the age of the mother is a factor in some cases, as are heredity and environmental exposures. Certain couples do have a greater than normal chance of having a child born with a physical abnormality. However, while the likelihood of some problems does increase with age, it remains low well into the thirties.

As with other age-tied problems, there's no abrupt jump in the rate of birth defects as a couple gets older. For example, the chances of having a child with Down's syndrome—a condition involving many mental and physical abnormalities—increase steadily as the mother ages. It is the only clearly age-related birth defect. Only 1 in 1,600 children born to mothers in their early twenties would be expected to have this problem. On the other hand, Down's syndrome occurs in 1 of 365 children born to women at the age of thirty-five. At age forty, the risk is 1 in 100; and at forty-five it's 1 in 32. Striking as this increased risk is, you should note that even at age forty a woman has a 99 percent chance of *not* having a baby with Down's syndrome; even at forty-five she has a 97 percent chance. Down's syndrome, also called trisomy-21, is caused by an extra chromosome along the twenty-first pair. (Remember, there are a total of twenty-three pairs, one of which determines the baby's sex.) Besides trisomy-21 (Down's syndrome), trisomy-13 and trisomy-18, which involve the thirteenth and eighteenth pairs of chromosomes, respectively, although very rare, increase in occurrence with advancing maternal age. These conditions are associated with profound mental retardation and physical abnormalities. In addition, abnormalities of the sex chromosomes, specifically Kleinfelter's syndrome (47 XXY) and Super female (47 XXX), also increase with advancing maternal age. Children born with Kleinfelter's syndrome are boys who are usually infertile, are mildly retarded, and develop breast tissue. The Super female may be indistinguishable from a normal girl, but she may have decreased fertility and learning disabilities.

The effect of the father's age does not appear to increase the risk of chromosomal abnormalities in offspring. However, older paternal age may increase the risk of certain genetic diseases like neurofi-bromatosis (the Elephant Man's disease) and Marfan's syndrome. Although these diseases cannot be screened by tests like amniocente-sis, they are extremely rare (only 1 in 5,000 to 10,000), so even a dou-bling of the risk constitutes a very small number.

Identifying your risk of having a child with a birth defect is one of the main reasons to work closely with your obstetrician in planning a pregnancy before you even try to get pregnant. Couples in the high-risk group, because of age or other factors, can still have normal, healthy children. And the doctor can increase the chances of that happening. But the partners need to be well informed about the risks that apply to them and should discuss their plans and any known problems with their obstetrician so that medical supervision can be provided.

If you are thirty-five or older, already have a child with birth defects, have a family history of genetic disorders, or have a personal history of miscarriages or stillbirths, your obstetrician may recommend genetic counseling (see chapter 1). This will allow you to assess your risks and make an informed decision about having a child. Such counseling is done by doctors, nurses, or health educators with special training in genetics. They can give you important information based on your family history, your personal history, and sometimes a physical exam and laboratory tests.

With the genetic counseling information obtained from these specialists and the guidance of your obstetrician, you can do every-thing possible to ensure a healthy pregnancy and birth. Health care before conception (preconceptional care) is especially necessary for women over thirty. The first eight weeks or so of pregnancy—when many women don't even know yet whether they are pregnant—are some of the most important for the baby. This is, as we've said, the time when the organs are being formed, for example. Women particu-larly concerned about these early weeks might want to consider preg-nancy testing at the earliest possible time.

ON BECOMING A FATHER

Becoming a father is an awesome event in a man's life. The sheer responsibility of having a baby can be frightening. It can also be chal-lenging. Yet the male experience is usually treated as insignificant compared to becoming a mother. As a result, the emotional strains and stresses of the father-to-be are not appreciated, and men are not prepared for pregnancy and fatherhood. The stereotype of the nervous father in the waiting room has been the butt of jokes in the past. This has changed.

Most men, upon learning that they will be fathers, have new and conflicting emotions. Happiness and pride coexist with doubts about the changes in their lives, the financial burden, and the change in their identity. The old easy way of life and the spontaneity of the close one-to-one relationship change. Life centers on the new baby's needs. Many men feel rejected as their spouses become more involved with the pregnancy and the needs of the new baby. Some men feel that the physical changes of pregnancy are unattractive.

These feelings, to some extent, are normal. Most men usually resolve these conflicts. Eventually, they take an active role in this special event in their lives and enjoy it to its fullest. In fact, research has shown that women who have active, supportive partners have fewer problems during pregnancy. The labor and the delivery are usually shorter for these women. The move into parenthood is smoother for both parents if the father takes an active role in the pregnancy.

How much a father chooses to participate is an individual decision. The more he knows, the more he can help. He can prepare by reading and attending childbirth classes. Of course, he needs encouragement from his partner.

How can a father help? During the first trimester of pregnancy, the woman experiences many discomforts. She may have mixed feelings about being pregnant. The father can help by understanding these changes, participating in the educational process, and being patient with the woman's needs and moods.

During the second trimester, women need reassurance about the changes in the size and the shape of their bodies. A husband may wrongly assume that his partner no longer wants to have sexual relations. Feeling desirable and wanted is even more important now. A woman should be physically loved during pregnancy. This may not necessarily mean sexual intercourse. Stroking, touching, and kissing are also part of this expression of warmth. In normal pregnancy, sex is generally considered safe. Most couples can have intercourse until shortly before labor. The comfort of the pregnant woman is the basic guide to having sex during pregnancy. A couple may want to try different positions to find a comfortable one.

The third trimester may be the most difficult. Fear of the delivery, exhaustion, discomfort, and impatience with the pregnancy are all common maternal feelings. The expectant father may feel left out at this point. By understanding that this is normal and not taking it personally, the father can be of great help.

During this period, childbirth preparation takes place. When partners attend classes together in preparation for childbirth, they share in the birth process. They can learn a good deal about the physiological process and the changes of labor together. The father can learn how to support and participate in the birth itself. Many different types of courses prepare for labor and delivery. Most programs give information about pregnancy and birth. They also teach exercises and breathing techniques to use during labor. In addition, the father learns how to be a coach during labor. The father's role as coach requires practice at home and attendance at classes. Its importance to the success of the childbirth experience cannot be underestimated.

In the last three months of pregnancy, a man can help his partner get more rest. The heavy jobs are now his. But this does not mean that the woman has to be treated like an invalid. They can go out together, shop for the baby, and help prepare the "nest."

Going to the doctor's office as a couple can be a satisfying part of the pregnancy experience. Hearing the fetal heartbeat helps the bonding process. Your physician may even point out parts of the fetus's body when examining the mother's abdomen. The amazing pictures of the fetus on the sonogram machine will make even the most hardened partners' hearts skip a beat. Your physician wants to build a good working relationship with both of you as a couple in preparation for labor.

It is a good idea for a couple to visit the hospital before labor. Familiarity with the equipment, the surroundings, and the personnel can make all the difference in promoting relaxation during the real event. Hospital machinery and masked figures in uniforms can be intimidating. A trial run helps to alleviate the anxiety of not knowing where you will park and how to find the labor room.

Most hospitals permit and welcome expectant fathers in the labor and the delivery rooms. During labor, the partner or coach guides and supports the laboring patient. The coach helps carry out the relaxation and breathing exercises that were learned and practiced in childbirth class.

The father takes an active role. He stands at the head of the delivery table, usually beside the mother, providing emotional and physical support. From this position, the birth can be observed and the father and the mother can share the birth experience. The father who knows how to help is in a much better position than one who is just observing. His guidance, support, and encouragement are important. It is a real pleasure as an obstetrician to watch partners share this most exciting event.

After delivery, most hospitals provide an opportunity for the mother, the father, and the baby to spend time together. This is a moment of special joy after a long wait. It is the launching of a new life for the baby and the couple. Having a baby is a family affair.

Chapter 4

Changes Caused
by Pregnancy

⸎

DURING PREGNANCY, your body functions like a highly efficient factory for the period of gestation. Myriad changes occur in every system of the body—some visible, others hidden. Pregnancy is also accompanied by mood changes; some women feel exhilarated, others depressed and irritable. In short, pregnancy is a highly individual experience. And the same woman may have very different experiences with each pregnancy. But there are enough similarities in physical and psychological changes during gestation that we can classify them. Doing so will help you and your partner understand some of what is happening during the nine-month preparation for birth.

PHYSICAL CHANGES

Moments after the fertilized egg implants into the uterine wall, the body undergoes dramatic changes. Although you may quickly notice these changes, most outsiders will not see any physical differences for some time. These physical changes will now be covered in detail.

Weight Changes

Prompted by hormonal secretions, your whole body metabolism changes to promote your continued good health while you nourish the fetus. The altered metabolism increases the body's efficiency in squeezing out every bit of nutritive value foods have to offer. This handy change allows you to fulfill the health needs of yourself and your developing baby without eating for two (see chapter 5), but it can result in a slight acquisition of body fat.

84

Generally speaking, however, most of the weight gain of pregnancy is caused by the growing fetus and all of its supporting systems. Statistics show that two-thirds of all normal women gain between 13 and 35 pounds during pregnancy. The average weight gain is 2.5 pounds during the first three months, 10.8 pounds the second three months, and 11.2 pounds the last three months, which adds up to an average of 24.5 pounds. A gain of about 1 pound per week is suggested as a realistic maximum during the last half of pregnancy. More rigorous weight restriction than this is not advisable and may be harmful, except under a doctor's orders and close supervision. At the same time, too much weight gain during pregnancy increases the possibility of complications and makes it much more difficult to reduce weight after delivery. Maintaining a balance will be covered in more detail in chapter 5, which discusses nutrition in pregnancy.

Fluid Retention

There is a general increase of about three pounds of body fluid in pregnancy. Most of this accumulation occurs toward the end of gestation and is often confused with swelling of the legs and the ankles. This latter type of swelling is caused by pressure on the veins of the mother's legs from the fetus, the placenta, and the amniotic fluid. The general increase in body fluid is spread out through the whole body.

Generalized water retention is caused by the increased circulatory needs of the mother, who is carrying the food and the waste products in her blood for herself and her baby. The placenta helps by secreting sodium-retaining hormones that chemically accentuate fluid accumulation. Doctors are not able to measure this retention directly, but they see it in swollen fingers and faces and in weight gain that cannot be accounted for by fetal growth alone. Finger swelling causes many women to abandon their wedding rings toward the end of the pregnancy, much to the chagrin of fathers-to-be.

Skeletal System

One of the most common characteristics acquired in pregnancy is the ducklike strut of the expectant mother. Although many women are able to maintain a graceful posture throughout gestation, they are in the remarkable minority. Because of the increased prominence of the uterus and the abdomen, the expectant mother tends to throw back her head and shoulders, exaggerating the curve of the small of the back and changing the body contour generally. In a woman carrying a very large baby or twins, this change of posture may be even more pronounced. The new posture may result in backache and strain in certain muscles.

Skin

Although it may seem totally unrelated to what's happening inside your body, the skin is affected in many ways as a result of pregnancy. Among the early changes in the skin is a darkening of the nipple area. Women who have any warts, moles, or scars may notice them darken as pregnancy progresses. There is also a line from the navel to the pubic bone that may become very dark and then gradually fade out at the edges. This *linea nigra* is much more visible on more darkly pigmented skin. These areas fade following delivery.

Another condition, referred to as the mask of pregnancy, or chloasma, may vary from small, yellow-brown spots to extensive dark-brown patches on the nose, the cheeks, and the neck. Although sometimes unsightly, these patches are no cause for worry since they disappear within a few weeks after delivery. (Some birth-control pills, which mimic pregnancy hormonally, may cause the same skin discoloration.) A sunscreen may decrease the pigmentation, which tends to increase in ultraviolet light.

Sometime during the second trimester, a woman may notice red spots on her face, neck, chest, and arms that look "spidery" because they have a tiny red center and threadlike branching "legs." These become more apparent as pregnancy progresses but disappear after delivery. A variation on these "spider spots" may appear on the feet, the palms, and the hands, causing them to become red and mottled. These skin changes are probably a result of hormonal changes.

Some women find themselves sweating more heavily during pregnancy, especially after the third month. To avoid annoying skin conditions, such as heat rash, try to stay cool and dry; a light dusting of talcum can be used, and clothes should be loose and comfortable.

Stretch marks, or striae, are common during pregnancy, probably also due to hormone changes. These occur mostly on the swelling belly, but some may also appear on the breasts and the thighs. On white skin, these start as thin pink lines but may become dense and white and brown and appear as loosely wrinkled skin. Striae are less common in black women. After delivery, the pink color fades but narrow ribbons of silver-white remain. It is difficult to predict who will or will not develop stretch marks during pregnancy. In most cases, there appears to a genetic predisposition.

Many studies have looked at both prevention and treatment of this condition. In one 1999 study, a reduction was found in the development of stretch marks in women who had developed them in past pregnancies when they used a cream containing *Centella asiatica* extract, alpha tocopherol, and collagen-elastin hydrolysates. As far as treatment goes, we recommend waiting until after pregnancy, because many times stretch marks will disappear with time. If they remain, however, fear not: A 2001 study using topical tretinoin 0.1 percent (retinoic acid) demonstrated, after twelve weeks of use, a reduction of striae by over 20 percent. Side effects included redness and scaling of the skin. This medication is available only by prescription and should never be used while pregnant or breast-feeding, as it may cause birth defects or health problems for the infant.

During the second half of pregnancy, there may be a gradual increase in the sensitivity of your skin to ultraviolet light. Be careful not to sunburn. Following pregnancy, you may experience some temporary hair loss, a condition attributed to withdrawal of the pregnancy hormones that have controlled hair growth for the past nine months. Hair grows in cycles, and as the hormones decrease after delivery, many cycles end abruptly. Loss of hair after birth, called postpartum alopecia, is described as a diffuse shedding of scalp hair that usually begins around two to five months after birth. A review of articles that examined various treatments from the 1960s until the year 2000 failed to reveal any positive results. Treatments have included birth control pills, topical hormones, and thyroid medication. Be reassured that hair that thinned during and after pregnancy will eventually return to normal.

The Uterus

Throughout pregnancy, the uterus, or womb, enlarges to make room for the fetus. Before conception, the uterus is the size and shape of a small pear and weighs about one and a half ounces. At the end of pregnancy, it weighs one and a half pounds. Its muscle fibers lengthen more than 100 times to support the developing baby. Uterine blood supply also increases to the point where veins carrying blood away from the uterus almost double their capacity.

There are two main parts to this primary organ of pregnancy. Its upper portion, called the *corpus*, is very muscular and expansive. The uterine mouth, called the *cervix*, is relatively inactive during fetal growth and development. But at the time of birth, both sections work in harmony and help deliver the baby.

The uterus is shaped so that the baby's head will probably settle near the cervix, its feet and buttocks in the upper portion of the corpus, the fundus. During labor, the fundus begins contracting, pushing the baby down. The cervix, meanwhile, dilates to allow the baby's exit.

The Uterine Cervix

The cervix is the entrance and the exit to the womb. Throughout pregnancy, the $1\frac{1}{2}$-inch-long "door" stays shut and sealed with a plug of mucus to keep germs away from the developing baby. For this whole period, the cervix is soft, thick, and passive. Then, just before labor, it begins a thinning, or effacement, until the whole length seems to disappear and the entire cervix is only a fraction of an inch thick. As labor progresses, the cervix opens, or dilates, to about the width of the hand to allow the baby to pass through. This dilation is coordinated with the contracting movement of the uterus.

Sometimes, the cervix fails to dilate, which may necessitate cesarean delivery. Once in a great while, the cervix fails to stay closed, a condition known as *cervical incompetence*. This is a rare cause of late abortion or miscarriage. The condition can be remedied by running a string or a suture around the perimeter of the opening of the cervix, which is then drawn and tied like a sack until labor begins, when it is removed.

The Position of the Uterus

The position of the uterus is a key factor in determining the length and the progress of pregnancy. For the first two months, it is situated below the pelvic bones and cannot be felt from the outside, but as it enlarges, it moves forward and lies on the bladder, causing more frequent urination than normal. As it enlarges, it rises out of the pelvis and in time lies against the abdominal wall, where the doctor's trained hand can feel it externally. It continues to move up until it has displaced the intestines and the stomach, which sometimes causes indigestion.

Each stage of growth of the uterus is accompanied by abdominal landmarks that help the doctor estimate the length of pregnancy. If the uterus is one-quarter of the way to the navel, you are two months pregnant; if it is halfway between the pubic bone and the navel, you are three months pregnant; three-quarters of the way marks four months of fetal growth. A uterus reaches the navel at about the fifth month of pregnancy. The uterus then rises one-quarter of the way from the navel to the end of the rib cage each month. Just before term, it sinks back to the eight-month level. This method of determining the length of pregnancy is called Bartholomew's Rule. It is really an approximation because of many variables in measuring, such as the thickness of the uterine wall, the amount of amniotic fluid, the size of the baby, or the presence of twins. But it is a fairly accurate and helpful tool for the doctor in confirming his or her original estimation of the date of delivery.

Lightening

About two weeks before birth, the uterus sinks. This sinking is caused by the fetus's head moving down into the pelvic cavity. It is called dropping, settling, or lightening and occurs in about 65 percent of all pregnancies prior to labor, although it is more common in women having a first baby.

Lightening may occur suddenly or gradually; in fact, it may occur without your even knowing it. It allows you to digest food more easily, to breathe a little easier. Your clothes will probably fit better, too. But because of the lowered position of the uterus, the early pressure symptoms of constipation and frequent urination may return. Yet lightening is usually a welcome sign because it means that the head is not too far away from eventual delivery.

Vagina and Vulva

For the purpose of reproduction, the vagina serves as the birth channel. Like the cervix, it stays relatively passive through the pregnancy, waiting to perform its special function at birth.

In preparation for birth, the veins enlarge enormously almost from the time of implantation, so that the vagina and its lips, the vulva, take on a deep port color. This purplish hue is known as Chadwick's sign of pregnancy. The vein engorgement may make intercourse a little uncomfortable, since the capacity of the vagina is diminished by the enlarged veins.

You may notice an increase in vaginal discharge, caused by the increased blood supply or by secretions from the cervix. If this discharge burns or has a disagreeable odor, report it to your doctor.

During pregnancy, the vagina stretches in length and increases in elasticity, so that at birth it can accommodate the body of a baby comfortably; then it shrinks back to its original size. Because the mouth of the vagina is not as elastic as the rest, it is common obstetrical practice in the United States to slit the opening of the vagina to accommodate the baby's exit and prevent unnecessary tearing. This incision is called an episiotomy and necessitates the stitches associated with delivery. There has recently been a large body of literature to support selective use of episiotomy. In other words, your doctor needs to make a decision at the time of delivery whether an episiotomy is necessary. Since all the data have surfaced, a major decline has occurred in episiotomy rates. A recent study looking at over 34,000 births in Philadelphia showed a decrease in the episiotomy rate from 69 percent in 1983 to 19 percent in 2000.

Abdomen

The greatest bodily change of all takes place in the abdomen. As the baby grows, you suddenly develop a great configuration that you may not be able to see over or lie on. Your navel may pop out, making it visible through thin layers of clothing. Stretch marks may also develop.

The stretching of the abdomen is made possible by the relaxation of the inner wall, especially in the area around the navel. In first pregnancies, the wall is very tense, and sometimes the baby grows faster than the uterine and the abdominal walls can stretch, so that the mother may periodically experience a tight feeling in the abdomen. For women who have had many babies, the abdomen may begin to droop, making it look very much like a sagging breast.

Breasts

Beginning in the second month of pregnancy, when the mammary, or milk-producing, glands begin to develop, the breasts grow. This growth, like most, continues throughout the period of gestation, reaching maximum potential during lactation. The breasts also become softer. Their veins enlarge and show up as bluish streaks. Striae gravidarum—stretch marks—may also be present.

During pregnancy, the nipples are more erect and the areolae (the darker pigmentation surrounding the nipples) may become even more deeply pigmented. Fluid may ooze out of the breasts quite early. In later months, this fluid changes to a diluted premilk called colostrum. This yellowish fluid nourishes the baby for the few days after birth before milk comes into the breasts of the nursing mother. Most doctors believe that colostrum is beneficial, in that it contains most of the mother's resistance to disease antibodies and offers the child equal immunity for the first few months of life. However, some feel that this factor is relatively unimportant since most of the antibodies are obtained while the infant is still in the uterus.

Ovaries

The ovaries that produced the egg that was fertilized play a different role during the pregnancy itself. One ovary usually becomes enlarged and grows a cyst or a fluid-containing structure called a corpus luteum. The cyst secretes hormones that signal the mother's body to prepare for gestation. The corpus luteum is the site at which the egg has broken away from the ovary during ovulation. It continues secreting hormones for six weeks, until the placenta is formed to take over the task.

COMMON SYMPTOMS DURING PREGNANCY

Pregnant women usually experience a range of symptoms, most of which are not threatening to their health. The following are the most common.

Braxton-Hicks contractions. These periodic uterine contractions may start as early as the first trimester. They begin as a tightening feeling at the top of the uterus, gradually spread downward, and then disappear. These contractions exercise and strengthen your uterus for the hard work of labor ahead. In the late third trimester, these contractions increase and may be responsible for early thinning (effacement) and opening (dilation) of the cervix before labor actually begins.

Breast swelling. The breasts may swell, tingle, and throb during pregnancy as milk glands develop. Lumpy breasts are also quite common in pregnancy. However, if the breasts feel suspicious in any way—if lumps are hard or fixed or cause dimpling—discuss this with your physician.

Wear a support bra right from the start: Most of the weight gain in the breasts comes during the first half of pregnancy. If your breasts get very large, it may be a good idea to wear a bra even at night. Lack of support during pregnancy may exacerbate sagging afterward. Hereditary factors also play a part in how much loss of tone you can expect in the breasts.

Nipple secretions. Colostrum, a sticky, yellowish, watery fluid that will be the baby's first food, may be secreted from the nipples during pregnancy. In the later months of pregnancy, drops may form spontaneously on the nipples and may be expressed (squeezed) from the nipples by hand.

Muscle cramps. Cramps are common during pregnancy and may be due to changes in the blood supply to various muscles or to changes in calcium metabolism (calcium is involved in muscle contraction). Shooting pains down your legs can be due to pressure of the fetus's head on certain nerves. Elevating your legs and using heating pads may help ease cramps.

Dizziness or faintness. During pregnancy, a dizzy or faint feeling can be due to (1) the enlarged uterus pressing on the major blood vessels, causing blood pressure to drop; or (2) hormonal changes that cause a relaxation or a widening of blood vessels so that blood pools in the legs. Move slowly to avoid sudden blood pressure changes; also assume new positions (especially from lying down to standing) slowly.

Gas. Flatulence is a common complaint of pregnancy. The stomach and the intestines may swell and give you a bloated feeling. Taking laxatives may help, as will avoiding gas-producing foods like beans, cabbage, onions, and fried foods. Regular bowel movements reduce gas.

Hemorrhoids. A well-known result of increased pressure on the veins in your anus is hemorrhoids. They are the lower bowel's equivalent of the legs' varicose veins. Avoid constipation and straining when moving the bowels. Cold compresses with witch hazel comfort hemorrhoids that do form. Hemorrhoids generally become worse just after delivery and then gradually recede in the postpartum period.

Shortness of breath. Pregnant women take in more air for various hormonal reasons. Also, by late pregnancy the fetus is so large it borrows some of the space that the lungs normally expand into. This shortness of breath is nothing to worry about and is not a sign of heart or lung disease.

Backache. This is one of the most common minor problems of pregnant women. It is caused by the changes in posture required by the growing, thriving fetus. Backache is usually best treated with heating pads, analgesics (check with your doctor first), a pillow to support the small of the back when sitting, a maternity girdle, and a firm mattress.

Special exercises may help alleviate backache by strengthening the back muscles and relieving excess tension. Consult your physician, however, before starting any exercise program. Severe backache may be incapacitating and should be treated.

Constipation. Pregnancy hormones produce a relaxation of the bowel and, along with decreased physical activity and pressure on the lower bowel by the growing fetus, increase the tendency toward irregularity. Most women who had very regular bowel habits before pregnancy can cope with the tendency toward constipation by drinking plenty of fluids, taking gentle exercise like walking, and using mild laxatives such as milk of magnesia, dried fruits, prune juice, and fibery whole-grain cereals. Avoid the routine use of harsh laxatives and enemas;

they may become habit-forming. Here, again, your physician is your best guide to the use of *any* medication, even those available without a prescription.

Excessive urination. Frequent urination may become a problem as the fetus grows and presses on the bladder. "Every five minutes—even during the night!" I've been told more than once in mock seriousness. This is normal. Burning or a constant urge to urinate, however, suggests a bladder infection and should be checked out by your doctor.

Swollen ankles and varicose veins. Many women develop varicose veins as the fetus grows and puts pressure on the veins in the legs. An inherited tendency may aggravate this condition, in which veins are distended and swollen and may be painful and tender. They are aggravated by long periods of standing and by large weight gains. Many women find that elastic support hose provide the best relief from discomfort. Support stockings vary in strength, from mildly elastic light support to surgical stockings that are expensive and require expert fitting. Ask your doctor for suggestions.

Fatigue. Pregnant women tire easily, especially in the first and third trimesters. Taking a nap during the afternoon or going to bed earlier may help. If you are a working woman, try to rest during lunch and breaks.

Headaches. Mild headaches of short duration are a common complaint, especially during early pregnancy. We do not know the cause, but most disappear by midpregnancy. Simple analgesics, such as Tylenol, are helpful. Check with your physician to see what he or she prescribes, and to be sure your headaches are not severe enough to suggest other problems.

Heartburn. The growing fetus pressing on the stomach causes your food to occasionally be pushed up into the esophagus, the tube that runs from the mouth to the stomach. Heartburn—irritation of the esophagus—causes a burning sensation in the lower chest or the mid-abdominal region. Treatment consists of taking antacid medication and eating bland foods like bread, pasta, and milk. Sleeping on two or three pillows may also help by enlisting gravity to help keep food down where it belongs.

Nausea and vomiting. These are among the most common problems of the first trimester of pregnancy: About 50 percent of women have them to some degree. Nausea may actually be your first clue to pregnancy—

it can appear as early as the second week, but usually develops about the fifth week or following a missed period. Symptoms may continue into the third month or longer. Most, but not all, women report feeling sick after getting up or after breakfast—hence the moniker *morning sickness*.

The cause of this nausea is not really known, although hormonal effects on the gastrointestinal tract are probably to blame. The treatment is quite simple: Most women find that frequent small snacks of dry foods (like graham crackers), small sips of liquids, and starchy foods (like rice and pasta) are helpful. Keep a couple of crackers at your bedside and eat them when you wake up. If vomiting is so persistent you can hardly keep anything down, let your doctor know.

Rhinitis. Pregnant nose is what many women who develop it call postnasal drip, a persistent feeling of nasal stuffiness caused by a swelling of the mucous membranes of the nose and the throat. The "pregnancy rhinitis" is due to the effects of estrogen on these tissues. If it is annoying, appropriate medication can be prescribed by your physician.

Tooth decay. The old theory had it that the mother's teeth decalcify to provide calcium and phosphorus for the fetus. It is now known that this theory is not valid. But while there is no evidence of an adverse effect of pregnancy on healthy teeth, chronic inflammation of the gums is common. This inflammation, due to the increase in estrogen, which boosts the blood supply to and thickens the gums, usually gets worse as pregnancy progresses. Routine dental visits should be scheduled during the course of pregnancy and any cavities filled. Local anesthetics for the treatment of dental caries will not harm the fetus in any way.

EMOTIONAL REACTIONS DURING PREGNANCY

Most women realize that in addition to physical changes, pregnancy can cause profound emotional reactions. Some of these are conscious feelings, such as the deep pleasure that comes from the confirmation of pregnancy; others are unconscious, such as the fear of bodily pain or death. When a woman realizes that she is pregnant, even if the pregnancy is much wanted and carefully planned, anxiety and ambivalence coexist. Pregnancy, delivery, and the postpartum period may be marked by physical strain and psychological stress. Fear and uncertainty are frequently experienced in the same way that they are in any other major life change.

Extreme anxiety can interfere with labor and delivery and with being a parent. It can stem from several different sources:

- Worry about the effects of the baby on your relationship with your partner
- Worry about not having the capacity to love and care for an infant
- A special deep preference regarding the baby's sex
- Dread of having an abnormal baby
- Ambivalence about giving up your personal freedom

It is important to recognize that some anxiety and ambivalence are absolutely normal. They do not mean you can't be a good parent, or that you weren't ready for pregnancy. Contrary to common sense, and probably against all evidence from friends and family members who have been there themselves, many people persist in expecting pregnancy to be an idyllic time. It won't be. Pregnancy is too momentous an occasion to be contained by one small part of your emotions. One patient commented, "I'm a successful banker, 200 people work for me, and I rise to every business challenge. But I'm scared stiff of having this baby." Another patient, a successful model, was vomiting a lot during pregnancy—it turned out she was scared of having an ugly child. A good doctor–patient relationship will make it possible for you to voice your fears: It is important to get your doubts out in the open (where a looming anxiety often shrinks to a more appropriate size), without feeling criticized or guilty.

Certain physical discomforts of the first trimester—nausea, vomiting, fatigue, and headaches—may bring a sense of disappointment if the expected feeling of excitement is not present. Moodiness is common. However, the second trimester is usually characterized by a sense of well-being. The unpleasant symptoms of the first trimester often disappear, and the excitement of feeling your baby move and seeing your belly swell contributes to this good feeling.

Often during the third trimester, some discomfort and fatigue occur. There is also increased anxiety, as well as insomnia. These normal fears center on the realities of being a mother, the inevitable changes in the marriage, concerns about labor and delivery (especially if there have been problems in the past), concern about the sex and the health of the baby, and concerns about death or injury to yourself and the child.

Emotional Aspects of High-Risk Pregnancy

A pregnancy following a period of infertility, the birth of an abnormal child, a spontaneous abortion, or the loss of a child may be accompanied by understandably heightened anxiety. If a miscarriage has occurred in the past, a woman may wonder if she can carry the current fetus to term. She may fear that she has physical problems or is somehow damaged. Listening to the fetal heart tones, seeing the fetus on ultrasound, and becoming involved with the progress of the pregnancy may all help to ease anxiety.

Pregnancy is generally a normal event. However, with high-risk obstetrical patients, pregnancy is not normal. Living with the fear of losing an unborn baby is highly stressful. Feelings of guilt and blame are common. Worries about hurting the fetus during sex may create tension with your partner. Talk to your doctor about these feelings; if they seem out of proportion or otherwise too difficult to handle, your doctor may suggest seeing someone specially trained to help couples through this very difficult time. One of our patients, who had three spontaneous abortions, was overcome by terrible anxiety. Her problem was handled by scheduling an appointment every week so that she could listen to the fetal heartbeat.

Sex during Pregnancy

There are marked individual differences in the effect of pregnancy on sexuality. Many women report increased desire, although pregnancy has also been reported to dampen sexuality. As a general rule, sexual interest and frequency of intercourse are reported to be higher during the first trimester than before pregnancy; above normal, but below the first trimester, during the second trimester; and decreased in the third trimester and after delivery. Fatigue, physical discomfort, and fear of harming the fetus are common interferences at the end of pregnancy.

Women may become anxious about their attractiveness before and after delivery. Many feel there's something not quite right about even showing their sexuality during pregnancy. Women who are pregnant—and facing the challenge of nurturing for the first time in their lives—may also experience an increased need for nurturing and physical contact themselves. If you are surprised by a disruption in your sex life and wonder whether this reaction is normal, a discussion with your obstetrician will help put things into perspective.

Fears about Labor and Delivery

No one doubts that women experience pain during childbirth. However, preparation, understanding, and a positive attitude can reduce that suffering.

For some women, delivery may be their first experience in a hospital. An earlier tour may help reduce fears associated with a hospital. Virtually all so-called psychoprophylactic techniques (Lamaze is a well-known one) contain elements of education, physical therapy, and psychotherapy and, for many women, reduce the need for pain relief and anesthesia. Women in such classes are educated in the anatomy and the physiology of childbirth, trained to relax mentally and physically, and taught to concentrate on breathing exercises, which distract them from the pain.

Many studies on the psychological factors relating to childbirth agree that underlying a positive childbirth experience is a woman's desire to be an active participant in labor and delivery. Prepared childbirth not only reduces pain, but also enhances the experience of birth and facilitates the bond between mother and child. Prepared childbirth has been shown to result in the use of fewer drugs and in higher levels of enjoyment of the process of childbirth.

Yet there are limits to what prepared childbirth can accomplish. If a woman sets very rigid standards or has unrealistic expectations about delivery, she could have a very difficult time when things do not follow a precise, predetermined course. If ideal labor is painless and the use of drugs represents failure, then a woman may feel that she did not "measure up" to natural childbirth if she didn't revel in every nonmedicated contraction. Women should be prepared for the potential need for medical intervention and drugs. Understanding the use of medications ahead of time will avoid help women needless anxiety and prevent their feeling inadequate and guilty if they need medication.

A difficult delivery can be traumatic and emotionally exhausting and may contribute to postpartum depression. Since women do most of the work involved in labor, even the most competent women require support, encouragement, and praise. That is where a husband, a friend, or a family member plays a critical role.

Fetal monitoring can both ease and create anxiety. Monitoring, although a major advance in obstetrical care, may present a dilemma: It transforms the labor room into an intensive-care setting at a time when couples are seeking a more personal childbirth experience. Many women find the monitor a reassurance of the baby's condition during labor, but others find it an uncomfortable annoyance that interferes with labor, detracts attention from them, and provokes anxiety. Women should be fully advised when it is needed, be familiar with the equipment before-hand, and have their views about it considered. Women who have had problems with labor and delivery in the past—with previous obstetrical losses—more readily accept fetal monitoring and respond more positively to it. Fetal monitoring, when used sensitively and intelligently, can be an asset in the management of childbirth.

Family-centered obstetric care includes the father in delivery. It treats childbearing as a normal and healthy process—a major family experience. Fathers are now present much more often in the labor and the delivery rooms, even in the cesarean section room. They have become actively involved in the delivery process, even to the extent of assisting in the delivery in some centers. A father's participation during labor and delivery provides emotional support to the mother, even during cesarean section. Some obstetricians may wish the father to leave should certain problems arise at delivery. In any event, the doctor's and the hospital's policy should be discussed in advance.

Home births may seem to be gaining in popularity, but their number has actually remained constant at about 1 percent since 1977. A major deterrent is the fact that a complicated labor can follow a perfectly normal, uneventful pregnancy: 20 percent of normal pregnancies may be followed by labor complications. The solution, therefore, would seem to be to make the hospital more homelike, rather than take delivery back to the home. Caring, warmth, and attention on the part of the medical staff will help this occur. Birthing rooms also contribute to a more home-like feeling in the hospital.

Recently, the option of having a baby delivered by a midwife in a hospital setting has become more widely available. Midwives are nurses who have taken special training in pregnancy and delivery. They are certified to do deliveries under supervision in most states. They provide another alternative method of care and may also offer the economic benefit of lower cost.

Chapter 5

Prenatal Care

———✸———

PREGNANCY AND CHILDBIRTH today are safer than ever because of the emphasis on prenatal care now given in this country. It is important that every woman visit a doctor as soon as pregnancy is suspected. This visit will mark the formal beginning of prenatal, or antepartum, care. The purpose of prenatal care is to ensure the delivery of a healthy baby to a healthy mother.

The fetus, throughout pregnancy, is not totally accessible to the doctor, who wants to know its condition but cannot see it inside the safe, cushioned environment of the womb. Your doctor can, however, monitor you on a regular basis, looking for signs and symptoms that might indicate trouble. The doctor is especially sensitive to signs in the early months, when the developing human is most vulnerable to outside influences, such as medications taken by the mother.

As discussed in chapter 1, good prenatal care should really begin prior to conception. By the time pregnancy is usually confirmed, about six weeks following the last menstrual period, most of the fetal organs are already formed; the circulatory system and major sense organs are well developed. Ideally, every woman should have a complete physical before she plans to become pregnant.

Although we do not live in a perfect world, you can safely rely on the skill of your physician to watch closely what will probably be a smooth and uneventful pregnancy.

THE FIRST VISIT

When you first visit the doctor, you will probably be anxious for him or her to examine you to confirm your suspicion that you are going to have a baby. Or, if pregnancy has been confirmed, you will want the doctor to give you some instructions to follow during this very special period of gestation. But before that, the doctor will probably want a complete medical history of you and your family. He or she will pay particular attention to your past obstetrical history, which includes a brief account of each former pregnancy and delivery, miscarriages, or abortions. You will also be asked about any prior infections and medical problems.

With this completed, you will be given a physical examination, starting with a measure of your blood pressure, which will be checked at each succeeding visit. An abnormal rise in blood pressure late in pregnancy may indicate the development of toxemia, a disturbance in the system that can occur only in pregnancy.

You will be weighed, and your doctor will use your weight at this visit as a reference point to know how much and how quickly you are gaining.

The doctor will take a blood sample, which will provide much information. First, he or she will measure the hemoglobin, the oxygen-carrying protein of red blood cells. Too few red cells will indicate anemia, which is very common among pregnant women. If you have anemia in pregnancy, chances are you will tire more easily and will not be able to support your own health and the growth of the fetus as well as you might otherwise. This condition is easily corrected with daily supplements of iron. The doctor may give you a prescription for iron, in addition to one for prenatal vitamins. From the same blood sample, the doctor will determine your blood type—especially your Rh status, which is discussed at length in chapter 12. He or she will also do a blood test to rule out syphillis, a venereal disease that can cause congenital abnormalities in the fetus. Other commonly performed blood tests look for a susceptibility to rubella or toxoplasmosis and the presence of abnormal blood antibodies and hepatitis.

You will probably be asked by the doctor to bring a specimen of your first voided urine on the day of your visit, and you will be asked to do so for each visit thereafter. By analyzing the specimen, the doctor can check for the presence of sugar or protein, which would indicate diabetes or kidney abnormalities, respectively.

The doctor will also perform a physical examination. A vaginal exam will yield a great deal of information. By feeling the uterus, the doctor can measure its size, which will confirm pregnancy. The birth channel or the pelvis will be measured to see if it is wide enough to allow the passage of a baby. Ask for a Pap smear, the cancer-screening test that every woman should have at least once a year. The doctor may take another smear for gonorrhea and chlamydia, venereal diseases.

While you are on the table, your doctor will examine your breasts and feel your abdomen for the growth of the uterus. The uterus with the fetus within can usually be felt through the abdomen after the third month of pregnancy.

After the physical, your doctor will outline the course of pregnancy and will ask you to return every three to four weeks until the eighth month, when you will probably visit the doctor every two weeks. In the ninth month, you will go every week and sometimes more often.

Fetal growth will be measured by feeling the abdomen, but occasionally a vaginal examination may also be performed to monitor fetal growth, position, and size more closely. Vaginal examinations during the ninth month are often a routine procedure to determine if the baby's head will pass through the pelvic cavity and to assess the condition of the cervix to predict the possible onset of labor. Sometimes this examination is followed by some slight vaginal bleeding, which should be no cause for worry.

Many physicians perform routine sonograms during pregnancy to determine the stage, the growth, and the health of the fetus. See chapter 7 for more information on sonography.

Instructions to patients vary from doctor to doctor, but basically, diet, sleep, bowel function, clothing, bathing, and dental care are reviewed. The main goals of the first examination are to check the health of the mother and the fetus; to determine the age of the pregnancy and the fetus; and to start a plan for continuing obstetrical care.

Don't be afraid to ask questions. The more you know, the less frightened you will be and the more you will enjoy your pregnancy.

POTENTIAL DANGER SYMPTOMS IN PREGNANCY

Your doctor will probably outline certain warning symptoms to watch for. If any of these are present, report them to your doctor immediately. Smoking and drug and alcohol use will be discussed, as well as diet and exercise.

- *Vaginal bleeding* is usually insignificant; 20 percent of all pregnant women report having it in some form during the first three months of gestation. Bleeding may be caused by a leaking blood vessel or a number of other factors. But it may also be a sign of impending miscarriage. Always report this to your doctor. If significant bleeding occurs in the first trimester of pregnancy, there is approximately a 50 percent chance of miscarriage; the other 50 percent of women will likely have normal pregnancies.

- *Swelling of the face or the fingers* may be a sign of fluid retention, but it may also signal the onset of toxemia, and it, too, should be reported to the doctor immediately.
- *Blurring of vision,* like swelling, may be a sign of fluid retention or of preeclampsia.
- *Severe and continual headaches* may result from rhinitis, a sinus condition often occurring in pregnancy, but they can also mean that an excessive amount of fluid is being retained or that toxemia is developing. They should be reported to your doctor.
- *Severe pain in the abdomen* is not normal. The abdomen may be a little sore during pregnancy from the rapid growth of the fetus. Intermittent contractions may also be normal. But constant or debilitating pain is not normal and should not go unattended.
- *Persistent vomiting* is dangerous. Some nausea and vomiting occur in 50 percent of all pregnancies and, by itself, vomiting should be no cause for alarm. But persistent vomiting should be reported to your doctor.
- *Fever* usually means that there is a foreign virus or bacteria in the body to which your system is reacting. Fever in pregnancy is no exception. A high temperature may result from a cold, but it may also mean an infection in the reproductive or the urinary tract, so it should be reported to your doctor immediately.
- *Fluid discharge from the vagina* can have several causes. Sometimes the fluid is actually a little urine leaking from the bladder due to pressure. This is normal. Vaginal discharge during pregnancy usually increases, becoming thick and sticky. A clear fluid discharge is not so normal. It may be just a secretion of the cervix, but it may also indicate a leakage of amniotic fluid, which means there is a rupture in the amniotic sac, the membrane surrounding the fetus and the fluid.

NUTRITION IN PREGNANCY

During pregnancy, the mother is the sole source of all the nutrients her fetus needs for growth and development. If this supply is too low, fetal growth may be affected—an infant may be born with a condition known as intrauterine growth retardation (IUGR). These small babies may have problems after birth. The dramatic result of severe food deprivation has been graphically demonstrated during famines in various areas of the world: During famine periods, average birth weight falls as much as 10 percent.

But IUGR doesn't happen only in remote Third World countries. Poor women in the United States whose food supply is limited and very underweight women are also at risk. Maternal malnutrition exists as well among pregnant adolescents and women who limit their food intake for reasons such as weight control or fad diets. Also, excessive physical activity can deplete the mother's energy intake and possibly deprive the fetus of needed calories for growth. It has been found that babies born in developing countries during the months of heavy agricultural labor are lower in birth weight than babies born at other times of the year. Although the food supply of these active pregnant women may not be limited, their nutritional needs differ from those of the sedentary pregnant woman.

Good maternal nutrition should begin even before you become pregnant. Women who start off too thin are more likely to deliver small babies, even if they eat right and gain weight normally during pregnancy. Women who are overweight when they conceive are more likely to have difficulties with delivery and to develop high blood pressure. However, pregnancy is *not* a time to diet. Along with depriving the fetus of the critical nutritional support it needs, extreme dieting, with the breakdown of fat that occurs, can release toxic substances, called ketone bodies, that could harm the fetus.

Basic Principles of Nutrition in Pregnancy

Because the baby's only source of nutrition comes from your diet, it is essential to have a good understanding of your nutritional needs.

Caloric Intake and Weight

The total number of calories consumed appears to be the single most important nutritional factor affecting infant birth weight. But "eating for two"—even for one and a half—is out. A typical sedentary pregnancy requires about 300 extra calories per day, assuming that you maintain your normal level of activity. Active pregnant women need more. Three hundred calories is only the amount in one generous scoop of ice cream. You obviously can't eat everything in sight. And you can't even just go for that ice cream every day. You have to spend those added extra calories wisely on the extra nutrients your baby needs: extra protein, calcium, iron, and B vitamins.

During the average pregnancy, twenty-four to twenty-six pounds is considered the appropriate amount of weight to gain. But the rate of gain is as important as the total amount gained. For the entire first three months, a pound and a half to three pounds gained is average. Thereafter, one pound can be gained every nine days. The most rapid weight gain occurs in the last three months, when the fetus is growing quickly.

A total weight gain of about twenty-four pounds breaks down the following way: The baby weighs about seven and a half pounds at birth; the placenta, one and a half pounds; the amniotic fluid, two pounds; the increase in the size of the uterus adds two pounds; increase in breast size, one pound; fat and water in the maternal tissues weighs about six to ten pounds; and the increase in the mother's blood volume is about four pounds. A week or two after the baby is born, you should have lost about eighteen to twenty pounds. Most women will lose the remainder within four months if they are not breast-feeding.

Women who start out underweight should gain about thirty pounds, or about six pounds more than the normal twenty-four. A weight gain of greater than thirty-five pounds is not recommended. Excessive weight gain may result in permanent obesity, with its resulting complications of high blood pressure, diabetes, and heart disease. Although many women who gain excessive weight during pregnancy do lose it after delivery, too many women retain the excess. Nutrition in pregnancy, therefore, is a delicate balance of taking in the right nutrients without overdoing the calories. Even women with minimal willpower find the idea of doing right by the baby a strong source of motivation to keep them eating right but without dieting.

Protein

Deficiencies in protein during pregnancy can be dangerous for the developing fetus. Recent studies looking at pregnant rats given a low-protein diet demonstrated their offspring developing more hypertension and heart problems. In this 2001 study, the researchers found that when the pregnant rat had insufficient protein in its diet, the developing fetus produced increased amounts of a chemical that led to higher blood pressure. Many other animal studies in the past have also established this result. An increase of 30 grams of protein per day is recommended for pregnancy. This makes the total desirable intake 75 to 100 grams of protein per day. That should be about 12 percent of your total calories. Most protein-containing foods are also excellent sources of many vitamins and minerals essential for the fetus, such as iron, vitamin B_6 and zinc. In addition to the milk products every pregnant women should have, you need at least three servings a day of protein-rich foods, such as meat, fish, poultry, or eggs.

There is no evidence that eating more than 100 grams of protein per day is of any value. A high-protein, low-calorie diet is *not* desirable during pregnancy. You need a steady supply of energy, which can best be provided by carbohydrates.

Vegetarian diets that exclude some or all animal proteins can provide adequate nutrition, but pregnant vegetarians need to be even more careful about food selection than the meat-eating pregnant woman. Lacto-ovo vegetarian diets—those that include dairy products and eggs—easily provide all the nutrients needed for pregnancy. But if all animal protein sources are avoided, it's hard to get enough vitamin B_{12} zinc, iron, calcium, vitamin D, and riboflavin into your meals. If vegetable protein is used to meet the day's requirements, the essential amino acids in the various foods must be properly balanced so that the protein intake becomes "complete" in terms of the body's needs. This is achieved by combining grains with beans or nuts, or combining any of these with dairy products in the same meal. Due to the low fat and the high bulk of vegetarian foods, pregnant women may have trouble consuming enough calories. Vitamin and mineral supplements are generally recommended, and added vegetable oils and fats may be encouraged if there is too little fuel in the diet otherwise.

Iron

Women whose diets are deficient in iron can develop anemia. A study done between 1998 and 1999, on women who had iron deficient anemia during their pregnancy, found that their babies also showed evidence of anemia at nine months of age. Extra iron is needed during pregnancy for the additional red blood cells the mother produces and for the fetus to produce its own entire blood supply. About 800 milligrams of iron are needed to accomplish this during the second half of pregnancy. This comes to about 5 to 6 milligrams daily, which many women's bodies cannot provide for the fetus without depleting their own stores. Therefore, a daily supplement providing 30 to 60 milligrams of elemental iron is recommended for all pregnant women. Folic acid may also be given as a supplement, since pregnancy doubles your folic acid requirement and because it helps iron metabolism.

Good food sources of iron include dried fruits, liver, kidneys, prune juice, and dried beans. The type of food selected not only influences the amount of iron you get, it also influences the amount of iron that can be absorbed by your body. Some foods enhance iron absorption, whereas others inhibit it. Animal proteins and vitamin C (ascorbic acid) enhance iron absorption. Tea and milk reduce this absorption and should be avoided at meals, especially when good iron sources are consumed. (Cast iron pans may provide significant amounts of iron, particularly if acidic foods like spaghetti sauce are cooked in them.)

A part of your prepregnancy and pregnancy counseling will include a complete blood count to rule out anemia. If you start a pregnancy with an iron deficiency or develop anemia during pregnancy, larger doses of iron will be required, and your physician will prescribe an extra iron supplement. If you find yourself constantly overtired, ask your physician to check your iron status again.

Calcium

A daily intake of 1,200 milligrams of calcium is recommended during pregnancy to provide the extra 30 grams of calcium required to build your baby's bones. An animal study conducted in 2002 showed that rats given a low-calcium diet produced offspring with high blood pressure problems later in life. If you don't like milk, you don't have to drink it. Milk products like cheese, yogurt, and cottage cheese are equally good sources of calcium. Whole, skim, or powdered milk can be added to soups and baked goods and even whipped into potatoes. Broccoli, spinach, kale, and mustard greens also supply calcium, but the calcium from vegetables is less easily absorbed by the body.

Four cups of milk or yogurt supply the daily recommended amount of calcium. The calcium equivalent of one cup of milk is supplied by one and a half ounces of cheddar cheese, one and three-quarter cups of ice cream, or two cups of cottage cheese. A quart of milk also provides the needed amounts of vitamins A and D and two-fifths of the day's protein needs. If you can't drink regular milk because of lactose intolerance (an inability to digest milk sugar), you should have no trouble with hard, unprocessed cheeses, like cheddar or Swiss, and you may be able to handle cultured milk products like yogurt and buttermilk.

Sodium

There is an increase in the total amount of water retained in a pregnant woman's body. To keep your chemical balance, you need to increase the total amount of body sodium—about twenty-two grams extra.

In the past, salt was forbidden to pregnant women, and diuretic ("water") pills were prescribed whenever fluid accumulation occurred. It used to be thought that high salt intake caused a serious condition known as toxemia of pregnancy, which could then be treated with salt restriction and diuretics. We now know that this is not true. In fact, toxemic women have too *little* total body water and salt. Diuretics should not be used in pregnancy unless prescribed by a physician, and even then only in very special cases.

Still, you should avoid excess amounts of salt. Salt your food to taste. A diet based on whole, natural foods can be safely salted within reason. Processed foods are usually heavily preseasoned with salt and should be eaten in moderation, without additional salting.

Other Nutrients

The body's dietary need for folic acid increases during pregnancy to support the growth of the fetus. Many vitamin supplements for pregnant women (often prescribed by a doctor) now contain folic acid. Foods rich in folic acid include eggs, leafy vegetables, oranges, whole grain cereals, and wheat germ. Whole grains and wheat germ also provide zinc, vitamin B_6, magnesium, and vitamin E. These nutrients are removed during the refinement of grains and are often not replaced during the enrichment process. A diet that includes whole grain cereals will be rich in nutrients and fiber, which adds bulk and aids bowel function.

Nutrition when Breast-Feeding

If you plan to nurse, you should know that a woman's nutritional needs are even greater during lactation than in pregnancy. A nursing mother has to produce about a quart of milk a day to satisfy her baby. To do this, she will probably need an extra 1,000 calories a day above her prepregnancy diet. Those calories should include an extra 40 grams of protein, at least a quart of milk a day, and additional eggs, cheese, butter, liver, and vegetables. Fluid intake should total 2 quarts to maintain the volume of milk produced.

Eating for Active Pregnant Women

Based on our knowledge of the nutritional needs of pregnancy and the effects of strenuous exercise, we can make some general recommendations for women who exercise during pregnancy.

A pregnant woman who exercises needs to consume more calories than a pregnant woman who does not exercise. That amount depends, of course, on how much exercise she is getting. Therefore, it is impossible to make a specific recommendation. As a general rule, however, a woman who maintains a thirty-minute daily exercise program during pregnancy should consume an additional 500 calories. Of course, every woman is different, and you should carefully monitor your rate of weight gain; if it begins to fall below normal at any stage, you should increase your calorie intake. In all cases, be alert to your appetite, so you can best adjust your food intake to match your physical needs.

A diet high in complex carbohydrates is recommended because carbohydrates best replace muscle glycogen burned during exercise. Pregnancy and physical activity increase the need for protein. However, since the usual protein consumption in the United States is well above the requirement for pregnancy, it probably also covers the additional needs of exercise. In general, the physically active pregnant woman's diet should be about 12 percent protein. If you consume 2,300 calories a day, about 69 grams should be in protein. A woman taking in 3,000 calories a day would need about 90 grams of protein.

The iron needs of all pregnant women are similar, since exercise does not appear to increase the need for iron. But a woman who starts an exercise program after becoming pregnant will need greater amounts of iron to accommodate the blood volume expansion associated with training. However, if you were not involved in an exercise program prior to becoming pregnant, it is *not recommended* that you embark on one now. The requirements of the training program on top of the developing pregnancy may simply be too much for the body to take at once without risking your good health.

Physically active pregnant women need to drink lots of water in order to replace that depleted during exercise. Taking care to drink extra fluids—and plain water is best—is important to maintain adequate hydration.

Sodium sweated off during exercise also has to be replaced. Most pregnant women take in more than enough salt, but the physically active pregnant woman may risk sodium depletion if her exercise is vigorous and her sodium intake low. Although prolonged outdoor exercise in hot weather is not recommended, those who do it should eat extra amounts of salty foods. Table 5.1 summarizes the various nutritional needs of active nonpregnant, nonactive pregnant, and active pregnant women.

TABLE 5.1
Comparison Study of Nutritional Needs

	ACTIVE NONPREGNANT WOMEN	NONACTIVE PREGNANT WOMEN	ACTIVE PREGNANT WOMEN
Calories	1. Increase to energy needs. 2. Complex carbohydrates important.	1. Increase 300 cal/day. 2. Increase protein sources.	1. Increase 500–600 cal/day. 2. Weight gain is good guide. 3. Increase proteins and carbohydrates.
Protein	Normal percentage of calories.	Increase to 75 g/day.	Increase to 75–90 g/day.
Iron	1. Increase required during training. 2. No increase after training.	Increase to 30–60 mg/day.	Increase 30–60 mg/day.
Water	During exercise, 10–12 glasses of fluids per day.	Increase fluids to thirst.	1. 8–12 glasses extra water during exercise. 2. Increase during heat.
Sodium	Increased needs, especially in hot weather.	Salt to taste.	Increased needs, especially in hot weather.
Calcium	Retention higher with activity, resulting in increased bone density; no additional requirement.	Additional 30 g calcium. Daily total of 1,200 mg calcium.	Same as nonactive pregnant women.

NOTE: *Active woman* means one who exercises for at least 30 minutes 3 times per week.

In summary, energy is the main nutritional need of the physically active pregnant woman. If you get enough total calories, most of the other nutritional requirements will be satisfied, as long as you try to eat a wide variety of foods and keep empty "junk" calories to a minimum. The athletic woman is urged to eat according to her appetite and to double-check the accuracy of this approach by tracking weight

TABLE 5.2
Basic Daily Pregnancy Diet

PREDOMINANT NUTRIENT	FOODS	NUMBER OF SERVINGS
Protein and iron	Lean meats, fish, poultry, lentils, dried beans and peas, eggs, nuts	3 or more (7 oz. total)
Protein and calcium	All milks, cheese, cottage cheese	4 or more
Vitamin C	Citrus fruits and juices, broccoli, brussels sprouts, tomatoes, peppers	1 or more
Vitamin A	Dark green and deep yellow vegetables, fortified margarine, kidneys, liver	1 or more
Energy and B vitamins	Whole grain or enriched breads and cereals	5
Other vitamins and minerals	All fruits and vegetables	2 or more
Energy	Fats and sugar	Only as needed for energy

gain carefully. We advise athletic women to buy a good scale and weigh themselves weekly. If your rate of gain deviates from the normal range at any time, you should adjust your calorie intake to get you back on your food track.

Menu Suggestions

As a general guide, remember: Everything you eat or drink, except water, has calories. For the period of pregnancy, your goal is to find foods with maximum nutritive food value per calorie. This does not mean that all carbohydrates should be removed from the diet. A small or moderate amount of starches is needed to satisfy your appetite and thus avoid overeating. The byword, though, is moderation.

The following plan may help you. It contains a sample diet for one day, based on a nucleus of protein-rich foods. These meals will be good for the whole family and can be altered easily to meet special dietary needs. Table 5.2 summarizes the basic daily needs during pregnancy and offers nutritionally sound choices.

BREAKFAST
Citrus fruit, 4 oz.
Cereal, 1/2 oz., and/or bread and butter
Egg, 1
Milk, 8 oz.

LUNCH
Protein dish (see table 5.2)
Bread, 2 slices as in a sandwich
Vegetables or salad
Milk, 8 oz.
Fruit, 1 cup

DINNER
Meat or equivalent, 4 oz.
Potato, 1
Vegetable, 1/2 oz. spinach, broccoli, peas, etc.
Butter
Milk
Fruit or dessert

BETWEEN MEALS
Milk and/or fruit

A two- to three-ounce serving of lean cooked meat, fish, or poultry without bones is

1/4 lb. hamburger after cooking
1/2 cup cooked diced lean meat, fish, or poultry
1 medium meat or fish patty
1 slice roast meat or poultry (5 in. × 2 1/4 in. × 1/4 in.)
2 frankfurters
2 slices of liver
2 slices of meatloaf
2 medium chicken drumsticks
1 chicken leg (including thigh)
1 medium-sized fish steak

A substitute for a two- to three-ounce serving of lean cooked meat, fish, or poultry without bones is

1/2 cup cottage cheese
3 ounces cheddar or jack cheese

1 cup cooked dried peas, beans, or lentils
1/2 cup shelled peanuts
4 tablespoons peanut butter
3 eggs

A serving of vegetable or fruit is

1/2 – 3/4 cup
1 medium apple
1 medium banana
1 medium orange
1 medium potato
1/2 medium grapefruit
1/2 medium cantaloupe

A serving of whole grain or enriched breads and cereals is

1 slice enriched or whole grain bread
1/2 – 3/4 cup cooked whole grain cereal (cracked wheat, oatmeal, brown rice, rolled wheat)
1/2 – 3/4 cup cooked enriched cereal (grits, cornmeal)
1/2 – 3/4 cup enriched noodles, macaroni, spaghetti
3/4 cup enriched ready-to-eat cereal
1/2 – 3/4 cup rice, enriched or converted
1 large enriched flour tortilla
2 small corn tortillas

EXERCISE DURING PREGNANCY

Pregnancy is quite a bit like a marathon. It is physically demanding, takes a long time to complete, and requires that you have a last burst of energy in reserve for getting over the finish line. Fortunately, you don't have to be in marathon form for pregnancy. But being in shape, having strength, stamina, and a feel for your body's responses to physical demands, can be a big advantage.

Although whipping your body into shape before pregnancy is challenging and demanding, when you exercise *during* pregnancy, you must also consider how the growing fetus may be affected. Pregnancy is a unique physical condition that brings with it special demands, challenges, and potential individual problems, so it's difficult to set accurate exercise standards for active pregnant women.

Most authorities agree that exercise guidelines during pregnancy should be based on the physical changes taking place. Based on those changes, general guidelines for the pregnant woman have been established. But keep in mind that general recommendations may not be appropriate for you. A very fit pregnant woman may tolerate a more strenuous program, whereas an overweight, out-of-shape woman may have to be much more cautious.

Pregnancy Changes That Affect Exercise

One of the most common questions we hear is whether exercise patterns should change after pregnancy. The American College of Obstetricians and Gynecologists (ACOG) Committee opinion of January 2002 states that

> the physiologic and morphologic changes of pregnancy may interfere with the ability to engage safely in some forms of physical activity. A woman's overall health, including obstetric and medical risks, should be evaluated before prescribing an exercise program. Generally, participating in a wide range of recreational activities appears to be safe during pregnancy; however, each sport should be reviewed individually for its potential risk, and activities with high risk of abdominal trauma should be avoided during pregnancy.

The committee goes on to say, "In the absence of either medical or obstetric complications, 30 or more minutes of moderate exercise a day, on most, if not all, days of the week is recommended for pregnant women."

The amount of oxygen your body needs increases as your pregnancy progresses—as much as 16 to 32 percent just before delivery. That means you will end up needing almost a third more oxygen just to do the things you normally do—watch TV, brush your teeth—because of the increased demands of the fetus, the placenta, and the uterus. Oxygen consumption also, of course, increases with exercise. Thus the most dramatic increases in oxygen consumption would occur during exercise late in pregnancy.

On the other hand, because all normal, weight-bearing activities during pregnancy require this higher energy output, some improvement in fitness seems inevitable unless you cut back activity. In other words, you'll get more fit just by being pregnant. The ability to produce this increase in oxygen consumption seems within the reach of most women, suggesting that they should be able to handle most of the same tasks they did prior to pregnancy. However, your capacity to work is affected by a variety of conditions, including your body build, environmental factors, what the work is, training and adaptation, and psychological factors, including motivation.

Pregnancy also requires a 50 percent increase in the work of the heart (cardiac output). This increase peaks at the seventh month of pregnancy and then holds steady until delivery. During labor, the heart has to work harder, too. A woman who has maintained aerobic fitness prior to pregnancy comes into pregnancy with a greater capacity to meet the demands of carrying and delivering a baby.

In general, target heart rates of pregnant and postpartum women should be set approximately 20 to 35 percent lower than would be appropriate at normal times. Women's cardiovascular systems vary a great deal in the nonpregnant state. When you exercise during pregnancy, you should measure your heart rate during the activities by taking your pulse, and stay below a maximum of 140 beats per minute. Women who are anemic, very out of shape, or overweight should be particularly careful about pushing themselves too hard during a workout—their heart rates can quite quickly shoot up past the safe zone.

Temperature: A Critical Exercise Factor

An elevated temperature during the first trimester of pregnancy seems to increase the risk of congenital abnormalities (teratogenesis). The critical core (deep body) temperature at which risk occurs is 102°F (38.5°C).

During exercise, your temperature goes up. Although most of the extra heat your body produces is lost into the air around you, some cannot be dissipated fast enough. This results in increased body temperature. The longer and harder you exercise, the higher your core temperature is likely to go. If heat loss through the skin is reduced because the weather is hot or humid, your body is even less able to get rid of the excess heat.

The temperature of the fetus averages about half a degree centigrade higher than that of the mother. Most of the heat the fetus produces is transferred to the mother across the placenta via the blood— much the way the body core is cooled by sending heat to the skin via the blood. If the mother's temperature is elevated, the fetus cannot transfer its heat. As maternal body temperature rises, so, too, does fetal temperature. As both increase, the transfer of heat from the fetus decreases. Therefore, the temperature rise during exercise may become critical. Studies on this effect are the basis for exercise recommendations at the end of this chapter.

One study of five pregnant women doing strenuous exercise—such as exercising during hot weather or exercising vigorously in an aerobic dance class for an hour followed by a session in a sauna or a hot tub—revealed they had core temperatures of around 0.9°F to around 1.3°F higher than had similar nonpregnant women. Strenuous exercise for fifteen minutes, however, will not usually increase the temperature over 38°C (100.4°F). Pregnant women should, therefore, be cautioned not to exercise when they have a fever or in hot weather. And they should certainly not linger in a hot tub or a sauna after exercise.

How the Fetus Responds to Maternal Exercise

The flow of blood to the uterus decreases the harder and the longer you exercise. But this does not mean that there is a reduction in the supply of oxygen and nutrients to the fetus, because the concentration of red blood cells in the blood increases during exercise, enabling the blood to carry more oxygen. The net result appears to be a fairly constant oxygen supply to the uterus and the fetus.

Fit people in general also have less of a reduction in blood flow to various organs during exercise, suggesting that the in-shape pregnant woman is better able to maintain blood flow to the uterus during exercise. How does the fetus respond to any changes in blood supply? Most studies show that the fetal heart rate rises *after* maternal exercise, but it may actually decrease during exercise. However, a great deal of variation exists in the findings of these studies. Results differ with different stages of pregnancy, the intensity and duration of the exercise, even the position in which the exercise is done. It is also difficult to monitor the fetal heart rate during exercise.

In general, it appears that upright, weight-bearing exercises (running and walking) cause greater changes in fetal heart rate (rising slightly) than do non–weight bearing exercises (swimming, rowing, and bicycling). However, no association has been found between such heart rate changes and subsequent problems in the newborn. And in no studies, even with moderately strenuous exercise, did the fetal heart rate show signs of distress.

Fetal health has been studied in relation to varying degrees of exercise. But because there are so many other factors in fetal health—genetic, socioeconomic, nutritional, environmental, and stress-related—it's very hard to pin down the effect of one single factor such as exercise. The effects of strenuous exercise during pregnancy have been studied mainly in women who were already highly trained before pregnancy. All these studies show normal or improved fetal health, and while that might be because those women began pregnancy in excellent condition and health, it does suggest that there are no major negative effects of strenuous exercise on the health of fetuses in active women. However, one 2002 study concluded that low-risk pregnant women who exercised regularly were more likely to have smaller babies, an increased number of inductions and augmentations of labor, and longer labors. They also had more frequent colds and flu. Another study showed that a great amount of moderate-intensity, weight-bearing exercise in mid- and late pregnancy makes for smaller babies. If exercise was decreased, this enhanced the growth, with a proportionally greater increase in fat mass than in lean body mass. In this study, working out produced leaner babies.

Among the negative effects of strenuous exercise during pregnancy, the most commonly noted is low fetal birth weight. Some studies have reported a decrease of as much as 400 grams (1 pound). However, this may reflect the poor nutritional status of the women studied or may involve factors other than just the physical activity.

If you follow the guidelines on the following pages, you should reduce the factors that lead to negative effects.

Psychological Benefits of Exercise during Pregnancy

In general, people who exercise report fewer feelings of anxiety and stress, as well as a greater degree of self-confidence, self-control, and self-esteem, than those who do not exercise. Exercise helps the pregnant woman feel physically and psychologically healthy, especially if she exercised routinely before pregnancy. Exercise may also help reduce the pregnant woman's anxiety about the birth process itself. A woman who feels strong and in control of her body before and throughout her prenatal period is more likely to feel secure during her labor and delivery.

Exercise Specifics

The goal of exercise during pregnancy should be to maintain the highest level of fitness possible, with maximum safety in mind. That means you shouldn't try to run faster or farther than ever before, or aim for the same level of strength training that would be reasonable if you weren't pregnant.

The following exercise program is designed for a broad spectrum of women. It incorporates modifications required by the physical changes of pregnancy and the postpartum period, and by a special concern for safety. Some women may be able to tolerate more strenuous exercise. Others may need to cut back even more, to, say, a simple walking program. There is enormous variability in the way different women will respond to the same activity, so no single exercise prescription can meet the needs of all women. Your obstetrician should assess your abilities and needs individually and help you construct a program that works for you.

The importance of this communication between you and your physician cannot be overemphasized. But you have to take responsibility for being alert to the potential hazards of exercise when you're out on the track or the tennis court, be aware of the warning signs, and report back to your physician if anything unusual occurs.

Of course, your exercise program is only one part of a healthy pregnancy lifestyle. A daily walk won't cancel out a junk food diet, smoking, or not getting enough sleep. But taken with all the other healthy approaches to pregnancy, exercise can help you feel better, stronger, and more energetic. And that can make a big difference.

ACOG Exercise Guidelines

The following guidelines are based on the unique physical and physiological conditions that exist during pregnancy and the postpartum period. They provide direction in the development of home-exercise programs and outline general criteria for safety. Check with your physician before starting an exercise program.

PREGNANCY AND POSTPARTUM

1. Regular exercise (at least three times per week) is preferable to intermittent activity. Competitive activity should be discouraged.
2. Vigorous exercise should not be performed in hot, humid weather or when you have a fever.
3. Ballistic movements (jerky, bouncy motions) should be avoided. Exercise should be done on a wooden floor or a tightly carpeted surface to reduce shock and provide sure footing.
4. Deep flexion or extension of joints should be avoided because of connective tissue laxity. Activities that require jumping, jarring motions or rapid changes in direction should be avoided because of joint instability.
5. Vigorous exercise should be preceded by a five-minute period of muscle warm-up. This can be accomplished by slow walking or stationary cycling with low resistance.

6. Vigorous exercise should be followed by a period of gradually declining activity that includes gentle stationary stretching. Because connective tissue laxity increases the risk of joint injury, stretches should not be taken to the point of maximum resistance.

7. Heart rate should be measured at times of peak activity. Target heart rates and limits established in consultation with the physician should not be exceeded.

8. Care should be taken to gradually rise from the floor to avoid lightheadedness from falling blood pressure. Some form of activity involving the legs should be continued for a brief period after rising.

9. Liquids should be taken liberally before and after exercise to prevent dehydration. When necessary, activity should be interrupted to replenish fluids.

10. Women who have led sedentary lifestyles should begin with physical activity of very low intensity and advance activity levels very gradually.

11. Activity should be stopped and the physician consulted if any unusual symptoms appear.

PREGNANCY ONLY

1. No study data for humans indicates that women who are pregnant should limit exercise intensity and lower their maximum heart rate because of potential adverse effects; however, a good maximum maternal heart rate should be around 140 to 150 beats per minute.

2. Strenuous activities should stop when and if you are fatigued, and you should never exercise to exhaustion.

3. No exercise should be performed while lying on your back after the fourth month of gestation is completed.

4. Exercises that employ the Valsalva maneuver (strong bearing down) should be avoided.

5. Caloric intake should be adequate to meet the extra energy needs not only of pregnancy, but also of the exercise performed.

6. While exercising, you should avoid getting overheated. Animal studies have suggested that prolonged temperatures above a threshold of 39.2°C (102.56°F) can cause birth defects.

WHEN NOT TO EXERCISE

Relative contraindications: A physician will need to evaluate each patient individually with respect to an exercise program. The following conditions may make vigorous physical activity during pregnancy undesirable:

- Poorly controlled hypertension
- Anemia or other blood disorders
- Poorly controlled hyperthyroid disease
- Poorly controlled diabetes
- Cardiac arrhythmia or palpitations that have not been treated
- History of precipitous (very fast) labor
- History of intrauterine growth retardation (cases where fetal and newborn size is smaller than average)
- History of bleeding during present pregnancy
- Breech presentation in the last trimester
- Excessive obesity
- Extreme underweight
- History of extremely sedentary lifestyle
- Orthopedic limitations
- Chronic bronchitis
- Poorly controlled seizure disorder
- Heavy tobacco use

Absolute contraindications: If you have any of the following conditions, you should not do any vigorous exercise during pregnancy.

- History of three or more spontaneous abortions
- Ruptured membranes
- Premature labor
- Diagnosed multiple gestation at risk for premature labor
- Incompetent cervix
- Bleeding that is persistent in the second or third trimester
- Placenta previa after twenty-six weeks
- Significant heart or lung disease
- Preeclampsia

You must be aware that complications arising during pregnancy may make vigorous activity dangerous for a woman who was previously able to exercise without restriction. Warning signs to terminate exercise while pregnant include:

- Vaginal bleeding
- Shortness of breath prior to exercise
- Dizziness
- Headache

- Chest pain
- Muscle weakness
- Calf pain or swelling (need to rule out a blood clot)
- Premature labor
- Decrease in fetal movement
- Leakage of amniotic fluid

In addition to the ACOG guidelines, we want to enlarge on some special points that in our experience have proven important:

- Prepare for pregnancy by increasing your aerobic fitness and building your cardiac reserve even before you conceive. By establishing a good exercise program beforehand, you will feel better and have an easier time continuing to exercise *during* pregnancy.
- Consult with your physician about an exercise program at your first prenatal meeting. Stress your exercise history, current exercise program, and exercise goals. Your exercise routine should be well within your physical limits. Do not push too hard.
- Consider decreasing weight-bearing aerobic exercises like aerobic dancing, rope jumping, jogging, and running. Concentrate on bicycling, swimming, calisthenics, and stretching. These non–weight bearing workouts cut down on bouncing, are a bit less strenuous, and may be better tolerated by the fetus. Even if you are an avid runner, it's probably best to decrease the length and the pace of your runs by your seventh month. This will probably feel natural to you, since this is when the fetus goes on a growing spree and your weight and balance will change quickly.
- Avoid risky activities such as mountain climbing, sky diving, motorcycle riding, strenuous horseback riding, gymnastics, and downhill skiing. As your pregnancy progresses, the increase in weight, the shift of your center of gravity, and the changes in your joints and ligaments will affect coordination and balance. Therefore, activities requiring very precise body control may be dangerous.
- Exercise regularly—at least three times a week, as long as you are healthy—to maintain your cardiac reserve and muscle tone. Sporadic exercise is much more stressful to your body.

- Exercise for shorter intervals. Start with a ten- to fifteen-minute interval; then rest for five minutes and resume exercise for another ten to fifteen minutes.
- Decrease your exercise level after seven months of pregnancy. Your increased body weight will demand a larger energy output, so you may feel more fatigued and reach your exercise limit sooner. A sensible rule of thumb is to forget everything about your old exercise regimen—how long, how fast, and how intensely you worked out—except for how it *felt*. If you keep the feeling of exercise intensity steady, or even a bit lower, you'll naturally cut time, speed, and duration as your weight increases and other body changes occur. If you are a runner, decrease your mileage and speed drastically during the last four weeks prior to delivery.
- Take your pulse every so often while you are exercising. If it is more than 140 beats per minute, slow down until it returns to 90, then build back up a bit. Your pregnancy maximum is 140.
- Avoid becoming overheated for extended periods. It is best not to exercise for longer than thirty-five minutes total, even less in hot, humid weather. Do not forget that as your body temperature rises, so does that of your fetus. Limit the time spent in hot tubs, saunas, and baths: Stay in a sauna (below 178°F) for less than five minutes; stay in a hot bath (water below 102°F) for less than fifteen minutes.
- Avoid extreme stretching of joints because of the softening of connective tissue during pregnancy.
- Always warm up and cool down. Five minutes of low-intensity exercise—walking, leisurely pool laps, easy biking—prepares the body gradually for more strenuous exercise. This is important to prevent strain or injury. A five-minute cool-down after exercise will let your breathing, heart, and metabolic rate ease back to normal gradually.
- Rest for ten minutes after exercise by lying on your left side. This takes the pressure off the vena cava, promotes return circulation from your extremities to the working muscles of your heart, and increases blood flow to your placenta and fetus. (Get up slowly to avoid dizziness or faintness after this or any other period of lying down.)

- Drink two or three large glasses of water after exercise to replace body fluids lost through perspiration. When exercising, stop to drink water every fifteen minutes. A few sips help even if you aren't thirsty, since thirst often lags behind your body's need for water.
- Increase your caloric intake to balance the calories burned during exercise, as stated previously.
- Wear a support bra and good sports shoes. Your increased breast size and overall weight gain mean you'll be much more comfortable—and safer—if you opt for good support gear.
- Stop exercising immediately if you have shortness of breath, excessively rapid heartbeat, dizziness, numbness, tingling, vaginal bleeding, passage of fluid from the vagina, or abdominal pain. Call your doctor to report the problem as soon as possible, and certainly before resuming exercising.

One last thought: By training and exercising during pregnancy, you may also be training your fetus for a better start.

Special Exercises for Pregnancy and the Postpartum Period

The weight of a growing uterus often adds unexpected stress to specific areas of your body. Identifying and strengthening these areas with special exercises may reduce the incidence of future injury.

Back Exercises

Exercises for the back are not recommended during pregnancy after the fourth month because they require a woman to lie on her back or bear down. The back is subjected to significant stress during pregnancy and the postpartum period, and many traditional back-strengthening exercises would add risk. As the fetus grows, it puts pressure on the major vein carrying blood back to your heart—the vena cava—on the right side of the abdomen. After delivery, back pain and injury remain significant problems because of the repeated bending, lifting, and arrying associated with child rearing. At this time, a full program of strengthening and stretching exercises for the abdomen, the back, and the legs can be incorporated into your daily program.

One exercise that can be done throughout pregnancy is the pelvic tilt, which strengthens abdominal muscles and reduces the arching of the lower back. Pregnant women are encouraged to perform this exercise as many times as possible throughout the day.

To do the pelvic tilt, lie on the floor on your back with your hands at your sides and your knees bent. Slowly flatten the curve at the small of your back, pushing your spine down against the floor. This move is called a "pelvic tilt" because to do this, you are tightening your abdominal muscles (they should feel tight to the touch) to tilt, or rotate, your pelvis and eliminate the normal curve in the lower back. After holding the tilt position for a couple of seconds, relax your abdominal muscles and allow your spine to return to its relaxed position, curved up slightly off the floor. Repeat several times. The pelvic tilt should be continued even after delivery.

Kegel Exercises

Exercises for the pelvic muscles (Kegel exercises) are simply the alternate tightening and relaxing of the pelvic and the vaginal muscles, an isometric technique. The physical and the hormonal changes of pregnancy cause relaxation of the pelvic-supporting tissues. Vaginal delivery stretches these tissues even further. Most women are not troubled by these changes, but some will complain of discomfort or of incontinence of urine. Others may be concerned about looseness of the vagina during intercourse.

In patients with mild pelvic relaxation, the regular use of Kegel exercises may be all that is necessary to provide symptomatic relief in the postpartum period. To get a feel for which muscles to squeeze, practice starting and stopping the flow of urine when you urinate.

IMMUNIZATION DURING PREGNANCY

In the last two decades the number of available vaccines has increased greatly. Special concerns relate to the vaccination of pregnant women. Because the effects of many diseases and vaccines on the pregnant woman or her fetus are unknown, current information is subject to change.

A systematic approach to vaccinating women of childbearing age is needed to ensure that every pregnant woman and her fetus are protected from preventable, serious diseases and from the possible risk that may accompany unnecessary or hazardous vaccines.

The use of immunization agents during pregnancy should be limited to a few specific situations. If possible, you should be protected from preventable diseases by vaccination *before* you become pregnant. Live virus vaccines, in particular, should not be given during pregnancy except when your susceptibility and exposure are highly probable and the disease to be prevented poses a greater threat to you or your fetus than does vaccination: Live viruses pass through the placenta and may affect the fetus. It might be desirable, for example, to give a yellow-fever vaccine to a pregnant woman who will be living in an area in which yellow fever occurs.

In the United States the only routine immunizations recommended during pregnancy are tetanus and diphtheria toxoids. Measles, rubella, and mumps vaccines should be given prior to pregnancy or in the immediate postpartum period. Pregnant women in the United States should receive their first vaccination against polio only when the risk of exposure is high. As with all adults, this should be done with inactivated polio virus (IPV) vaccine when available. Live, attenuated oral polio virus vaccine can be used if time does not allow the administration of at least two doses of IPV or if IPV is not available.

Most women of childbearing age in the United States are immune to measles, mumps, rubella, tetanus, and diphtheria. Most women born prior to 1957 were infected naturally with measles, mumps, and rubella and thus developed immunity. For women born since 1957, a reliable indicator of measles immunity would be a history of physician-diagnosed measles, documentation of vaccination with live measles vaccine on or after your first birthday, or positive blood test results for measles antibody. A documented history of vaccination on or after the first birthday or evidence of any detectable antibody in your blood specific for rubella is considered evidence of immunity to rubella. A history of physician-diagnosed mumps or mumps vaccination on or after the first birthday is adequate evidence of immunity to mumps.

You are considered immune to tetanus and diphtheria after receiving at least three doses of each vaccination, with the last dose administered at least six to twelve months after the preceding dose. A booster dose is required every ten years. Other vaccines are indicated for adults in the United States only under special circumstances. For example, hepatitis B vaccine is recommended for women at risk for hepatitis B. These women include workers in the health-care field, those with a history of IV drug use, those with a history of STDs, women with multiple sexual partners, people in contact with hepatitis B carriers, those who work in an institution for the developmentally disabled or in a hemodialysis unit, or those who have received clotting-factor products. Pneumococcal vaccine is safe and recommended for women at high risk for this infection and its complications. This includes women who have had their spleens removed. Influenza vaccine is also safe and is now recommended for all pregnant women after the first trimester.

Because of the theoretical risk to your fetus with live vaccine, you should not receive measles, rubella, and mumps vaccines if you are pregnant. You should not get pregnant for three months after receiving these vaccines as well. Nonpregnant women of childbearing age should be questioned about their history of having chicken pox. Varicella vaccine (chicken pox) has been available since March 1995 and has been approved for use in healthy susceptible people of twelve months or older. This is a live vaccine, and women who receive it should not get pregnant for at least one month after receiving the second of two required doses.

In summary, you should be immune to measles, rubella, mumps, tetanus, varicella, and diphtheria prior to pregnancy. Tetanus and diphtheria vaccinations are the only immunizing agents routinely indicated for susceptible pregnant women. Other vaccines such as influenza vaccine are being used more regularly during the flu season and are becoming the standard of care. Other vaccines may be indicated for pregnant women under special circumstances.

The following are the recommendations of the ACOG regarding the safety of various immunizations during pregnancy.

Tetanus-diphtheria	Give if no previous vaccination or no booster in last ten years
Polio	Not recommended routinely for adults
Mumps	Not safe during pregnancy
Rubella	Not safe during pregnancy
Typhus	Recommended if traveling to high-risk regions
Smallpox	No need; disease has been eradicated
Yellow fever	Immunize only before travel in high-risk areas
Cholera	Immunize only before travel in high-risk areas
Hepatitis A	Immunize after exposure or before travel in developing countries
Rabies	Recommendations do not change for pregnancy
Influenza	Safe and recommended in pregnancy after the first trimester

Chapter 6

Problems of Early Pregnancy: Miscarriage and Ectopic Pregnancy

⊶∾⊷

MOST PREGNANCIES proceed normally. However, the purpose of prenatal care is to watch out for certain conditions that may be unpleasant to contemplate but are crucial to be aware of. Knowing what they and their danger signs are will help you to understand the nature of pregnancy and what can be done to ensure the best health for mother and child.

MISCARRIAGE

During the early part of pregnancy, most commonly during the first three months, there is a possibility of losing the pregnancy. This is called a *miscarriage* or a *spontaneous abortion*. If a pregnancy is not progressing normally, for reasons we shall discuss, the lining of the uterus may begin to shed, and bleeding may occur. Eventually, the pregnancy separates from the uterine lining and passes out of the body. Spontaneous abortion—a naturally occurring miscarriage—should not be confused with a planned therapeutic abortion, which is a voluntary procedure to end a pregnancy.

Medically, miscarriage is defined as the premature delivery of a nonviable fetus (one that could not live) before it weighs about one pound. This generally can occur up to about twenty weeks of pregnancy, although over 90 percent of miscarriages occur within the first three months. Amazingly, the incidence of miscarriage may be as high as *half* of all conceptions. Most of these early miscarriages occur before women even know they were pregnant. A very heavy, maybe slightly late, menstrual period associated with severe cramps may actually be a very early miscarriage. Studies done on women who were trying to conceive, in which pregnancy tests were given every month—*before* a missed period—revealed that many pregnancies aborted very early and without the women's knowledge. Of the pregnancies documented after a missed period, the incidence of miscarriage is approximately 15 percent. In women over forty, the miscarriage rate may be as high as 30 percent.

A miscarriage is always a traumatic event in any family and may be followed by depression in both partners. (Postmiscarriage depression is discussed later in this chapter.) Spontaneous miscarriage, however, is most often followed by another pregnancy, which results in the birth of a healthy baby. The vast majority of the causes of miscarriage will not occur again.

Usually, two signals indicate that something is wrong and there is a chance of miscarriage: one is vaginal bleeding without the passage of tissue; the other is cramping pain in the lower abdomen. The cramps may come and go and are felt right above the pubic bone. Sometimes vaginal bleeding stops and pregnancy goes on without any problem whatsoever. At other times, the bleeding and the cramping may continue, becoming increasingly stronger until miscarriage occurs. In some ways, a miscarriage is a less-intense version of labor. The pain is usually stronger than menstrual cramps. If the bleeding is heavier than a menstrual period and the cramps are worse, it probably indicates a miscarriage. Any bleeding during pregnancy should be reported to your doctor.

At the beginning of pregnancy, a few women may have slight bleeding when the fertilized egg attaches itself to the lining of the uterus. This is normal. Some women may confuse this implantation bleeding with a normal, but light, menstrual period. A pregnancy test, however, will show early pregnancy.

Twenty-five percent of all pregnant women experience bleeding or spotting during the first three months of pregnancy. Only slightly more than half of these end up having a miscarriage; the others go on to deliver healthy babies.

If bleeding stops and the pregnancy goes to term, the baby is as likely as any other baby to be completely normal. This is a very important point, to reassure the many couples who fear—unnecessarily—that bleeding in pregnancy means that something is wrong with the baby.

The Causes of Miscarriage

The causes of miscarriage are largely random and hard to foresee. In spite of all the wonders of modern medicine, doctors have absolutely no control over the vast majority of these causes. Not all the seeds you plant in your garden grow; not every fertilized egg can result in a normal baby. There may be something wrong with the sperm cell or the egg cell, or something may happen when they are joined that keeps the fertilized egg from growing properly.

Chromosome and Structural Abnormalities

A large number of miscarriages are caused by a spontaneous defect arising in a growing embryo during its early stages of development. Since most of the fetus is formed in the first three months, any serious problem will manifest itself by that time and the body will reject fetuses that have problems. In one analysis of 1,000 miscarriages (the ejected tissues were studied), it was found that over half were caused by what is called a blighted ovum. In these cases the embryo stops growing and dries up, and the amniotic sac ends up empty. Something was intrinsically wrong with that fertilized egg that did not allow it to develop.

Often there may be a month between the time the embryo stops growing and the actual miscarriage. The extreme is a "missed abortion"—when the body holds on to the dead embryo for two months or more. Once the fetus has failed to develop normally, it is only a matter of time until the miscarriage occurs.

The causes of these abnormalities, which are forty times more frequent in spontaneously aborting fetuses than in normal full-term babies, are not known. They are just random accidents of nature. Given the many millions of sperm produced, and the thousands of ova, it is not really surprising that this can happen.

Genetic Causes

Couples who have had three or more miscarriages might choose genetic counseling. Although rare, an abnormality of the chromosomes in one of the partners may allow pregnancy to begin but may end in recurrent miscarriages.

Other Causes of Miscarriage

Several factors influence the frequency of spontaneous abortion. One is maternal age. The miscarriage rate doubles from an average of 15 percent in women ages twenty-five to forty to over 30 percent after age forty. Certain maternal conditions can result in miscarriage: abnormalities of the uterus (double uterus, septate uterus, uterine fibroids); an incompetent cervix; hormonal dysfunction (such as an inadequate luteal phase, related to a deficiency of progesterone); thyroid dysfunction; and other hormonal imbalances.

Some infections—herpes, toxoplasmosis, rubella, cytomegalovirus, chlamydia, and mycoplasma—have been implicated in causing miscarriage. Several acute infections associated with high fever, such as pneumonia and typhoid fever, sometimes can lead to spontaneous abortion. Teratogens (substances such as radiation and certain drugs and chemicals that cause fetal malformations) can increase the miscarriage rate.

Immunological factors have been extensively studied as a cause of miscarriage. The theory is that the mother may make certain antibodies or specialized proteins that may attack the developing embryo. Much work has been done in regard to the value of immunizing the mother with a specially derived vaccine to protect the developing embryo. Unfortunately, no studies have really shown any positive results using these methods.

Small blood clots, or microthrombi, may lead to miscarriage. Some women with certain conditions, like lupus, have a propensity to form clots. In those women, giving a blood thinner like baby aspirin or heparin may save future pregnancies.

Pregnant women commonly fall or trip, probably because of a change in their gait or balance. In general, the fetus is well protected from these bumps. The uterus acts as a fluid-filled buffer if the woman is jostled during pregnancy. It is unusual for trauma of this nature to cause any problems. Remember that most miscarriages are due to random factors that will not occur again. Rarely does trauma result in damage to a pregnancy.

The Course of Miscarriage

The course of miscarriage depends on whether or not the pregnancy is viable. A miscarriage is called a *complete abortion* if all the fetal tissue is passed spontaneously and none remains in the uterus. This is usually associated with strong laborlike pain of increasing severity, followed by the expulsion of a complete fetus and other pregnancy tissues. Bleeding and pain subside once the tissue is expelled, and the uterus reverts to normal size. Your physician will usually have you in for several follow-up checks without requiring any further procedures.

An *incomplete miscarriage*, which is more common, occurs when some fetal tissue remains in the uterus. With this type of miscarriage, vaginal bleeding continues from the tissue that remains. That tissue, if left in the uterus, may be the trigger for severe infection. For this reason, a dilatation and curettage (D&C), or opening of the cervix and scraping of the uterus, is required to remove the tissue left behind. This can be done either in the doctor's office or in a hospital, with either regional or local anaesthesia. Women with Rh-negative blood must also receive a shot of Rh immunoglobulin after a miscarriage (see chapter 12).

A *missed abortion* occurs when an embryo dies but is not expelled from the uterus. Diagnosis is made by ultrasound studies and blood tests that measure pregnancy hormone levels. A D&C can be performed in order to avoid the heavy bleeding that might have occurred when the body finally expelled the no longer viable pregnancy. Recently, certain studies have treated missed abortions with medication instead of the traditional D&C. In a 2002 study, women diagnosed with missed abortions were given a medication called misoprostol vaginally. Within a few days, 80 percent of those women were able to safely pass the pregnancies without needing a D&C.

A *threatened abortion* is a situation in which bleeding occurs with some mild cramps but the pregnancy is still viable. Bleeding itself does not mean a definite miscarriage. However, the bleeding plus cramping is a more ominous sign. The treatment of threatened miscarriage is very individual and depends on the woman and her physician. The classic approach is bed rest and restriction of physical activity and sex. Some physicians use vitamins, hormones, and sedatives. Ultrasound and pregnancy hormone levels may differentiate threatened abortion with a healthy fetus from an inevitable abortion with a fetus that would not survive.

The use of ultrasound after vaginal bleeding has proven to be of great value. As early as six to seven weeks after the last menstrual period, a fetal heart can be seen. If the fetal heart is beating healthily, it is much more likely that a miscarriage will not occur. However, if a woman has bleeding after seven to eight weeks of pregnancy and ultrasound shows no fetal heart, then miscarriage is inevitable and a D&C can be performed.

Keeping track of blood hormone levels is useful in the early stages of pregnancy before the fetal heart can be detected. A healthy, viable pregnancy will have increasing levels of these pregnancy hormones during the first four months of pregnancy. This test is called a "quantitative beta sub unit HCG pregnancy test." Normally, the level of hormone doubles every two to three days. If this is not the case, further testing may be desired.

Late miscarriages, occurring after ten to twelve weeks of pregnancy, are much less common, especially if the fetal heart has been heard and a missed abortion is ruled out. One cause of late abortion is a condition called *cervical incompetence*: The cervix cannot hold itself closed once the fetus grows to a certain size in the uterus; it slowly opens, eventually resulting in the loss of the pregnancy. The causes of cervical incompetence include previous surgery to the cervix, malformations of the uterus, and exposure of the mother to the drug DES when she was in her own mother's uterus. Sometimes no cause is discernible.

Treatment of cervical incompetence is very simple once the diagnosis is established. The doctor sews a stitch around the outside of the cervix, draws it tight, and knots it. This "purse-string suture" is left in place until the end of pregnancy, when it is removed to allow the birth of the baby. The procedure can be repeated with each pregnancy, after twelve to fourteen weeks and once a viable fetus has been established.

Treatment of Multiple Miscarriages

Since most miscarriages are due to random factors that will not usually repeat themselves, a workup for miscarriage is usually not necessary until a woman has had three successive miscarriages. Of course, this is a general rule, and each case needs to be individually studied.

A workup for habitual abortion or miscarriage will include an X ray of the reproductive system, called a hysterogram, which will reveal abnormalities or growths in the uterus. Hormone studies, including thyroid function tests, are also performed. Genetic abnormalities and infections in the couple need to be ruled out. Cultures for infections such as chlamydia and mycoplasma can be done.

Women who have had miscarriages, with or without a D&C, should wait two menstrual cycles before trying again for pregnancy. This allows the lining of the uterus to heal enough to be fully ready to receive and nurture the next pregnancy.

The Emotional Impact of Miscarriage

A miscarriage is often so shattering that many couples blame themselves, even though spontaneous abortion is a natural event and most of them are due to an intrinsic abnormality of the egg or the sperm.

In the great majority of cases, the embryo was simply unable to survive. Like any accident, a miscarriage is regrettable, upsetting, but unavoidable.

Most couples review their lifestyle to see if something they did caused the event. Some even interpret a miscarriage religiously, as divine punishment. This is unhealthy and unnecessary. Healthy pregnancies remain intact even after strenuous activity and severe emotional disturbances. It is nobody's fault if a woman miscarries. The best thing a couple can do following a miscarriage is to look to the future: This pregnancy loss will, very likely, be followed by a successful birth.

The experience of a miscarriage may be frightening for you and your partner, and mutual support and compassion are very important.

Following a miscarriage, a period of grieving is normal; you and your partner may feel a sense of loss and emptiness. Our society has no accepted ritual to support you during this kind of crisis. Talking with friends, physicians, and other people who have had a similar experience may provide comfort. "I didn't understand how I could be so wiped out by losing a baby I never even felt move inside me. But other women—some of them friends I never knew had miscarriages—told me they had felt that way, too. That helped John and me tremendously," a woman who is now the mother of a healthy newborn commented.

PREGNANCY LOSS AND GRIEVING

Despite all the advances of modern obstetrics, and despite the overwhelming odds of a successful outcome, occasionally a pregnancy is lost.

The grief you feel over the loss of your baby is a natural process of healing. The impact of this loss may be as great as the death of a spouse or an older child. The memory will always be with you and should not be downplayed or denied.

Communication between you and your partner, your family, your doctor, or possibly a counselor may help you understand the intense and confusing emotions you feel and will feel for some time.

Grief is a normal and necessary response to the loss of your baby. Through grieving, you gradually learn to let go of the ties you have formed with your fetus or newborn and go on with your life.

For a mother, this bond can be very strong. It often begins well before birth, sometimes even before conception, and grows throughout pregnancy. Your baby becomes a person in your mind.

A father can also feel a strong tie to his unborn child. His feelings may be different from a mother's, because he does not experience the pregnancy in the same way, but a father also feels the death as a profound loss. Both of you may have intense feelings of grief, even if you lose a pregnancy in the first few months.

The grieving may last a long time and follows a common pattern in many people.

Shock and numbness are the mind's way of protecting itself when first faced with a great loss. Parents often think, "This is not really happening."

Searching and yearning begin when the initial shock phase of grief has begun to pass. You begin looking for a reason. You search for who or what caused the death. You may imagine that you were somehow responsible for your baby's death, but this is seldom the case. Mothers often feel anger toward their partner, the doctor, or the hospital staff, or they may question their religious beliefs.

Depression and loneliness are a part of the next phase, during which the most intense emotions begin to ease. You may feel tired and run down, sad, disoriented, and helpless. But somehow, you slowly begin to get back on your feet and accept your loss.

Acceptance is the final phase of grieving. You begin to have renewed energy, and your baby's death no longer dominates your thoughts. Although you will never forget, you begin to think of the loss less often and with less pain. You find yourself resuming activities and social contacts and making plans for the future. Before thinking about starting another pregnancy, allow time for you and your partner to work through your feelings about this one. Often couples feel that having another baby right away will fill the emptiness or take away the pain. Of course, a new baby cannot replace the baby who was lost. Grieving takes a lot of energy, and the process of healing is not helped by another pregnancy soon after the loss. Talk to your doctor or a counselor about future pregnancy plans before making any decisions. It is important for you to know that the chances of losing another pregnancy are almost always very small. Still, you may be very anxious and concerned during your next pregnancy. It is important for you and your doctor to talk about the reason for the first baby's death (if known), the chances it will happen again, and the measures that can be taken, if any, to reduce these chances. Your doctor may recommend certain tests before or during your pregnancy to find potential problems as early as possible.

The loss of a baby is a traumatic event. Grief is the normal reaction to such a loss, and through grieving you can come to terms with your baby's death.

Everyone grieves in a different way and at a different pace. It may take anywhere from several months to a few years to learn how to cope with a loss. Counseling can greatly help you and your family come to terms with this sad and painful event and to go on with your lives.

ECTOPIC PREGNANCY

Ectopic pregnancy occurs when the fertilized egg implants and grows outside of the uterus. Most often (95 percent of the time, in fact) this occurs in the fallopian tubes, although ovarian or abdominal pregnancies are not unheard of. Misplaced, or ectopic, pregnancies appear to be on the rise: Now 1 in every 100 pregnancies is ectopic. This increase may be related to the increased use of intrauterine devices in the last thirty years; the rise in the number of pelvic infections; or the widespread delay in the age of childbearing, which allows a longer period of time for such gynecologic problems as endometriosis to occur.

Tubal ectopics occur when there is some kind of erratic trip-up in the passage of the fertilized egg through the fallopian tube. There may be blockage in the tube due to scars left from an infection, endometriosis, tubal surgery, pregnancy with an IUD in place, or a tubal abnormality with which the woman was born. If the fertilized egg is delayed, it may simply implant where it's stuck, since the environment in the tube will allow implantation and development, at least for a short time. The uterus, however, is the only organ that can accommodate healthy implantation and full growth of a fetus. A growing ectopic pregnancy will eventually burst or rupture the tube and often cause severe internal hemorrhage. If an ectopic pregnancy is not diagnosed or if treatment is delayed, the result can be fatal.

Symptoms of Ectopic Pregnancy

During the first few weeks, an ectopic pregnancy usually appears to be a perfectly normal pregnancy. As the pregnancy progresses, however, aches and twinges of pain may occur on the side of the ectopic pregnancy. Vaginal bleeding may start, due to the insufficient hormone production of this abnormal pregnancy.

If you experience pronounced pain on one side of the lower abdomen, associated with a missed period or slight vaginal bleeding, consult a doctor right away. The seriousness of ectopic pregnancy requires the physician to consider its possibility, do a pregnancy test and an ultrasound examination, and follow you very closely. Women who are at increased risk for ectopic pregnancies—who have had a previous ectopic, tubal surgery, or a pelvic infection—should be followed even more closely during a pregnancy.

The development of sensitive measurements of pregnancy hormones and ultrasound allows the diagnosis of ectopic pregnancy much earlier than in the past. When a woman seeks medical attention shortly after a missed period, especially if she has worrisome symptoms, often the diagnosis of ectopic pregnancy can be made early, before the tube ruptures and is destroyed.

Treatment of Ectopic Pregnancy

The treatment of ectopic pregnancy depends on the size of the embryo at the time of diagnosis. If an ectopic pregnancy is discovered early enough, it may be possible to treat it successfully with medication and avoid surgery. This underscores the importance of seeking medical attention very early in your pregnancy, especially if there are ectopic warning signs. If the diagnosis of ectopic pregnancy has been made, and if the ectopic pregnancy is less than three centimeters in size by ultrasound, most women can be given an injection of a drug called methotrexate. This drug is widely used to treat some forms of cancer and can have many side effects if given at high doses. When used to treat ectopic pregnancies, methotrexate is given at very low doses, so the side effects are extremely rare. Once the injection is given, the patient must be followed very closely since the treatment may not always work, and ectopic pregnancies can be life-threatening. Most patients will experience some pain approximately four or five days after the injection, as the pregnancy tissue dies, and then slowly the pregnancy will regress and dissolve. Usually, your doctor will follow the levels of pregnancy hormones in the blood until the levels go to zero. The methotrexate method of treatment is the best way to preserve fertility.

When an ectopic pregnancy is larger or begins to rupture, treatment should be surgical. The procedure can be either complete or partial removal of the tube (salpingectomy), or the tube can be opened and the pregnancy can be extracted (salpingostomy). Generally, if the tube appears to be destroyed, it will be removed. If the tube is not removed and the pregnancy is extracted, the doctor must carefully follow blood levels of the pregnancy hormones postoperatively, as there is a risk of regrowth of the pregnancy. Rh immunoglobulin should also be given to Rh-negative women with ectopic pregnancies.

The woman who has had an ectopic pregnancy, even if her other tube seems to be normal, has an increased risk of another ectopic pregnancy—perhaps as high as 10 to 15 in 100, compared to the normal woman's 1 in 100. However, the good news is that 50 percent of women who have had an ectopic pregnancy will go on to successfully bear a child.

Chapter 7

Perinatology— the Fetal World

PERINATOLOGY IS the study of human development from a microscopic cell to a fully formed infant, floating gracefully in the liquid prenatal environment, awaiting birth. As a science, perinatology has been of interest to biologists for many years. But within the last three to four decades it has become a useful tool for the practicing obstetrician.

In 1963, Dr. A. William Liley performed the first recorded intrauterine blood transfusion, which marked the beginning of modern perinatology. The New Zealand physician, faced with a fetus severely weakened by Rh disease (a mother/fetus blood incompatibility problem) but too premature to survive early delivery, passed a needle through the mother's abdominal wall, through the uterus into the baby's abdomen, giving the fetus new blood and new strength to live. While this procedure might sound very matter-of-fact in today's chronicle of medical miracles, Dr. Liley's transfusion represented the first intrusion into the womb to help a developing fetus. Since then, doctors have come from this relatively simple procedure to opening the uterus during pregnancy, performing surgery on the fetus, and replacing the developing baby to continue gestation.

These are special uses of the science of perinatology, reserved for the few problem pregnancies. But the knowledge gained from this special work has contributed an invaluable amount of information about the normal growth and development of the fetus. That is why a lengthy discussion of this subject is included in this book. It is our hope that the information in this chapter will help you, as a mother-to-be, marvel at the intricacies, as well as the beauty, of birth and that this understanding will make the experience much less mysterious.

FETAL GROWTH AND DEVELOPMENT

Throughout most of pregnancy, the fetus is completely formed, with all its organs: a miniature human being who is active and quite lively. The unborn baby has senses of touch and hearing. It responds to pain, pressure, and loud noises. It sucks and swallows.

By the third month of gestation, the fetus has developed all the systems needed to maintain life after birth. It then spends the next six months letting those systems mature and get used to working together under the direction of its master conductor, the brain. Toward the end of pregnancy, the fetus develops a layer of fatty tissue just under the skin for warmth. This pattern of growth is truly amazing, but it is also quite deceiving. While the third trimester growth is most obvious, the fetus actually grows at a much faster rate in the early months. During the first month of pregnancy, fetal weight increases 10,000 times. In the second month, it increases another 74 times. In the third month, growth increases only 11 times. In the last few months of pregnancy, the rate of growth falls to 0.3 times. But even if this rate of increase were maintained after birth, your child would weigh about 160 pounds by his or her first birthday.

Chapter 2 shows the average height and weight of the fetus at the end of the various lunar months of pregnancy. In general, the length of the fetus is a more accurate measure of its age than is its weight. The average birth weight of American babies is about seven pounds. Boys tend to be about three ounces heavier than girls at birth. Besides the baby's sex, birth weights are influenced by the socioeconomic status of the mother (which often determines her nutrition), the race and the size of the parents, the number of children previously born to the mother, and a number of other factors. So that while seven pounds is the average, a normal, healthy full-term baby may weigh anywhere from five and a half to eleven pounds at birth, although weights over ten pounds are considered excessive. The infant weighing less than five pounds is considered growth restricted.

Along with physical growth, the developing fetus is sharpening its five senses, which will help it sort out its environment and negotiate its way in the world. If the fetus were not confined to the darkness of the womb, it would probably be able to see and distinguish gradations of light. Doctors suspect this from observing the behavior of premature infants, who have this ability at birth.

More fascinating is the development of the fetus's sense of hearing. While in the uterus, the fetus is bombarded with many different sounds: its mother's heartbeat, the grumbling of her digestive tract, the echo of her voice. Some specialists believe that loud outside noises penetrate the closed uterine environment of thin women. An interesting experiment grew out of the suspicion that the fetus hears and reacts to sound during gestation. A nursery in one hospital decided to play a recording of a slow, steady heartbeat in one room to see what effect it had on the babies. The newborn infants who were exposed to the amplified heartbeat seemed to be calmer and better eaters than the infants in an adjacent nursery, in which the heartbeat was not played. Many young mothers are applying the results of the experiment themselves by placing a soft-ticking clock in the cradle or the crib of their newborn infants.

Fetal movement occurs very early in pregnancy but is not usually perceived by the mother until after the fourteenth week. This early perception can be influenced by such factors as the amount of fat the mother has in her abdomen. While most of the early movement is reflex action, later movement may be caused by discomfort or pressure. During prenatal examinations, when the doctor measures fetal growth by feeling the abdomen, the fetus inside often changes position. A more dramatic illustration of the fetal sense of touch can be seen during a diagnostic procedure called *amniocentesis*. Amniocentesis, an analysis of the amniotic fluid, requires the insertion of a small needle into the uterus through the abdominal wall. Sometimes, the fetus is struck inadvertently and responds with violent kicking, amply demonstrating its displeasure.

The Placenta and Umbilical Cord

The placenta is a perfectly marvelous organ. This smooth, glassy barrier serves two main functions for the fetus, which depends on the placenta for its existence. First, the placenta produces the hormones needed to keep your body primed for pregnancy. Then it serves as a kind of border patrol — selectively letting substances come and go from mother to baby, and vice versa. It transfers respiratory and nutritive materials to the fetus and collects the wastes of respiration and metabolism, all the while keeping two separate circulatory systems between mother and baby.

The placenta enhances the passage of gamma globulin from mother to baby. Gamma globulin, a blood protein, contains the antibodies against disease, so that the fetus receives its mother's immunity.

The placenta also acts as a physical barrier between the mother and the fetus. In other words, the fetus is actually a transplanted foreign element within the mother, which she will tolerate for nine months before expelling it. In fact, some people hypothesize that labor is initiated by the mother's body rejecting this "foreign transplant."

In addition to its very basic functions, the placenta changes throughout pregnancy to adjust to the size and the needs of the fetus. For instance, as the fetus gets bigger and needs more food, the cells of the placenta thin out, allowing nutritive material to pass through more easily. This thinning phenomenon is called the "increasing permeability" of the placenta.

The placenta seems to possess certain selective powers that allow it readily to pass calcium, gamma globulin, and proteins — all essential for fetal growth — into the fetus at concentrations higher than those in the mother. The placenta also easily passes most substances composed of small molecules. From a practical standpoint, you should be aware that almost all drugs are made up of small molecules and pass readily from the mother into the fetal blood and tissues. It is also believed that some bacteria and viruses pass through the placenta, resulting in an occasional infection of the fetus. Rubella, or German measles, virus can result in fetal malformation if it is contracted during the first trimester of pregnancy.

Fetal Circulation and Respiration

Fetal circulation differs from circulation after birth for several reasons. First of all, very little fetal blood passes through the lungs. Instead, blood is purified of carbon dioxide and filled with oxygen and nutritive material in the placenta and is carried to the fetus through the umbilical vessels.

The lungs are collapsed until a few seconds after birth, when blood is forced in with the baby's first breath. Special ducts that were used by the fetus to bypass this pulmonary circulation are simultaneously closed. There is a small opening from the right side of the heart to the left side called the foramen ovale. This also closes once circulation in the lungs has been established. If the foramen ovale remains opened, circulation disturbances can result, which may require treatment after delivery.

The Fetal Head

All of fetal development can be considered a marvelous engineering feat. But the best-designed feature in the overall body structure is the fetal head. The head is composed of bony portions not firmly united but separated from one another by spaces filled with membranes called sutures. The design allows the head, the largest single part of the fetus, to compress, change shape, and adapt to the contours of the birth canal during labor. The compressibility is called molding and will be discussed in more detail in the next chapter.

The two most important spaces are the frontal suture and the sagittal suture in the base of the skull. The frontal suture is covered with a membrane called the fontanel, which is more commonly known as the "soft spot" on top of the baby's head. After birth, as the baby gets older, the sutures fuse, giving the child the closed skull of the adult.

As labor approaches, the head of the fetus usually settles into the narrow opening of the uterus, with legs, feet, thighs, and buttocks filling out the wider portion of the pear-shaped organ. Ninety-six percent of all babies conform to uterine contour this way, using the shape of the womb in the most efficient manner for labor.

Amniotic Fluid

Throughout the pregnancy, the fetus floats in a liquid called amniotic fluid. This fluid serves several purposes. It helps the developing fetus maintain body temperature. It serves as a shock absorber against injury. It allows the fetus easy motility. It is also known that the fetus continually drinks the fluid. Since amniotic fluid contains protein and carbohydrates, it may also provide some nutrition for the fetus.

The actual source of amniotic fluid is not completely clear, but very early in pregnancy it begins to collect in the space left between the wall of the placenta and the fetus itself. This space is called the amniotic cavity. The amount of fluid may be as little as a cup at three months' gestation and as much as a quart at term. The composition of the amniotic fluid changes throughout pregnancy, and it reflects the sum total of any one time of fetal swallowing, urination, circulation, and the size or the stage of pregnancy.

Because the amniotic fluid also contains cells shed by the fetus, an analysis of the fluid can give us much information about the health and the well-being of the growing baby. For example, the sex of the fetus can be determined by an analysis of cells within the fluid. Other tests may help tell fetal age. Still other tests allow doctors to detect many genetic abnormalities early in pregnancy.

Teratology

Teratology is the study of abnormal fetal development. About 3 percent of babies are born with major defects. By the age of five, an additional 1.5 percent will demonstrate abnormalities. Although we will determine the cause of the defect only about half of the time, several agents have been found to be directly related. These agents are called *teratogens*. Teratogens can be substances in the environment, a drug that is ingested, or an organism like a parasite or a virus. (See chapter 1.)

Several factors may influence whether a particular agent may cause a birth defect. Three important factors are the quantity of teratogen that is present, the time during development when the teratogen is around, and the ability that the particular woman and her fetus have to fight off the teratogen.

PRENATAL TESTING

One of the most exciting advances in all of medicine during the last few decades has been our ability to evaluate the health of the fetus while it's still snug in the uterus. Before these new tests were developed, we really couldn't tell much about what was going on in the fetus's small self-contained world. We could listen to its heartbeat with a stethoscope, estimate roughly its size and age by feeling the expanding uterus within the abdomen, and, if necessary, use various types of X rays to determine the fetus's developmental stage and viability.

A wide range of tests has been developed that can reveal much about the fetus at many different stages of pregnancy. And these tests are continually being improved—made faster, safer, and more accurate. Genetic defects can sometimes be diagnosed in the uterus, as can some developmental problems of the brain and the spine, Rh disease of pregnancy, intrauterine growth retardation (slowed fetal growth), and much more.

Of course, keeping an eye on fetal health is important in every case so that special attention, which includes employing the previous tests, can be given in situations where the baby is clearly at increased risk. Women with these conditions are carefully watched throughout pregnancy and labor so that any problems can be taken care of swiftly, efficiently, and with the least possible harm to mother and child.

Although "high-risk" has been defined in various ways, we feel that the following conditions place a woman in a category requiring special care. This doesn't mean something will go wrong. In fact, it probably won't. But since the chances here of developing a problem are higher than in women who don't fall into one of these groups, it's wise for women, their partners, and their doctors to be prepared, just in case.

- Maternal age over thirty-five
- Maternal age under eighteen
- Anemia
- High blood pressure
- Diabetes
- Obesity

- Malnutrition
- Previous cesarean section
- Past obstetrical problem (such as miscarriage, prematurity, or stillbirth)
- Infections (kidney, liver; viral, bacterial, etc.)
- Fibroid tumors of the uterus
- Cancer
- Epilepsy
- Family history of genetic disease

The techniques that allow us to measure fetal health include maternal serum screening, amniocentesis, chorionic villus sampling, electronic fetal monitoring, fetal blood sampling, and ultrasonography.

Maternal Serum Screening

Maternal serum screening is a method used to gather information about the fetus through analysis of the mother's blood early in pregnancy. Originally, a blood test called a maternal serum alpha-fetoprotein (MSAFP) was used to single out the small number of women whose unborn babies might have a problem called a "neural tube defect." Multiple blood tests are now used in conjunction with the MSAFP to help identify women at risk for other fetal abnormalities, including chromosomal abnormalities such as Down's syndrome.

The purpose of this testing is to take a large population of women and find in it a smaller group of women that may be at risk for problems. Those women at high risk can then be offered more specific and possibly invasive testing. It is important to be aware that this test has several limitations. For example, a normal test (negative result) is not a guarantee that the baby will be perfect, and an abnormal test (positive result) is not indicative of abnormal but just indicates the need for further testing.

Currently, multiple serum markers are looked at in the blood of pregnant women between approximately sixteen and eighteen weeks of gestation. Depending on the laboratory used, up to five markers are analyzed: MSAFP, human chorionic gonadopropin (HCG), unconjugated estradiol (uE3), pregnancy-associated plasma protein A (PAPP-A), and inhibin-A.

Maternal Serum Alpha-Fetoprotein

Neural tube defects are so named because the central nervous system—the brain and the spinal cord—develop from a structure in the embryo called the neural tube. Normally, the neural tube closes completely. However, if it fails to close, it may leave a defect, or an opening, somewhere along the central nervous system. In some cases, the opening in the spinal cord may be covered with bone and skin (a closed neural tube defect); in others, it may be completely uncovered (an open neural tube defect). Two common and serious types of neural tube defects are *anencephaly* and *spina bifida*. Anencephaly occurs when the brain and the skull do not develop normally. Such a fetus cannot survive. In spina bifida, the opening is in the spinal cord, a problem that varies from somewhat minor to very serious, depending on its type and location.

Alpha-fetoprotein (AFP) is a substance produced by the fetus. If the neural tube is not closed, large amounts of AFP can spill into the amniotic fluid and, from there, into the mother's blood. Measurement of the mother's blood and the amniotic fluid for AFP can detect elevated levels that may be due to a neural tube defect.

As mentioned, included in your maternal serum screening is a test for AFP. If that shows elevated levels, the test will be repeated immediately. If your blood test has normal levels of AFP, there is no need for further tests. However, the test is not infallible. The first AFP test may miss as many as 20 percent of neural tube defects.

If the second test is also elevated, there is still only a 4 to 10 percent chance that the fetus actually has an open neural tube defect. After two high AFP levels, additional tests will be performed to determine the cause. The most common reason for an elevated MSAFP is underestimation of the fetal age. Also, although much less common, twins could falsely elevate the MSAFP levels. A sonogram or an ultrasound will determine whether the dates are correct and there is only one pregnancy. If this is the case, a comprehensive ultrasound evaluation should be performed. Many centers throughout the United States and around the world possess trained specialists qualified to perform such an examination. If done in such a manner, ultrasound can rule out approximately 95 percent of neural tube defects. If no obvious defect is seen on the ultrasound, the dates appear correct, and twins are ruled out, amniocentesis can be done to increase the detection rate to close to 100 percent. Many people will opt not to do this more invasive procedure in the face of a normal ultrasound. Some investigators have suggested that ultrasonography alone may be an acceptable alternative to amniocentesis for diagnosis of neural tube defect.

If amniocentesis is performed and detects a high AFP level in the amniotic fluid, the fetus is very likely to have a problem. Another enzyme called acetylcholinesterase can also be measured in the amniotic fluid to add certainty to the diagnosis of a neural tube defect. At that point, a couple may be faced with the difficult decision of whether or not to continue the pregnancy. If the AFP levels are high and this enzyme is not detected, defects other than neural tube defects are suggested in the fetus. On many occasions, the mother's blood test (MSAFP) is elevated, the ultrasound shows no defects, and the amniocentesis is perfectly normal. This last subgroup of women, as well as those women with elevated MSAFP tests who have normal ultrasound evaluations and who decline amniocentesis, are considered to be at higher risk for certain problems related to the pregnancy, such as poor growth of the fetus, low levels of amniotic fluid later in the pregnancy, and even fetal death. For those patients, increased surveillance is suggested.

The cause of neural tube defects is not known. Genetic and environmental factors (including diet) may play a part, but no one really knows for sure. In the United States, 1 to 2 live births per 1,000 involve a neural tube defect, half of which are spina bifida. Most occur in couples with no special risks. However, risks are higher in women who have previously had a child with a neural tube defect and in couples in which one partner has a neural tube defect or a family history of a neural tube defect. As mentioned previously, deficiencies of folic acid in a woman's diet right around the time of conception have been associated with an increased risk for neural tube defects. Many food products and all prenatal vitamins are now supplemented with folic acid. In addition, women with a history of a neural tube defect are instructed to take extra folic acid before and after conception to reduce the recurrence risk.

MSAFP and Other Serum Markers for Identifying Chromosomal Problems

Low levels of maternal AFP have been reported to occur in some pregnancies in which the fetus has Down's syndrome. This finding was first reported in 1984 and then verified by a larger study in many centers in 1989. Occurring in about 1 in 800 live births, Down's syndrome leads to severe mental retardation and is associated with heart defects, intestinal problems, and the development of childhood leukemias.

Currently, other serum markers, as mentioned previously, are also analyzed to improve detection rates. Human chorionic gonadotropin (HCG) is produced by fetal tissues and is first detectable in the mother's blood about eight days after ovulation. This chemical marker is used by standard home pregnancy tests to confirm pregnancies. It has been noted that fetuses with Down's syndrome produce higher levels of HCG. A large study in 1991 demonstrated that HCG levels are the most sensitive serum marker for the detection of Down's syndrome. Another serum marker called unconjugated estradiol (uE3), produced by the placenta and other fetal organs, tends to be lower in fetuses with Down's syndrome. This marker, in conjunction with MSAFP and HCG, adds to the detection rates of the maternal serum screening. Using all three serum markers, we still can pick up only around 60 percent of the Down's syndrome fetuses. With the recent addition of new serum markers such as PAPP-A and inhibin-A levels, detection rates have increased slightly; still, almost 30 to 40 percent of fetuses with Down's syndrome have normal markers.

If a woman has an abnormal maternal serum screen and the Down's syndrome risk is increased, an ultrasound should be done to confirm the dates of the pregnancy. Unlike with neural tube defects, detailed ultrasound fails to detect Down's syndrome most of the time. Therefore, amniocentesis is recommended to improve detection rates to close to 100 percent. Of note, patients should be reassured because most women with an abnormal screening test have falsely positive results and will have normal babies.

Maternal serum screening is also useful in identifying another much less common but very lethal chromosomal defect called trisomy-18. With this anomaly, all three markers are lower, and an amniocentesis can rule out this defect. Serum marker screening will identify some patients carrying fetuses with other chromosomal abnormalities as well.

First-Trimester Screening for Down's Syndrome

One of the main drawbacks of maternal serum screening is that the test is usually performed at around sixteen weeks in the pregnancy. Often a positive screen leads to an amniocentesis being done, and the results may not come until close to twenty weeks. If there is bad news and a patient is faced with the decision of whether to terminate the pregnancy, the trauma may be increased by the mother's awareness of fetal movement. Another problem with maternal serum testing is that despite the new multiple markers, detection rates are still not much better than 60 percent. Two very large investigational trials have recently been completed in the United States and the United Kingdom. Those trials looked at a combination of nuchal translucency (NT), an area seen at the back of the fetal neck on ultrasound, and several serum markers. These tests are performed very early in the pregnancy, usually between ten and fourteen weeks, and hold much promise in achieving very high detection rates for Down's syndrome. Using the NT with two blood markers (pregnancy-associated plasma protein-A and free beta-human chorionic gonadotropin), detection rates for Down's syndrome are around 80 to 90 percent. The false positive rate, however, is approximately 5 percent. If these values are integrated with the second-trimester serum markers, the false positive rate will drop to about 3 percent.

Ultrasound

Sonography, or ultrasound, is probably the single most successful method of intrauterine diagnosis that has evolved in recent years. A variation on ultrasound—sonar—was developed during World War II to scout out submarines lurking deep in the oceans. After that, sonar began to show its strengths in medicine. Recent technological advances have raised picture quality from merely remarkable (i.e., a trained technician could translate the blurry black and white lines and blobs into a recognizable baby) to simply amazing (so clear, doctors and parents gaze in wonder together at the absolutely unmistakable humanity of the tiny form). Ultrasound has enhanced almost beyond measure our ability to evaluate the health of the fetus, with no known risk at this time—no X rays, no needles, no pain.

The "magic" is in the method of ultrasound: sound waves of high frequency, above the range of human hearing. Sound is a physical force that is in no way related to X rays. Therefore, it does not have any of the tissue-harming potential of X-ray exposure during pregnancy. These sound waves are sent out by a scanner, or transducer, held over the abdomen, and travel into the body as vibrations. Echoes from the sound waves are reflected off the various surfaces within the body as the waves pass through; a fetus in the uterus, fluid, bone, tissue, and organs. The echoes are translated into electrical signals that, when projected onto a TV-like screen, reveal a detailed picture of these normally hidden structures.

Ultrasound is used in a number of ways. It can measure size, as of the bones in the fetus's arms or head. It can identify the shape and the location of structures like the uterus and the placenta. Movements, such as the fetal heart beating, can be seen, and still photographs can be made to record permanently what was revealed.

During pregnancy, ultrasound can be used in many specific ways.

- Pregnancy can be confirmed. The fetal sac can be seen in the uterus as early as three weeks after conception.
- The fetus can be proven to be alive, by demonstration of its beating heart, as early as six or seven weeks from the last menstrual period.

- Multiple births—twins, most often—can be identified with accuracy by the second or third month.
- The width of the fetal skull and the length of the femur bones in the legs can reveal the age of the fetus, so due dates can be checked. Several scans of these bones over time can determine if the fetus is growing normally.
- Major physical abnormalities (of the kidneys, the intestines, the limbs, or the spine, for example) can be visualized.
- The placenta can be scanned for clues to the cause of abnormal bleeding.
- Problems with the amount of amniotic fluid (polyhydramnios is too much; oligohydramnios is too little) can be diagnosed.
- Fibroid tumors of the uterus and ovarian masses can be tracked during pregnancy.
- Rare placental pregnancies, such as molar pregnancies (a rare placental tumor), can be diagnosed.
- A biophysical profile of the fetus can be done to measure its overall well-being. This profile includes fetal movements, fetal muscle tone, the amount of amniotic fluid, and fetal breathing movements.
- A "comprehensive ultrasound" can now be performed by a specially trained individual, when a more critical evaluation of the fetal anatomy is required.
- Doppler velocimetry, a noninvasive sonographic evaluation of blood flow through the umbilical cord, can be evaluated in high-risk patients to see if the baby is having trouble.
- Fetal echocardiography can be performed by specialized pediatric cardiologists to look at the fetal heart in the greatest of detail.
- Three- and four-dimensional ultrasound now exists and is best known for its ability to generate spatial 3-D and 4-D views and therefore produce spectacular imagery of the unborn baby.

Concern about the possible long-term effects of ultrasound on the fetus has been raised. No damage has been documented to a single mother or fetus after twenty-five years of ultrasound use in medical centers throughout the world; however, since even this extensive use leaves sonography still categorized as a relatively new procedure, it should be used only when there is a medical need for it, not simply out of curiosity. If the examination is needed to diagnose or rule out a suspected problem, almost every obstetrician would agree that the very real benefits obtained from this test outweigh a risk that is purely theoretical at this time.

If you have an ultrasound, your physician may ask you to have a full bladder during the examination. This may make you somewhat uncomfortable but does make the results clearer. Otherwise, the procedure does not entail any discomfort—no needles, drugs, or special diets are required. The examination is performed by either your physician or a trained ultrasound technician in a hospital or an office. You lie on your back on an examination table and an oily substance is rubbed on the skin of your abdomen so that the transducer can slide across it easily and smoothly. The oil also improves the penetration of the sound waves into your body by sealing the transducer to your skin and eliminating any air pockets between the two.

The exam itself will take less than thirty minutes. The image of the fetus will be visible on a TV screen, and still pictures may be taken of the screen image at various points. The sonographer may be able to tell you the baby's sex, if you want to know it before birth. Bonding, which normally occurs between the parents and the newborn just after birth, may also occur to some extent even before birth once ultrasound reveals your tiny offspring swimming and kicking in its little underwater world.

"From the second I saw our baby on the scanner, she was real in a way that had not struck me before, for all the pregnancy tests and doctors' visits," one woman commented. "She was no longer a fetus, she was my child. My husband was just as bowled over as I was."

What Do We See on a Basic Ultrasound Examination?

Unless technically impossible, the following should be determined during a basic ultrasound examination of a pregnant patient:

- Number of fetuses
- Fetal presentation, breech or head (in second and third trimester)
- Documentation of fetal life
- Placental localization
- Amount of amniotic fluid
- Date and age of pregnancy
- Detection and evaluation of maternal pelvic masses (best done in the first trimester)
- Survey of fetal anatomy for gross malformations (in the second and the third trimesters)

ULTRASOUND IMAGES

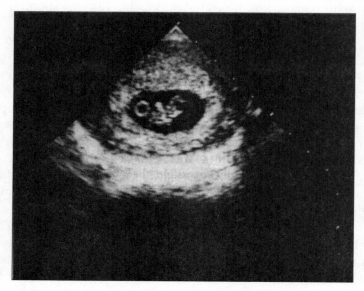

Twin embryo sacs, six weeks' pregnancy

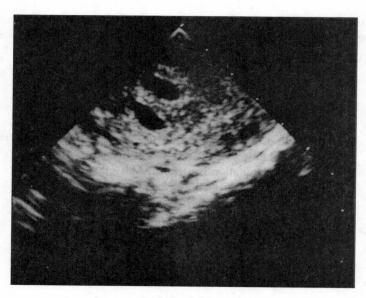

Eight-week fetus

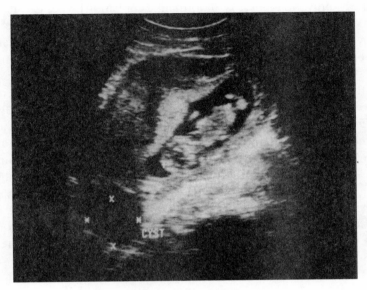

Eleven-week fetus

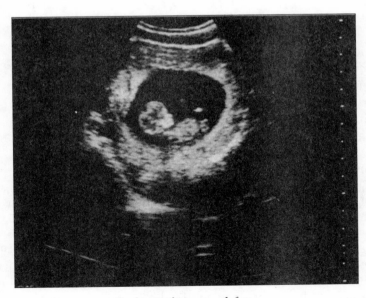

Twelve- to thirteen-week fetus

The basic ultrasound will not detect 100 percent of fetal abnormalities—only large obvious abnormalities of various types can be seen.

Many ultrasound scans are performed to document the pregnancy age when clinical dating is unsure or when there is a difference between the uterine size and the dates according to the last menstrual period. The most commonly used fetal measurements are the head and the leg bone measurements. Ultrasound dating is most accurate before twenty-six weeks of pregnancy. A comprehensive ultrasound examination, as the name implies, consists of a more critical view of the fetal anatomy. Requirements for this type of study include appropriately trained individuals, sophisticated sonographic equipment, and some good luck. For example, during the evaluation, if your baby is a little stubborn and hides from the sonographer, certain things may not be seen. The technician may insist that you return at a later date for another viewing. The following is an example of a list of anatomical areas that the sonographer needs to visualize during a comprehensive ultrasound done at our institution:

Calvarium	Fetal heart motion	Left hand
BPD level	Thoracic spine	Right hand
Lat ventricles	Lumbar spine	Left fingers
Cerebellum	Sacrum	Right fingers
Nose/lips	Four-chamber view	Left humerus
Orbits	Left ventricular	Right humerus
Face	outflow tract	Left forearm
Cervical spine	Left kidney	Right forearm
Choroid plexus	Right kidney	Left foot
Cisterna magna	Bladder	Right foot
Neck	Lungs	Left toes
Nuchal fold	Diaphragm	Right toes
Profile	Ventral wall	Left femur
Right ventricular	Stomach	Right femur
outflow tract	Liver	Left lower leg
Cardiac axis	Bowel	Right lower leg
Cardiac position	Genitalia	

Although somewhat controversial, most obstetricians insist that all pregnant women, both low and high risk, undergo comprehensive ultrasound evaluation at around twenty weeks' gestation. This gestational age is chosen because the fetal size is large enough for good visualization, and timing is early enough for termination of the pregnancy if a major anomaly is detected and the choice has been made.

The first trimester is the best time to examine the maternal uterus and the ovaries for abnormalities. The following fetal characteristics should be visible at the indicated weeks of gestation. A vaginal ultrasound alters some of these dates, allowing slightly earlier diagnosis.

- Five to six weeks: Fetal sac.
- Six weeks: Fetal mass itself.
- Seven weeks: Fetal heart is seen — rules out 95 percent of miscarriages.
- Seven to twelve weeks: Measurement of the length of the fetus, from the top of the head to the end of the spine, is a very accurate method for dating pregnancy.

At midpregnancy, it is possible to evaluate much of the fetal anatomy. The head, the spine, the heart, the abdomen, the sex organs, the limbs, and the growth rate are examined.

Often it is difficult to fully examine some fetal areas late in the third trimester, usually because of the relative decrease of amniotic fluid in the third trimester and the position of the fetus. Maternal obesity can also make sonographic evaluation difficult at any time during pregnancy.

In the third trimester, it is often useful to evaluate fetal behavior, in addition to surveying the fetal anatomy. This would include a brief appraisal of the frequency and the type of fetal movement, as well as a gross evaluation of fetal tone by noting the degree of flexion of the extremities and the volume of amniotic fluid. The presence of fetal respiratory movements is a reassuring sign of well-being. In high-risk patients, an assessment of fetal behavior may be useful. In those cases, a basic ultrasound examination is also performed.

Should All Patients Be Screened?

Controversy continues about whether ultrasound screening of all obstetric patients is beneficial. In 1984, a task force supported by the National Institutes of Health was convened to evaluate this issue. Based on the evidence available at the time, the task force concluded that no benefit in perinatal outcome was demonstrated by such a practice. More recent clinical studies, however, have suggested some benefits of routine screening. More studies with large numbers of patients are needed to address the question of the role of routine ultrasound screening. We find it very valuable in the practice of obstetrics, and almost all of our patients have ultrasounds. Currently in the

United States approximately 70 percent of women undergo ultrasound evaluation.

Amniocentesis

Amniocentesis has become one of the main tools of the obstetrician. Although it sounds frightening and is a bit disconcerting to undergo, it is generally safe and simple in the hands of an expert. Amniocentesis is performed by passing a long, thin needle straight through the skin of the abdomen and the uterine wall and into the amniotic sac—the structure that holds the fetus and its protective fluid, like a swimming pool. A small portion of the amniotic fluid is then drawn up into the needle to be studied.

Amniocentesis is quite safe. It's done after sixteen weeks (once sufficient fluid has formed) either in the office or in a hospital, depending on where the ultrasound equipment is. The location of the fetus and the placenta is determined by ultrasound so that they will not be harmed by a stray poke of the needle. However, as with any medical procedure, the risks of the amniocentesis should be weighed against the seriousness of the potential problem it is being used to detect. Minor complications for the mother include cramping, bleeding, and leakage of amniotic fluid from the vagina. Fortunately, these problems occur very rarely, and they usually require no treatment. Serious complications of amniocentesis, such as miscarriage and fetal injury, occur very infrequently, in fewer than 1 in 200 cases. Some recent studies have compared loss rates after amniocentesis, by studying those done by perinatal specialists and those done by general obstetricians. A 2001 study found that a group of perinatologists had a significantly lower loss rate than the matched group of general obstetricians. A more recent review of very busy general obstetricians in Detroit was found to have an extremely low loss rate. One could probably conclude that the loss rate may be partially related to operator experience, and that you should be sure that your obstetrician has appropriate training and experience. Women with Rh-negative blood require Rh immunoglobulin after the procedure, to prevent Rh sensitization (see chapter 12).

The Uses of Amniocentesis

The frequency of Rh disease has been markedly diminished by the development of the immune vaccine that keeps the Rh-negative mother from ever developing the antibodies harmful to her Rh-positive fetuses.

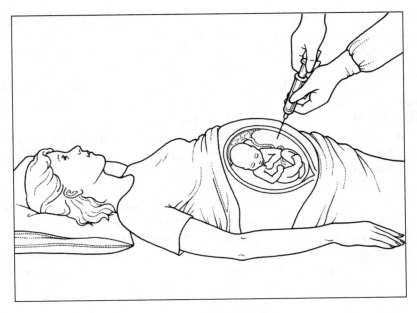

AMNIOCENTESIS

Tests such as amniocentesis can greatly aid in the care of those few cases that still do occur.

Studying the amniotic fluid of an Rh-sensitized woman (as explained in chapter 12) enables a physician to determine how seriously affected the fetus is. The levels of bilirubin, a sign of the destruction of the fetus's red blood cells, can be measured in the amniotic fluid. The degree of anemia of the fetus can then be determined and treatment given if necessary. A severely affected fetus is given an intrauterine transfusion or, if close to term, is delivered.

Respiratory distress syndrome is a lung condition that many premature infants develop. Because it leaves the newborn unable to breathe properly, it can lead to death. It is caused by the lack of a particular substance, surfactant, which normally forms on the surface of the lungs and facilitates the exchange of oxygen and carbon dioxide. The cause of hyaline membrane disease (an older name for respiratory distress syndrome) is not well understood, but it develops only after birth and does not occur in utero. Amniotic fluid can be tested for the presence of surfactant in order to zero in on babies who could develop the disease if delivered too soon. This may be necessary in complicated pregnancies when a decision has to be made whether to deliver the fetus or hold off a while longer. The surfactant test has proven to be very accurate and has greatly enhanced the ability of the perinatologist to make the best decisions about high-risk pregnancies. It is also used many times prior to performing a nonemergency cesarean section, to make sure that the fetus's lungs are mature.

Amniocentesis has become a valuable tool in—and is probably best known for—the prenatal diagnosis of birth defects. This now well-established procedure is critical to diagnosing the presence or the absence of more than 100 different chromosomal abnormalities. Genetic amniocentesis may be done if either parent or a previous child has chromosome abnormalities, if the mother is thirty-five or older or has had a child with Down's syndrome, if the parents are carriers of sex-linked diseases such as hemophilia or of autosomal recessive diseases such as Tay-Sachs, or if a neural tube defect is suspected (see chapter 1 for information on genetic counseling). Some women are electing to have amniocentesis done at ages under thirty-five because they feel that the total risk for all chromosomal abnormalities is less than the risks associated with amniocentesis (see table 7.1).

Chorionic Villus Sampling

Although amniocentesis has proven extraordinarily valuable, it does have several limitations. One is that the procedure cannot be done before sixteen weeks of pregnancy and often requires a two-week wait for the result. Therefore, a woman may not get the results until twenty weeks of pregnancy—the fifth month. If termination of the pregnancy is then elected because of fetal abnormalities, it is much more traumatic at this point, both psychologically and medically. Therefore, if a safe and reliable test existed for diagnosing fetal problems early—during the first trimester—it would be of enormous value.

One such technique, called chorionic villus biopsy or chorionic villus sampling (CVS), is a viable alternative to amniocentesis. Using ultrasound as a guide, it is possible to pass a small tube into the uterus through either the cervix or the abdomen at about eleven weeks of pregnancy. A tiny bit of tissue from the layer of the placenta known as the chorion can be drawn into the tube and removed for study. (Ultrasound will also be done before the test to confirm the presence of a good, healthy fetal heartbeat. If there is no heartbeat by ten to eleven weeks, it usually means that the woman is going to have a miscarriage and is, therefore, not a candidate for the CVS.)

Just about every disorder that can be found with amniocentesis can be diagnosed by CVS much earlier (except neural tube defects, which are diagnosable only by amniocentesis and alpha-fetoprotein tests).

TABLE 7.1
Chromosomal Abnormalities in Liveborns

MATERNAL AGE	RISK FOR DOWN'S SYNDROME	TOTAL RISK FOR ALL CHROMOSOMAL ABNORMALITIES
20	1/1,667	1/526
21	1/1,667	1/526
22	1/1,429	1/500
23	1/1,429	1/500
24	1/1,250	1/476
25	1/1,250	1/476
26	1/1,176	1/476
27	1/1,111	1/455
28	1/1,053	1/435
29	1/1,000	1/417
30	1/952	1/385
31	1/909	1/385
32	1/769	1/322
33	1/602	1/286
34	1/485	1/238
35	1/378	1/192
36	1/289	1/156
37	1/224	1/127
38	1/173	1/102
39	1/136	1/83
40	1/106	1/66
41	1/82	1/53
42	1/63	1/42
43	1/49	1/33
44	1/38	1/26
45	1/30	1/21
46	1/23	1/16
47	1/18	1/13
48	1/14	1/10
49	1/11	1/8

NOTE: Compare to the risks of amniocentesis, which are between 1 in 300 and 1 in 800, depending on various studies.

One of the problems at this point is the risk of miscarriage. Recent data from several centers indicate that CVS is a relatively safe procedure. Two large studies done in 1989 showed that CVS had a slightly higher loss rate compared to amniocentesis. One study showed 0.6 percentage points higher loss, and the other showed 0.8 percentage points higher loss. A large Canadian study in 1992 failed to show any significant difference in loss rate compared to amniocentesis. Several years ago, there were studies indicating an increased risk of babies born with limb-reduction defects in women undergoing CVS. Subsequently, this finding seemed to occur only in women who had had CVS prior to ten weeks. It is now recommended that CVS be performed only after ten weeks. One large case-controlled study conducted by the Centers for Disease Control and Prevention from 1988 to 1992 showed no overall increased risk of limb deficiency in infants born to women who had CVS but did see a sixfold increase in a specific type of limb defect called a transverse digital deficiency. The absolute risk of this, however, is only about 1 per 3,000 births. At this time, women who have a relatively low risk of having a baby with detectable defects may want to wait for amniocentesis, instead of having CVS. However, in very-high-risk situations, it might be worth taking a chance, despite the dangers of miscarriage and limb deficiencies. As of this publication, countless numbers of women have undergone testing by this technique.

Another prenatal use of this procedure will be by couples deciding to have a child of a particular sex. For example, someone with a family history of a disorder like hemophilia, which affects only male fetuses, would be a candidate for CVS, which could determine the fetus's sex early, still timely for an early abortion. Of course, if this were possible, parents would also have the ability to abort a child for reasons of sexual preference alone—if, for example, they had three boys and wanted a girl. This raises difficult ethical questions for both patients and physicians.

In summary, transcervical and transabdominal CVS, when performed by expert operators, is a relatively safe procedure and may be considered an acceptable alternative to midtrimester genetic amniocentesis. CVS requires appropriate genetic counseling before the procedure, an operator experienced in performing the technique, and a laboratory experienced in processing the specimen and interpreting the results.

Fetal Therapy

Now that it is possible to diagnose fetal anomalies, therapies can often be initiated prior to delivery. When the defects are severe or lethal, pregnancy termination may be considered. When less severe, correction of the underlying problem may be possible. Over the last few decades, fetal therapy has evolved in many areas; for example:

Open fetal surgery. The uterus is opened, the fetus is removed, and the problem is corrected surgically, then the fetus is replaced. This has been performed for a limited number of indications, primarily at the University of California, San Francisco. There is a high rate of fetal loss, and this should only be done in desperate situations.

Closed endoscopic surgical approaches. Using thin fiberoptic endoscopes, many of the same invasive procedures can be done with slightly less risk.

Ultrasound guided therapy. Many new techniques have been developed that use ultrasound guidance to correct specific problems, such as fetal kidney blockage or anemia.

Drug therapy. Often a condition is diagnosed where drugs can be given to the mother to treat a condition that exists in the fetus. An example is when an infection is detected that can cause defects, and the mother is given treatment to reverse the effects.

Genetic therapy. It may be possible to inject DNA into the fertilized egg to correct genetic defects that are detected.

Fetal Monitoring

Over the last three to four decades, we obstetricians have increased our understanding of how our second patient, the fetus, functions. We are no longer concerned just with delivering a baby to a healthy mother. We now want each child to be born well and the quality of life for that newborn to be optimal. We have entered an era in which the fetus is now rightfully treated as our second patient. As a result, we have improved our abilities to diagnose and take care of your unborn child.

Various tests of fetal well-being have evolved and are now used extensively. The most popular tests are used in the last three months of pregnancy and during labor; they involve accurate ways to keep track of the fetal heart rate. This technique is called fetal monitoring.

There are two general types of fetal monitoring. Before labor, we use the antepartum fetal non-stress test (NST). During labor, electronic monitoring is used to watch and record the fetal heart rate and the contractions of the uterus.

Both of these types use two main techniques. One picks up the fetal heartbeat, using ultrasound or an electrocardiogram, either through a device called a transducer on the mother's abdomen or by electrodes directly attached to the fetal head during labor. The other technique shows the duration and the strength of contractions and uses a pressure device either on the mother's abdomen or within the uterus.

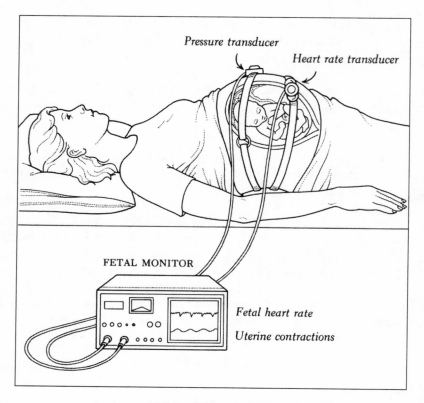

FETAL MONITORING

The development of the NST occurred because of the interesting observation that the fetal heart rate increases when the fetus moves. This heart rate acceleration shows a healthy fetus—and conversely, its absence is cause for suspicion. If the NST suggests that the fetus is having some problems, other more clear-cut and elaborate tests are performed to evaluate the situation further.

Another test, called the biophysical profile, is used with the NST to determine the health of the fetus. It consists of four other observations made by ultrasound—fetal breathing movements, fetal muscle tone, general fetal movements, and the quantity of amniotic fluid.

The NST has become the routine screening method for monitoring fetal well-being before labor in cases where a problem is suspected. Some of the indications for testing include conditions such as maternal high blood pressure, diabetes, poor fetal growth, Rh disease, long pregnancy (forty-two weeks or more), anemia, and other high-risk pregnancies. The reactive or positive NST is the best predictor of fetal condition yet devised.

In many centers, electronic fetal monitoring during labor has become almost routine. When active labor begins, transducers are placed on the abdomen of the mother to monitor contractions and fetal heart rate. These patterns of external monitoring show how your fetus is handling labor. The electronic machines provide a continual flow of information that is read to figure out fetal well-being. Labor may be an additional stress to the fetus, especially if a problem existed before labor began.

Internal monitoring can be used only if the fetal amniotic membranes are ruptured and the cervix is somewhat open or dilated. A small device called an electrode is attached to the scalp of the fetus to record the fetal heart rate. This does not harm the unborn child.

Information from these monitoring techniques is recorded on a long strip of paper. Various patterns of the fetal heart rate, in relation to uterine contractions, relay the state of fetal well-being. Certain patterns are possible warning signs of fetal problems. When fetal distress is suspected, additional tests can be performed and therapy can be given to help the situation.

Fetal monitoring is also used to determine the strength, the frequency, and the duration of uterine contractions. This is helpful in diagnosing premature labor, treating poor labors, and inducing labor.

If fetal monitoring suggests a problem with your fetus during labor, an additional test called fetal scalp blood sampling can be performed if the cervix is partially dilated. A small instrument is used to obtain a minute sample of blood from the fetus's scalp, from which the acid-base balance of the fetus is measured (the pH test). A trend toward an acid pH level indicates fetal distress. This may suggest the need for immediate delivery, often by cesarean section. There is no question that fetal monitoring has saved the lives of some infants who previously were not expected to present problems during labor.

With the increased use of electronic fetal monitoring, there has been an appreciable increase in the number of cesarean sections performed. Whether these two are related is not clear. However, more healthy infants have been born during this period than ever before.

Controversy exists as to whether routine fetal monitoring is required in low-risk pregnancies. Some studies have shown that good results can be obtained with clinical monitoring alone by well-trained professionals. But these studies were performed under perfect conditions that don't always exist in a practical setting. Recently, a medical task force concerned with the difficult problem of predicting fetal distress during labor reached the conclusion that the routine use of monitoring should not necessarily diminish the human experience of childbirth, if properly used and explained by supportive people. Its use should not necessarily increase the cesarean rate if the use of scalp blood sampling may provide additional diagnostic help with fetal distress. The task force concluded that the routine use of monitoring in low-risk pregnancies is not necessarily beneficial, but its use when risk factors increase seems beneficial.

We have come a long way since the mother was the patient for whom care was given and the fetus was simply a transient maternal passenger. The fetus is no longer just along for the ride but can be actively diagnosed and treated. The challenge is to use this technology appropriately to ensure the health of the mother and the fetus without compromising the natural beauty of childbirth.

Part III

LABOR AND DELIVERY

Chapter 8
Labor and Delivery

—⎯⎯⎯⎯—

LABOR

While standing at the stove one Friday evening, preparing a hearty roast beef dinner, Barbara Nichols sensed a "funny feeling" in her abdomen. "Could it be the beginning of labor?" she asked herself. Her baby was due in two days. After working into her ninth month of pregnancy, she had just completed household preparations the day before: The house had been cleaned thoroughly; the baby's furniture had been delivered and assembled. And, since she was an impatient person generally, she was ready for delivery.

But was this really labor? The feeling was not a pain. It more resembled a mild charley horse—a muscle tightening that increased in intensity and subsided. If this were truly labor, the feeling would have become progressively stronger, occurring more frequently. It did.

After dinner, Mr. Nichols asked about the evening plans: "Are we going to the movies or not?"

"We can," she replied, "but I think you should know I've been having these feelings for the last two hours. They have come regularly every fifteen minutes. I think they're contractions, but I'm not certain."

"Well, when were you going to tell me?" her husband asked in mock outrage. "Are we going to the movies?"

"Yes," she answered.

So, taking her prepared hospital bag along, they drove to the movies and relaxed for two hours. Mrs. Nichols remembered that her childbirth class instructor had told her that first babies do not just fall out—and she was in no hurry to go to the hospital.

When the movie was over, the contractions were coming about every four minutes. Mr. Nichols called the doctor from the theater, and the doctor suggested they go to the hospital. Five hours later, the baby, an 8¼-pound boy, was born.

165

Mrs. Nichols's approach to this process known as labor was a very relaxed one, for good reason. While labor is one of the most dramatic points in the pregnancy, it is really just a period of adaptation. There is a baby at one end of the birth canal, and the body is trying to expel it. The physical process that allows this to happen is called labor. The three important factors in this passage are the expulsion from the uterus, the passage through which the fetus must pass, and the fetus itself.

The Components of Labor

Labor can be evaluated by what we often refer to as "three 'p's'": the passenger or the fetus, the passageway or the pelvic canal, and the power or the expulsive forces of labor. A problem with any one of the three 'p's' may interfer with a successful vaginal birth.

The Fetus

The position of the fetus in the uterus is a crucial factor in the course of labor. Most babies—96 percent, to be exact—settle head down in the uterus and are born that way. The head-first birth is called a vertex presentation. In a small percentage of all deliveries, the feet or the backside of the baby presents itself first. This position is called breech presentation. Since the moment of birth is marked by the delivery of the shoulders, breech babies are the only ones whose sex can be determined before they are actually born. Even more rarely, a baby will settle across the abdomen, rather than up and down, which requires operative delivery if the fetus cannot be coaxed into a vertical position.

There is variation in the fetal position even in the vertex presentation. Three-quarters of all babies born head first come out of the birth canal facing the mother's back. The remainder face the front of her body. In this latter position, called a posterior position, the baby's bony skull is in contact with the mother's spine; she may feel labor pains in her back, rather than in the abdomen.

The prevalence of the vertex, or head-first, presentation is not totally understood by doctors. As mentioned in the previous chapter, one theory suggests that the fetus tries to use uterine space economically, choosing the position that best fits the shape of the uterus. Another theory says that the force of gravity is responsible for the head assuming the downward position. The two theories are not necessarily incompatible.

Another indication of the natural tendency for babies to be born head first is the construction of the head itself. The fact that it is made up of small bones joined by membrane, rather than one mass of bone, would tend to support this assumption. The construction of the head makes it somewhat compressible so that it can adapt to the shape of the birth canal. This process is called molding. Molding can affect the appearance of the fetus at birth. It is quite common for firstborn infants to have marked molding. The head's shape returns to normal a few days after delivery.

The Pelvis Passage

The diameter of the pelvis passage must be wide enough to accommodate the birth of the baby. Most pelvises are. Occasionally, however, a woman has an unusually narrow pelvis or has suffered some change in contour in an accident, in which case the baby is delivered by a cesarean section. Measurement of the pelvis can be taken by internal examination. More accurate measurement can be made by a special X ray called pelvimetry, usually performed if there is a breech presentation and a vaginal delivery is being considered.

The Expulsion Process

The baby is pushed out of the mother by two forces: the involuntary contractions of the uterus, and the involuntary and voluntary contractions of the mother to push the baby out.

True labor begins when the individual muscles of the uterus begin to contract together, acting like one big muscle. In early labor, contractions can be very irregular, occurring every fifteen or twenty minutes. The interval between the contractions gradually decreases so that toward the end of labor, they are occurring every two or three minutes. Each contraction lasts from thirty to ninety seconds; early contractions are usually shorter, later contractions longer. Certain breathing exercises aid the contractions by supplying more oxygen to the abdominal muscles. This, in effect, relieves tension in the muscles, lessening the feeling of tightening of the contraction (see chapter 9).

In addition to these factors, birth is helped by the pressure of the descending baby on the pelvic floor and the rectum. The pressure causes a bearing-down reflex, which is similar to that involved in defecation. The reflex can be controlled to some extent by conscious attempts of the mother to push the baby out.

The uterus and the cervix play a role here, too. As term is approached, the lower part of the uterus begins to get thinner. The cervix, the door to the uterus, loses its long thick character; it gets shorter and thinner in a process called effacement. This process helps the dilation, or opening, of the cervix.

The Stages of Labor

While most women think of labor as one continuous process, labor really has three distinct stages, each with its own landmarks and characteristics. The first stage begins with the first contraction and ends when the cervix is fully open or dilated. The second stage begins at full dilation and ends with the delivery of the baby. The third stage consists of the delivery of the placenta (see table 8.1).

First Stage

During pregnancy, the cervix undergoes continuous change in preparation for labor. It gets progressively softer and spongier. It also gets shorter and the cells become thinner in order to facilitate dilation. This shortening and thinning of the cervix is called effacement. Before effacement, the cervix is about 1½ inches long. After effacement, it has virtually disappeared.

Once the cervix becomes this thin, the contraction force of the uterus and the pressure from the baby's head gradually force the opening wider, until it is big enough to permit the baby's head to pass through. This is similar to trying to put your head through a turtleneck sweater, but slowly. The widening of the opening is called dilation.

TABLE 8.1
Summary of Stages of Labor

First Stage: Onset of Contractions to Full Dilation of Cervix

Latent phase
1. Onset to 3–5 centimeters cervical dilation
2. Contractions every 5–15 minutes
3. Last on average 8 hours (first pregnancy)

Active phase
1. 3–5 centimeters to full dilation of cervix
2. Contractions 3–5 minutes apart
3. Lasts on average 4 hours (first pregnancy)

Second Stage: Full Dilation of Cervix until Delivery of Infant

1. Lasts up to 2 hours or longer
2. Pushing begins with contractions and the urge to bear down

Third Stage: Birth

1. Begins with birth of infant, ends with delivery of placenta
2. Lasts up to 15–20 minutes

Full dilation is set at 10 centimeters, about the width of a hand. Women who have had babies before may be slightly dilated (2 centimeters) before the onset of labor.

Second Stage

Several forces are at work to aid the passage of the baby through the birth canal. Uterine contractions, which help dilate the cervix, are now even stronger, forcing the baby down and out. The contractions, which were coming about fifteen minutes apart in the beginning of labor, are now occurring every two to three minutes, lasting sixty to ninety seconds each. As the baby descends, the mother begins an involuntary bearing down, more commonly known as pushing. The head descends and emerges slowly, followed by a rapid expulsion of the rest of the baby's body.

Third Stage

After the baby is delivered, the uterus sheds the placenta, which nurtured the fetus during its nine months' gestation. The uterus continues to contract even after the birth of the baby. It begins to get

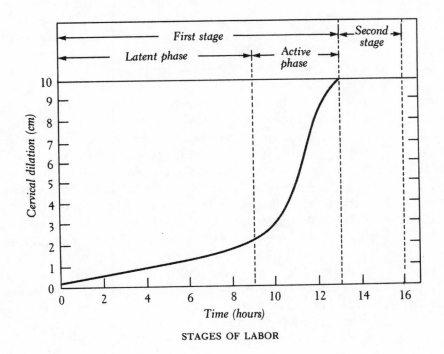

STAGES OF LABOR

smaller, and its wall becomes thicker, reducing the surface to which the placenta was attached. The placenta separates or tears away and is pushed down and out of the vagina. Blood clots immediately begin to form at the site of separation, preventing any excessive bleeding. Bleeding after delivery of the placenta is also controlled by the uterus contracting and closing the blood vessels that had previously supported the placenta.

WHAT HAPPENS IN LABOR AND DELIVERY

One or two weeks before you actually begin labor, you may notice intermittent contractions of the uterus. The contractions will feel like a tightening of an abdominal muscle, a dull ache, or a pressure in the lower pelvis or the lower back. You may feel the baby drop down into the pelvis at this time. This settling-in is called engagement because the baby has fixed itself in position for birth. From the mother's perspective this same phenomenon is called lightening, because the baby's new position is giving her a little more space to breathe and digest food.

During this period, the mucous plug of the cervix, which protected the baby from vaginal germs, may dislodge. You will be able to tell this has happened because vaginal discharge will be thicker and pink or a little deeper red. The membranes of the amniotic sac may also rupture as the baby settles down. While the rupture of membranes most often occurs rather late in labor, in about 20 percent of all women the membranes break before labor. If this occurs, you may expect as much as 2 pints of clear, watery liquid to leak from your vagina. If this does happen, you should call your doctor, who may advise you to go to the hospital. A tear in the amniotic sac means that the baby is more susceptible to infection. You will have no doubt about whether or not your membranes have broken. There is no discharge that can be confused with this watery fluid. Either of these two events—the dislodging of the mucous plug or the rupture of the membranes—is a welcome sign to pregnant women, who can be pretty certain that labor will start relatively soon. If the amniotic fluid is greenish in color, you should notify your physician. This may mean the baby has some distress because of the passage of meconium.

But the question most mothers-to-be have is: How do you know when you are in labor? The answer is: You might not know at first.

It is often very difficult to distinguish the intermittent contractions that occur before the beginning of true labor from the contractions of real labor. As a rule of thumb, remember that true labor pains are regular and persistent. They gradually increase in frequency, duration, and strength.

So-called false labor—prodromal labor contractions—are irregular and tend to disappear if you lie down or walk around. They do not increase in frequency or duration (see table 8.2).

Early in the first stage of labor, when the cervix is starting to dilate, contractions are most often felt in the back. You will be aware of them, but they will not interfere with normal activities. If it has not happened already, the mucous plug will soon dislodge.

As labor progresses and the contractions increase in frequency and length, the cervix slowly dilates. The rate of dilatation varies, being slower in women having their first babies than in women having second, third, or fourth babies.

For new mothers-to-be, it will take an average of eight and a half hours for the cervix to dilate 2.5 centimeters, one-fourth the amount of dilatation necessary for birth. Do not panic about the length of time. It most often goes unnoticed, which is why it is called the latent phase of the first stage of labor. You probably will not even know you are in true labor until the latent phase is completed.

TABLE 8.2
True Labor versus False Labor

CONTRACTIONS	FALSE LABOR	TRUE LABOR
Timing	Irregular; no increase in frequency or duration	Regular intervals, closer together
Change with motion	Stop and start, irregularly	Continued progression
Location	Abdomen	Back, radiating to front
Strength	Weak and don't get stronger	Increase over time
External manifestation	None	May pass mucous plug; rupture of membranes; bladder pressure; bloody "show"; or discharge
Occurrence	Association with fatigue, often in the evening	Anytime

DELIVERY

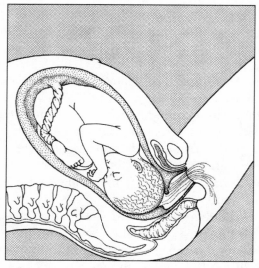

Contractions and breaking of the bag of waters

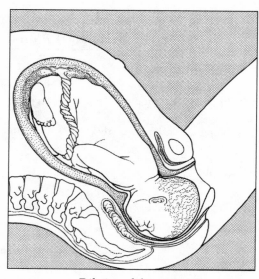

Dilation of the cervix

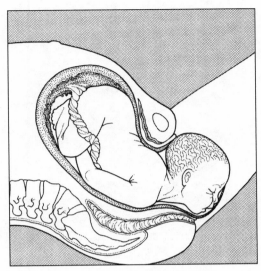

Episiotomy at this stage if needed

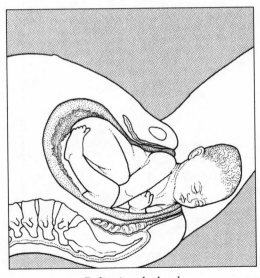

Delivering the head

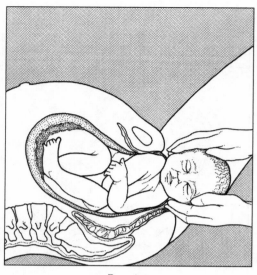

Rotation

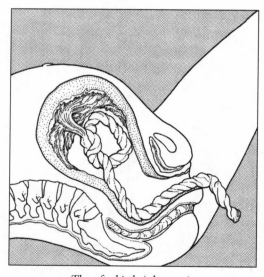

The afterbirth (placenta)

The latent phase is followed by an accelerated or active phase, during which time the cervix dilates from 3 to 10 centimeters (full dilatation). This phase takes an average of two to four hours. This is the phase of greater discomfort, and, usually, you will be in a labor room by now.

The average length of the total first stage of labor for a woman having her first baby is about twelve hours. For women who have had a baby before, full dilatation takes about seven hours.

After full dilatation, the second stage of labor automatically begins. The pressure of the baby on the pelvic floor will start the involuntary pushing reflexes described earlier. These can be aided by the voluntary efforts of the mother to bear down. It will take a first baby close to an hour to make its way down the birth canal, through the vagina to the vulva. When the baby's head can be seen at the mouth of the vagina, it is said to have crowned.

Following crowning, the doctor may make a small cut into the area between the vagina and the rectum. This cut is called an *episiotomy.*

Episiotomies are performed in more than 50 percent of all births in the United States today. Two types of episiotomies can be performed by your doctor. The first is called a midline or a median episiotomy. An incision is made directly between the vagina and the rectum. The second type is called a mediolateral episiotomy. With this, an incision is made at a 45-degree angle from the most inferior aspect of the vagina. The median episiotomy is much more commonly performed in the United States. The repair is quicker, there is less blood loss, and the postdelivery pain is much less. The downside to the median episiotomy is that there is a much higher risk of injury to the rectum and its surrounding tissues. Although very rare, even if the injury is repaired perfectly, there is a risk of future fecal incontinence. Usually, the mediolateral episiotomy is performed if much more room is needed to avoid rectal injury, such as may be the case with a forceps delivery. Today, the main reasons for performing an episiotomy are if the head is essentially stuck or if there is fetal distress and the baby needs to come out quickly. In both cases, an episiotomy may facilitate delivery.

Controversy exists as to the use of a prophylactic episiotomy. Should all women have episiotomies during vaginal births? In the 1970s and 1980s, many physicians believed in routine episiotomy for several reasons. It was felt that a straight incision versus a ragged tear was easier to repair and would heal better. The episiotomy might shorten the pushing stage so that the baby and the mother would be better off. Finally, many believed that the episiotomy reduced trauma to the muscles in the pelvic floor. These muscles are important for maintaining urinary continence.

Many studies over the last decade have disputed these assertions. One study that came out in 2001 looked specifically at the issue of the straight incision versus the ragged tear and actually found that when a median episiotomy was performed, there was a higher risk of fecal incontinence than in women who were allowed to tear spontaneously. Other studies have shown that spontaneous tears heal just as well as episiotomies and are less painful, according to patient questionnaires. In terms of urinary incontinence, most recent studies fail to show that an episiotomy prevents this occurrence. At the time of writing this book, we feel that an episiotomy should be performed only if necessary and should not be done routinely.

Once the head is delivered, the baby turns one shoulder to the side, then eases out the other. The rest of the body slides out easily. When the newborn enters the outside world, many things happen, and many changes occur within the first five to ten minutes of birth. The newborn infant begins to cry almost immediately upon its exit from the vagina. Crying causes the baby to begin active breathing. Certain changes also occur in the circulatory system of the newborn.

What causes an infant's crying and first breath has been a source of speculation for many years. It still remains something of an enigma. Some suggest that it results from physical stimulation—that is, the handling of the infant during delivery. Others suggest that crying is a response to the accumulation of carbon dioxide, due to oxygen deprivation. Whatever the cause of the first cry, it certainly is a welcome sound to those present in the delivery room.

The mother may receive medication to facilitate delivery of the placenta. After that happens, the episiotomy is sewn up, and the new mother can relax.

Going to the Hospital

Once you determine that you really are in labor, you should call your doctor about going to the hospital. You will probably be consciously aware of contractions for about two hours before you call him or her. Even if contractions are coming every fifteen minutes for an hour, it will still take some time to confirm the criteria for labor—regular, progressive, increasingly stronger. It is wise during this time to limit food intake to Jell-O or liquids. Solid foods or an excessive amount of fluid may cause vomiting during labor, which could be hazardous if anesthesia is being used.

When contractions are coming about every five minutes, your doctor will probably tell you to go to the hospital. Exactly where in the hospital you report to should be worked out with the admitting office beforehand, if possible. After admission, you will be sent to the labor floor, put in a separate labor or birthing room, and examined internally by a nurse or a resident physician, who will be able to tell the amount of cervical dilatation and the position of the fetus. This professional will listen to the baby's heart by placing you on the fetal monitoring unit. The normal fetal heart rate varies between 120 and 160 beats per minute. A rate of less than 100 may indicate some problems; this is why the fetal heartbeat is listened to so often during labor.

Following this initial examination, which is reported in full to your doctor, an enema may be given to remove all fecal material from the rectum. Many centers have stopped giving enemas. Although many people generally shudder at enemas, some women in labor welcome them. By removing a source of pressure in the pelvic area, the enema makes labor more comfortable.

As a sanitary measure, the pubic hair may also be shaved from the vulva. Most hospitals are eliminating this measure as standard procedure because the whole perineal area is doused with an antiseptic before birth anyway. An alternative procedure called a "mini-prep"— the removal of the small amount of hair at the episiotomy site—serves the purpose just as well.

During labor, your doctor will examine you vaginally several times to check the progress of dilatation and the position of the baby. Doctors perform only the minimum number of these examinations necessary to cut down on the possibility of infection.

When you are fully dilated, you will be taken to the delivery room for the actual birth, then to a recovery area, where bleeding and postdelivery contractions are checked. You may remain for up to two hours in the recovery area, during which time the nurse may press on your abdomen frequently to check on uterine tone, before you are taken to your room. Many hospitals have instituted special labor and delivery suites called birthing rooms. These all-inclusive rooms have special labor beds that can be turned into delivery setups so that you do not have to be moved. Birthing rooms also tend to be less antiseptic in nature, and some have even the amenities of TVs and telephones. You can call your family yourself with the news.

Pain Management

There are basically two ways of making labor more comfortable. A number of analgesics or anesthetics are perfectly safe to use during labor. Or a mother, with the help of her partner, can practice what is commonly called natural childbirth. This term is a misnomer because it implies no participation by the mother. Actually, natural birth in this country has come to mean psychoprophylactic childbirth, of which the most common form is the Lamaze method. This approach involves a number of breathing and body-building exercises, as well as a secondary conditioning to labor. This method is discussed in detail in chapter 9.

These two ways of managing labor are not mutually exclusive. Many women who take painkillers or anesthetics know and practice parts of the Lamaze approach. Likewise, Lamaze-trained mothers need not be wedded to a drug-free labor. Many go through the childbirth course to involve their partners more actively in the birth process. They are not necessarily committed to the whole regimen.

Analgesics for Labor and Delivery

Today, we use a variety of drugs to relieve pain during labor. The need for such relief is, of course, highly individual and variable, depending on a number of factors, such as the woman's ability to withstand pain, the size of the baby, and the size of the mother's pelvis and birth canal. Currently, various drugs can be given by injection, either directly through the IV or into the muscle, which can provide some pain relief. Many patients get only limited relief from this method of pain control. Most studies have failed to demonstrate pain relief unless the drugs are given at such high doses that the women become essentially unconscious. At these higher doses, there may be significant effects on the baby.

Two categories of drugs are currently used today. They are classified as either opioid agonists or opioid agonist-antagonists. These drugs can be ordered by the doctor during labor and administered in intervals to help with the pain of labor and delivery. One new method of administration that may be available in your hospital is called patient-controlled analgesia (PCA). This allows the patient herself to administer medication when she feels discomfort. The patient is hooked up to a machine that she controls and by her pressing a button, pain medicine is released into her system. There is no need to fear overdose; safety mechanisms are in place to prevent an overdose.

Various drugs are commonly used today during labor and delivery. Although these drugs decrease pain, they may also lead to respiratory depression and arrest, plus aspiration in the mother. Since these drugs cross the placenta, they can also depress the breathing of the baby. Therefore, it is helpful to have stopped administration of the drugs well before delivery and to have on hand at delivery a drug that reverses the effects, to administer to the baby. Drugs commonly in use today are

Meperidine (Demerol). This is probably the most commonly used. Once given in the IV, it takes effect within minutes and can last for around one to two hours. This is a relatively safe drug if used correctly, but its main disadvantage is that it can stay in the baby's system for up to twenty-two hours.

Fentanyl (Sublimaze). This is similar to Demerol but much more potent and is given in much smaller doses. It takes effect within a minute and lasts for about an hour. The main advantage over Demerol is that it is cleared from the baby's system much quicker.

Nalbuphine (Nubain). In use today, Nubain takes effect in two to three minutes and clears from the baby's system in a similar manner as Fentanyl.

Butorphanol (Stadol). This is also very quick acting and effective, but not much is known about the length of time in which it clears from the baby's system.

Morphine. Commonly used, morphine has a very quick onset of action and is cleared from the baby's system in about seven hours.

Often a tranquilizer will be added to one of the previously mentioned drugs to reduce nausea and vomiting. Such drugs often have a calming effect and may increase the effectiveness of the opioid without an increase in dosage. They are well tolerated by the mother and have little, if no, effect on the newborn. They may produce a state of relaxation that increases the mother's ability to participate in labor and delivery.

Anesthetics

Besides analgesics, or pain relievers, the obstetrical bag of tricks includes *anesthesia*—drugs that cause a loss of feeling, either all over the body or just in the affected area. This usage can be traced to 1853, when John Snow administered chloroform to Queen Victoria during the delivery of her eighth child, Prince Leopold.

Various inhaled and injected substances are now used as general anesthesia for delivery. General anesthesia had once been very popular but now is used only for cesarean delivery, when an epidural or a spinal cannot be performed. When general anesthesia is used, it is important to deliver the baby quickly, as prolonged exposure to these drugs can cause significant depression in the newborn. One recent study showed a significant increase in neonatal depression in babies exposed to more than eight minutes of general anesthesia. In addition, if vomiting occurs while the mother is under the influence of general anesthesia, she may breathe vomit into her lungs, causing pneumonia. Currently, most of the pain management during labor is through regional anesthesia. Today, this method of anesthesia is the most effective form of pain relief for labor and delivery in the United States.

The most common regional anesthesia techniques today are the epidural, the spinal, and the combined spinal epidural. In addition to the benefits of allowing the mother to see the birth and avoiding the danger from vomiting, regional anesthesia techniques do not pass significant quantities of drugs into the fetus. They can thus be used in labor, as well as in delivery.

There are some disadvantages with these techniques. They require an experienced, skillful doctor, often an anesthesiologist who specializes in obstetrical anesthesia, to be effectively administered. They also require cooperation of the mothers. Occasionally, some mothers have toxic reactions to the regional drugs, which means a mother must be carefully supervised after the drugs are administered.

Epidural anesthesia is extremely common in the United States during labor and delivery. When appropriate, you may decide to have an epidural placed during labor. At that time, your obstetrician will likely consult with an anesthesiologist. If there are no contraindications, the process will begin. This generally involves your getting an intravenous (IV) line inserted and receiving one to two bags of fluid. When appropriately hydrated, you will be placed on your side or will sit on the edge of the bed. Your back will be washed with antiseptic and your skin numbed with a local anesthetic. A small plastic tube called a catheter is placed into the canal surrounding the spinal column. This tube is taped to your back and left in place throughout labor and delivery. Through this tube, the anesthesiologist can administer medication as a bolus (one shot), in a continuous manner, or using a combination of both. The outgoing and incoming spinal nerves pass through this canal and receive the effects of the drugs. When effective, this method of anesthesia can almost completely eliminate pain without affecting consciousness.

The medications that are administered through the epidural catheter have been refined over the years but consist of two categories of drugs: local anesthetics and the opioids. The local anesthetics work by numbing the nerves, in a similar way that novocaine numbs your mouth before the dentist drills a cavity. In the case of the epidural, numbing the nerves that come out of the spinal canal can deaden the sensation of pain throughout the entire uterus and pelvis. The mechanisms of the effects of the opioids are not as clear, but these drugs are extremely effective in eliminating the pain of labor and delivery. The downside to local anesthetics is that they may also affect the patient's ability to move around. With the use of very dilute local anesthetics and opioids, it may be possible to have full motility. These are the so-called walking epidurals, which have become more popular today. Because these medications can have various effects on different women, not everyone is a candidate for a walking epidural.

Some studies have shown that women receiving epidurals may have a higher risk of needing a cesarean section, a forceps delivery, or a vacuum extraction; they may also be prone to prolonged labors, Pitocin use, and fever. A 1995 study looked at over 1,300 women who received either epidural or IV Demerol and found a two- to fourfold increase in cesarean sections. In addition, there was an increase in uterine infections and forceps deliveries. A more recent study, which compared epidurals using dilute local anesthetics plus opioids to those using IV Demerol in labor, found no increase in the cesarean section rate in either group. The implication may be that the older traditional epidurals, which used mostly strong local anesthetics that significantly blocked motor ability, may have given the newer walking epidural a bad rap, in terms of its supposedly increasing the cesarean section rate. Another factor may be the time period when the epidural is placed. Some studies have found that epidural placement before 4 to 5 centimeters of dilatation may also increase the cesarean section rate.

Spinal anesthesia involves injecting medication directly into the spinal canal, eliminating pain in the pelvic area and the legs. Spinal anesthesia is extremely effective and the onset of action is almost immediate, unlike with epidural anesthesia, which needs around twenty minutes to take effect. Because this can only be administered as a single shot, this will be effective for only a limited time, because it will wear off. Therefore, spinal anesthesia is usually done only in the case of a cesarean section or if delivery will occur very soon.

Combined spinal epidural has become extremely popular in modern obstetrical anesthesia. The same type of needle that is used to introduce the epidural catheter is used to locate the epidural space. Before the catheter is placed, a special needle is used to enter the spinal canal. Medication is then placed into the spinal canal, the needle is removed, and a catheter is placed in the epidural space. The big advantage of this method is that the pain relief is immediate because of the spinal, along with the epidural, so when the spinal starts to wear off, the epidural can be activated. This is particularly useful if labor is proceeding very rapidly. With this method, it's almost never too late for an epidural.

Regional anesthesia can have some side effects. It may cause the mother's blood pressure to drop, which in time may slow the baby's heartbeat. However, certain steps may prevent these complications, such as giving the mother lots of IV fluids and using certain IV medications. Also, positioning the mother on her side after the epidural is placed will aid circulation and prevent this temporary problem. Serious complications from regional anesthesia are rare in experienced hands.

Local anesthetics are also available. A drug, usually novocaine, is injected into the area where the episiotomy is to be performed. This drug is very useful for an uncomplicated, simple, spontaneous delivery. The drugs have no effect on the fetus and wear off very soon after delivery. They are used only for delivery and are of no help during labor.

While all of these methods of making labor more comfortable are available to most practicing physicians, each physician has his or her favorite. It would be wise for you to talk with your doctor about labor and delivery, and the use of medication during each, to make certain that your preferences are in sync. If possible, you can map out a primary approach, flexible enough to change during labor if you decide it is necessary.

How to Deliver a Baby in an Emergency

The likelihood that you will not deliver in the hospital is remote. However, virtually every physician has had at least one patient who unexpectedly gave birth outside the hospital, with no doctor present. These patients are usually women who have had many children before and just can't make it to the hospital in time. Taxis, elevators, ambulances, and hospital lobbies are well-known sites for these events.

The best way to avoid an emergency childbirth is to recognize the physical signs that announce the delivery is coming. Often your physician will do weekly pelvic examinations in the last month of pregnancy. If a woman has had previous fast or early labors, the presence of some cervical dilatation will warn you and your physician of the possibility of a quick labor. Certainly heightened awareness of a history of fast, painless, early labors will help prevent this problem from arising. If a mother in labor leaves for the hospital when her contractions are coming every ten minutes or less, under normal circumstances she should have no trouble getting there in time. However, if the occasion should arise when it is not safe to speed the mother to the hospital, and the baby's head can be seen, preparations should be made for an emergency delivery.

The qualifications required to deliver a baby under emergency conditions are common sense, a calm attitude, and patience. Ambulance attendants and police officers are trained to be good emergency midwives. Clean, if not sterile, conditions are desirable. Clean linens or even clean newspapers will do. If possible, sterile scissors and clean or sterile shoelaces, cord, or string should be available. The person who is going to deliver the baby should wash his or her hands and arms thoroughly.

Patience is not just a virtue in delivery, it is a necessity. No attempt should be made to hasten the delivery by pulling the baby or by yanking on the cord. Just let the baby come out naturally. As the head appears in the birth canal, the deliverer should stand to the left of the mother, place his or her left hand just below the infant's head, cradling it as it emerges but not interfering with this motion or attempting to turn it. If, as occasionally happens, the baby's umbilical cord is wrapped around its neck, the cord should be loosened, but it need not be untangled until after delivery. Once the baby's head is delivered, the rest of the body will follow naturally and quickly.

The baby's first breath often requires some assistance. If possible, the most efficient way to clear the infant's air passages is to clean out its nose and mouth with an ear syringe. But the traditional method of holding the baby upside down by the feet and smartly spanking its bottom is still effective. If at all possible, the deliverer should clear the nasal and the throat passages as soon as the baby's head is delivered.

Tying and cutting the umbilical cord take place after the baby has fully emerged. No attempt to cut it should be made until the cord has become limp, pale, and pulseless. One shoelace, a strip of cloth, or a string is tied firmly around the cord, halfway between the mother and the baby, and the other is tied about 4 inches away from the first. The cord is then cut halfway between the ties with sterile scissors.

The mother will usually expel the placenta about fifteen minutes after the birth. To help bring about this natural process, place the baby on the mother's breast with its face to the nipple. The baby's sucking triggers a reflex reaction that causes the uterus to contract and push out the placenta. The delivery of the placenta is usually followed by some vaginal bleeding. However, this will slow down sooner if the mother lowers her legs and places them together and the uterus of the mother is massaged through the abdominal wall. The uterus can be felt just above the pubic bone as a large firm mass. Massaging will quickly produce a tightening of this mass and a decrease in the amount of vaginal bleeding.

The mother may be taken to the hospital—in an ambulance, if possible—as soon as the placenta has been expelled. Remember to take the placenta along so that the doctor can examine it to make sure it is complete. The vaginal area should be carefully cleaned with water and covered with a sanitary napkin.

We hope this information is not necessary, but if it is, remember, don't panic. Healthy babies were born thousands of years prior to the invention of midwives and obstetricians.

OTHER TYPES OF DELIVERY

Thus far, when we have referred to birth, we have meant vaginal birth. As mentioned, most babies are born through the vagina, head first. Not all babies come into the world this way, however, and not all vaginal births are the same.

Some vaginal births need to be aided by the obstetrician. Currently, the doctor may use two types of instruments to help deliver your baby. The first is called forceps. This is a metal instrument that resembles salad tongs. It can be used to remove the baby's head from the mother's pelvis without injury to either baby or mother. It can also be used to help rotate the fetal head to put the baby in a better position for birth. The second type of instrument is called a vacuum extractor. Traditionally, the vacuum extractor was popular only in Europe. It consisted of a metal cup connected to a suction device. The cup was placed on the fetal head, suction was applied, and, with traction, the baby was removed from the birth canal. The fear in the United States was that this device would lead to trauma in the newborn. Eventually, the metal cup was replaced with a softer synthetic cup. Currently, vacuum extraction is a common form of operative vaginal delivery.

The incidence of operative vaginal delivery in the United States is estimated to be approximately 10 to 15 percent. Don't let the idea of a forceps delivery or a vacuum extraction frighten you; it should not. The use of these instruments in obstetrics got a very bad reputation because doctors in the past used them to reach high into the birth canal, which required a good deal of force to extract the baby. Today, however, neither forceps nor vacuums are used unless the cervix is completely dilated and the head is within 2 inches of the mouth of the vagina.

Operative deliveries are done in the following instances:

- Prolonged second stage—if a patient having her first baby has been in the second stage for more than three hours and has had regional anesthesia, or more than two hours if she has had no anesthesia, or, if a patient is having her second, or later, baby and she has been in the second stage for more than two hours with regional anesthesia or more than one hour without. A prolonged second stage may be due to poor contractions, a large fetus, a small pelvis, or any combination of these.
- Maternal emergency—such as shock or exhaustion.
- Fetal emergency—slowing of the fetal heart rate, indicating potential fetal distress.

Operative delivery, as practiced today, is very safe. A large study of more than 83,000 births between 1992 and 1994 looked at the use of forceps delivery, vacuum extraction, cesarean section, and spontaneous vaginal delivery. When compared to a cesarean section performed during labor, an operative vaginal delivery (either forceps or vacuum) showed no increased incidence of birth injuries. Another study looking at the long-term follow-up of babies delivered by either forceps or vacuum found no difference in cognitive development after ten years. Therefore, when appropriate, an operative vaginal delivery can be a safe alternative to a cesarean section.

Cesarean Section

Cesarean section is the delivery of the baby through an incision made in the mother's abdominal wall and then in the uterus. The term comes from the *lex caesarea*, which required an abdominal postmortem delivery of any woman who died in childbirth. It has come to mean delivery of any child by abdominal operation.

Back in the 1960s, obstetricians accepted a cesarean section rate of 3 to 5 percent as normal. Over the last three decades, certain factors have led to an increased cesarean birthrate. The rate peaked at around 23 percent in 1987. Recognizing this alarmingly high number, physicians exerted much effort to reduce the rate. Despite the attempts, we saw only a modest reduction, to around 21 percent in 1997. One reason for this change may be an increase in operative vaginal deliveries, from 9 percent in 1987 to 9.4 percent in 1997. The medical-legal climate may also have something to do with this. Physicians' fear of lawsuits due to adverse outcomes has certainly contributed to the continued high C-section rates.

Cesarean deliveries were once feared. But the improvement in surgical techniques and in preoperative and postoperative care, along with reduced infection, has made the cesarean section a safe procedure.

We have become increasingly aware that a cesarean birth results in a healthier infant than does a prolonged labor and a difficult vaginal delivery. Advances in monitoring the baby during labor have permitted earlier detection of infants who will not tolerate a vaginal delivery.

A C-section is a major surgical procedure, which may have to be performed unexpectedly. It should not be viewed as a failure on the part of either the mother or the obstetrician. The ultimate goal is having a healthy mother and child.

The most common reasons for cesarean delivery are the following:

1. The mother's pelvis is too small to allow the passage of the baby.
2. The baby is positioned abnormally, such as breech or across the abdominal cavity, rather than vertical to it.
3. The uterus is not contracting with enough force to push the baby down.
4. A previous cesarean has increased the chance of uterine rupture.
5. Pelvic tumors interfere with normal delivery.
6. Fetal distress makes vaginal delivery dangerous for the fetus.
7. An abnormality of the placenta, such as placenta previa or placenta abruption, causes an acute emergency.
8. Maternal diabetes and preeclampsia complicate pregnancy.
9. Rh disease endangers the fetus.

These subjects are discussed in detail in chapter 12.

As mentioned previously, attempts have been made to lower the cesarean section rate. One of the main efforts to accomplish this task has been through vaginal delivery after cesarean (VDAC). The first edition of this book spoke of the dangers of vaginal birth after cesarean delivery and suggested the phrase, "Once a cesarean, always a cesarean." The fear was that during labor the uterus would be more likely to burst open (rupture), putting the mother and the baby in grave danger. The mother could suffer large quantities of blood loss, making an emergency transfusion necessary and possibly a hysterectomy as well. The baby would immediately lose contact with the mother's supply of oxygen and could suffer brain damage and possible death.

The second edition mentioned the overwhelming evidence supporting the safety of vaginal birth after cesarean, provided the right circumstances existed. The evidence suggested that the risk of uterine rupture was no greater than if there had been no cesarean. At the time of the release of this book's second edition, the number of VDACs dramatically increased. Subsequently, there have been studies reevaluating the safety of the VDAC. The most influential study appeared in the *New England Journal of Medicine* in 2001, which looked at over 20,000 pregnant women with a history of one prior cesarean section and followed their delivery outcomes. Although the risk of rupture was very low in patients who electively had repeat cesarean sections (1.6 per 1,000 births), the risk tripled when the patients were allowed to labor, and was five to fifteen times higher when the patients' labor was induced. The study also found that the risk of fetal death was ten times higher if the uterus ruptured. Although the study has been met with some criticism, the criteria for offering a vaginal trial after cesarean section have been affected; they can be briefly summarized as follows:

1. The previous cesarean section was a so-called low-segment type of operation, that is, the incision was in the lower part of the uterus. If a classic cesarean section has been performed—that is, if the incision was made in the top of the uterus—it is absolutely necessary to deliver all subsequent babies by cesarean prior to labor to prevent the uterus from rupturing.
2. The medical indication for the first cesarean section is no longer present, and, of course, no new reason is present.
3. The trial of labor for vaginal delivery is closely monitored, and facilities are available for emergency care, such as blood transfusions and surgery.
4. Labor should not be induced, as there is a much greater risk of uterine rupture. In special circumstances, it may be possible for your doctor to perform induction of labor after you both carefully discuss the risks and benefits.

With these criteria, it may be possible to safely deliver vaginally after a prior delivery by cesarean section. The risk of uterine rupture should be extremely low, and even if there is a rupture, it is usually not catastrophic for the mother or the baby. Discuss this with your physician.

Preparation for Cesarean Delivery

Before the operation is performed, a nurse will prepare you. Certain medications may be given to help dry the secretions in your mouth and upper airway, and the lower part of your abdomen will be washed and may be shaved. A catheter is placed in the urinary bladder before surgery to keep it empty. This decreases the risk of injury to the bladder during the operation and aids delivery of the infant. An intravenous will be started, permitting fluids to be given during the operation. Certain medications that might be required are also given through the IV.

If there is time and no emergency is present, the anesthesiologist will discuss the various types of anesthesia available and may allow you to indicate your preference. Most anesthesia for cesarean section is either epidural or spinal anesthesia. Rarely is general anesthesia used today. It is normally used only if there is a contraindication for a regional block, such as a problem with your spine. The epidural or the spinal allows you to be awake but numb from just above the waist to your toes. If you are having an epidural or a spinal, ask your doctor about a relatively new method to control postoperative pain, called Duramorph. Recent studies show that the use of a small amount of preservative-free morphine placed into the spinal or the epidural before the cesarean can control pain for up to twelve to twenty-four hours after delivery. Side effects include itchiness for up to twenty-four hours, which may require treatment 35 to 56 percent of the time. If general anesthesia is used, you will be asleep throughout the operation. Either method is safe in the hands of a competent anesthesiologist.

In many hospitals, the patient's partner may accompany her to the operating room and may be present during the cesarean birth. If the father is to be present at a cesarean birth, he will be expected to change into appropriate clothing provided by the hospital before he enters the operating room.

The Operation Itself

The surgeon makes an incision through the wall of the abdomen. It may be a vertical, or midline, incision from the navel to the pubic bone, or it may be transverse, extending from side to side just above the pubic hairline, a so-called bikini incision. The choice of incision is the surgeon's. After the abdomen has been opened, an incision is made in the wall of the uterus in order to deliver the baby. This incision, too, may be either vertical or transverse. The transverse incision is used more frequently since it is made in the lower part of the uterus. The vertical incision, however, is sometimes needed for certain positions of the baby and certain other medical emergency situations. After the baby is delivered through these incisions, the placenta immediately follows. After the baby and the placenta are removed, the incisions in the uterus and the abdomen are closed with sutures.

Following surgery, you will usually be taken to the recovery room. During this time, your blood pressure, pulse rate, and respiration rate will be checked regularly, and you will be observed for excessive vaginal bleeding. If regional anesthesia was given, you will see your baby at delivery and will probably be allowed to hold him or her for a while before the infant is taken to the nursery for observation. Early contact between the parents and the baby following a cesarean birth is beneficial to everyone and allows early bonding. That is one reason why we prefer regional anesthesia for cesarean deliveries.

Postoperative Care

You will usually be kept in bed for the first day after delivery. During this time, you will be encouraged to move about. After the first day, you will be advised to get out of bed with the help of a nurse or other responsible people. The bladder catheter is removed soon after surgery, and you should be able to resume urinating without difficulty. IV fluids are continued until you are able to take fluids and nourishment orally. IV fluids are usually required only for the first twenty-four to forty-eight hours.

For several days after the operation, the abdominal incision will be uncomfortable. You may ask your physician to prescribe medication for relief of pain. How long you stay in the hospital following a cesarean birth depends on how soon you are able to resume your normal functions. In most instances, you can expect to be discharged within four to five days. The stitches or clips on the abdominal incision will usually be removed between the fourth and fifth day after surgery.

Complications and Risks

Cesarean section in the last thirty years has become an increasingly safe operation to perform. The advances in anesthesia techniques, blood banks, surgical care, and antibiotics have reduced the risks to the mother. Care of the newborn infant has also improved, making this method safer and more suitable for the baby. But there are risks involved that any mother should be aware of. Infection, blood clots, excessive blood loss, and occasional complications from anesthesia can occur. However, treatment is available, and these complications are usually temporary.

Following a cesarean delivery, you will rapidly regain normal body function and after four to six weeks should be able to resume full activity without real limitations. Breast-feeding should not be limited by cesarean delivery. Because of the increasing percentage of cesarean births, many centers have set up special antepartum classes, programs, and support groups for couples anticipating a cesarean delivery. A cesarean birth costs more than a vaginal delivery because of the longer hospital stay, the necessity for anesthesia, and the cost of using an operating room and its personnel and equipment. In the last analysis, your physician can best answer your questions and concerns regarding a cesarean section.

Induction of Labor

Sometimes, doctors have to induce labor artificially. Often, it is done for certain medical reasons, which include toxemia (preeclampsia), diabetes, postmaturity, and high blood pressure. Frequently, inductions are done for purely elective reasons. Labor induction is very common today. It occurs in approximately 15 percent of all deliveries.

The decision as to why, when, and how must be carefully evaluated by you and your doctor. A 2000 study confirmed the belief that compared to natural labor, induced labor has twice the risk of cesarean section being needed in first-time mothers. It is therefore important to have a clear understanding of why induction is done before the decision is made. Once the decision is made to induce, the second decision is when this should be done. As mentioned earlier in this chapter, the cervix undergoes changes during labor. Often the cervix will undergo changes before labor. If this happens, the cervix may be more "favorable" for induction. Sometimes, when the decision to induce is made, it is not an emergency, and you can wait for the cervix to be more favorable. One way that your doctor will decide how ready you are is by determining your "Bishop score." With this method of scoring, your doctor will use a point system, in which your cervical exam receives points for various factors, such as how open it is, how effaced it is, how many babies you have had before, and other determinants. If your exam total is more than 8 points, the chance of induction working to allow a vaginal birth is about the same as with natural labor.

Because induction of labor is so common and the cervix is not always favorable, many methods of inducing have been introduced. These include mechanical methods, various drugs, and nonmedical methods, all of which have various degrees of success. Most commonly, drugs are used. If the cervix is not so favorable, a synthetic prostaglandin can be used; the most commonly used today is called misoprostol. It was used in 90 per 1,000 live births in 1989 and in 184 per 1,000 live births in 1997. It comes in a tablet form that is placed deep in the vagina behind the cervix. This medicine helps the cervix become softer, thinner, and more favorable. Often a patient will go into labor from this medicine. The patient must stay in the hospital and be monitored because of the potential risk of fetal distress when she receives this medication. If the cervix is more favorable, labor is generally induced by injecting a synthetic hormone called Pitocin into the mother, which brings on uterine contractions and labor. Pitocin is one of the most commonly used drugs in the United States. The same hormone is used for women who are in labor but whose contractions are not strong enough to dilate the cervix or push the baby down. Pitocin increases the intensity and the frequency of contractions. It is quite powerful and must be supervised at all times. Pitocin is very valuable in the management of labor, when used correctly.

Some nonmedical ways of induction have fallen out of favor. The old fashioned use of castor oil usually just gives a woman diarrhea and abdominal cramps but doesn't put her into labor. Nipple stimulation will lead to uterine contractions, but it is unreliable and variable and is rarely successful in inducing labor. Finally, your doctor may want to "strip your membranes." Here the examiner places a finger inside the cervix and rotates it around. This is often uncomfortable and is also unreliable. A recent study looked at 195 normal pregnant women past their due date. In one group the membranes were stripped, and in the other they just had an exam. In the group that was stripped, 75 percent went into labor within seventy-two hours. In the other group, 33 percent went into labor within seventy-two hours.

ALTERNATIVE BIRTHING PROCEDURES

Traditionally, women in labor were isolated from their partner, heavily sedated, and delivered their baby in a delivery room in the hospital. Today there are a variety of birthing options for the pregnant woman.

Birthing Room

Many hospitals in the United States offer the option of having your baby in a birthing room. In it, a woman can go through labor, delivery, and recovery without the physical strain of changing rooms. Birthing rooms are sometimes decorated with all the comforts of home—paintings on the walls, curtains, comfortable chairs, a TV, phones—and your partner and maybe even your children will be allowed to be there for support.

The advantage is that the birthing room eliminates some of the psychological stress of a hospital environment and seems more like having a baby in your own home. The room is still in a hospital, with all the proper backup medical equipment and talent nearby in case of emergency.

Childbearing Maternity Centers

An alternative to the traditional hospital maternity section is the childbearing maternity center. These facilities are run by trained nurse-midwives and are usually located close to a maternity hospital. To cut the risks of childbirth, such centers carefully screen and monitor patients to ensure that no high-risk pregnancies or difficult deliveries will be encountered. Adequate screening and good transport facilities are basic to these programs.

One of the main attractions of these centers is that costs are generally lower than in a hospital.

Their use and safety are still being evaluated by the medical community. Some physicians worry that complications to mother and child may be higher at these centers. However, the best centers have to be evaluated in the context of their location, the service they give to the community, and the alternatives in their area.

Chapter 9

Psychoprophylaxis—
the Lamaze Method

⊶⊷

"I'VE ALWAYS BEEN prepared for big events in my life," said Elizabeth with some hestitation. "But I'm about to go through the most important event, and I'm completely unprepared."

Many of our patients express anxiety while anticipating labor and delivery. Often their anxiety stems from fear of the unknown. While it is true that all birthing experiences are unique, preparation, to some extent, is possible. Once you are prepared, labor and delivery can be a wonderful experience.

This chapter describes in detail various exercises, both physical and mental, that can be practiced. We have found these techniques quite helpful for the laboring couple.

THE DEVELOPMENT OF THE
LAMAZE METHOD

The psychoprophylactic method of prepared childbirth (PPM) originated in the Soviet Union and was based largely on the work of J. P. Pavlov and his theories of the conditioned response. In 1950, the method, which was already being used extensively in Russia, was presented by Dr. A. P. Nicolaiev of Leningrad to the World Congress of Gynecologists held in Paris. That presentation greatly interested a French physician, Dr. Fernand Lamaze, who visited Russia the following year to study the method and witness its successful use by Russian women in labor. He was so impressed with what he saw and heard that on his return to France he began dedicated efforts to introduce the method there, making only slight modifications that he felt were suitable for Western European culture.

The popularity of the method spread rapidly in France; it was well established in China and the communist countries, and, following sanction by Pope Pius XII in 1956, began to be used in the Catholic countries of southern Europe and South America.

Thus, in less than a decade, PPM was common in many countries around the globe, with the remarkable exception of the United States. A Swiss physician, Dr. Isador Bornstein, made a brief attempt to introduce PPM in Cleveland, Ohio, but because of illness, he had to abandon his work prematurely. In 1958, Dr. Bornstein's book, *Psychoprophylactic Preparation for Painless Childbirth*, was published in the United States.

Shortly after this came the first real introduction of the method in the United States, in New York. Marjorie Karmel, an American mother and a writer, had used the method with the birth of her first baby while living in Paris. The first experience had been so satisfying to Mrs. Karmel that when she became pregnant the second time, while living in New York City, she could not understand why the method was not familiar to anyone she sought out. After training herself and delivering her second child through Lamaze, Mrs. Karmel wrote *Thank You, Dr. Lamaze*, published in 1959, recounting her experiences with her two Lamaze deliveries. Although the situation is quite different now, this book remains one of the most widely used today by expectant mothers and teachers of the Lamaze method.

Marjorie Karmel was also instrumental in organizing a group of interested obstetricians and other professionals into what was to become incorporated, in 1960, as the American Society for Psychoprophylaxis in Obstetrics, usually referred to as ASPO. With the increasing popularity of the method, various chapters of ASPO were created throughout the United States, until today when ASPO chapters and affiliates can be found in virtually every major city in the country.

Functioning as a nonprofit organization, the society actively continues to encourage and support the use of the method by supplying information to interested parents, hospitals, and professional groups; by sponsoring teacher-training courses for interested professionals; and by making literature, film rentals, teaching aids, and so forth available for use by instructors throughout the country.

Even though the United States was relatively late in adopting the use of the Lamaze method, it has become amazingly popular, with many institutions sponsoring courses of instruction for couples, and every year more and more hospitals allowing fathers and mothers to participate together in the labor and the delivery rooms.

While much of this advance has been due to doctors and nurses becoming aware of the advantages of the method, a great deal of the increase in popularity of the Lamaze method has come about because of word-of-mouth influence from one couple to another—in other words, "satisfied customers" telling their friends.

Lamaze training falls into two major categories: (1) deconditioning, that is, learning correct information about what labor is really like, so that you can rid yourself of an accumulation of misinformation you have stored up for years; (2) conditioning, that is, learning a set pattern of breathing and relaxation techniques that are reinforced with daily practice so that they become conditioned responses, allowing you to control your labor, rather than having it control you. When your uterus starts to contract, it will signal your conditioned responses of breathing and relaxing, which will have become strong enough to minimize the perception of the contraction as painful. In addition, you will have gotten your body in shape for labor by specific, daily body-building exercises.

If at all possible, starting about eight weeks prior to your due date you should receive a course of instruction given by a responsible professional instructor with an organized group. Taking a course has several advantages: The exercises and breathing techniques are demonstrated and explained; the spontaneous exchange of questions and answers is informative; and it can be very helpful and encouraging to share your hopes and sometimes your fears and anxieties with people who are all in the same boat.

It is possible, however, for you and your partner to train yourselves, if no classroom instruction is available. If you elect to do this, you should first do sufficient reading to become thoroughly familiar with the Lamaze method. Then make out a schedule for yourself, listing the dates during that eight-week period when you will begin each individual exercise. Finally, practice each session every day until your labor begins.

Ask whether it's possible for you to have a tour of the hospital where you are to deliver, so that you know beforehand where you should go and what you should do when labor begins. Do not hesitate to ask questions about policies, procedures, and anything else about the hospital's routines that is not clear in your mind.

The rest of this chapter will outline specific exercises for women interested in using the Lamaze method and will discuss their biological or psychological benefit. There are seven categories of exercises, each designed for a different purpose.

Body-building exercises
Neuromuscular control (concentration-relaxation) exercises
General breathing techniques
Breathing for early labor
Breathing as labor progresses
Breathing for transition
Breathing for the second stage—expulsion

BODY-BUILDING EXERCISES

While these exercises are not something you will actually do in labor, they are designed specifically to prepare the parts of your body that will be involved. They are simple, few in number, and in no way harmful for the normal, healthy pregnant female. They also help to prevent or alleviate some of the annoyances and discomforts frequently associated with the last month or two of pregnancy, such as low backaches, leg cramps, and the feeling of heaviness of the abdomen. These exercises provide a purposeful form of routine daily physical activity, improve your circulation, and help to create a sense of well-being.

Daily Exercises

The body-building exercises should be practiced every day, as many times as your schedule will permit, but no less than five times a day for each exercise. They should be done on the floor, cushioned only by the softness of a bathmat or a scatter rug. For the exercises done in a supine position, a pillow may be placed under the head, with a smaller pillow under each knee.

Tailor Sitting

Sit on the floor cross-legged with your back slightly rounded and relaxed. Sit in this position not only when exercising but also as often as possible during the routine daily activities that you usually perform sitting in a chair. You will find it quite a comfortable position for such things as reading, watching TV, and sewing or knitting.

If you begin to experience the discomfort of low back strain, sit on the floor in the tailor position. Let your head hang loosely forward and gently rock back and forth until your back is a rounded arch (like a Halloween cat's) to straighten out the hyperaccentuated lordotic curve in your back.

Tailor Stretch

Sitting on the floor, place the soles of your feet together in front of you and then pull your feet toward the groin, as close to your body as possible. Now take your hands and push your knees down toward the floor. If your feet start to slide away from your body, put your hands on your ankles to hold them in place, and use your elbows to push your knees down toward the floor. At first, the muscles in your thighs may feel uncomfortably tight doing this exercise, but in a few weeks, you should easily be able to pull your feet all the way back to your groin and have your knees loosely go all the way to the floor. The Lamaze-trained woman who has been doing this exercise for six to eight weeks feels no uncomfortable strain when her legs are placed in the stirrups during delivery, or when her obstetrician asks her to separate her legs for examinations.

The Pelvic Rock

This exercise benefits two areas: the abdomen and the back. When you have progressed to the second, or expulsive, stage of labor, one of the forces you will use to help the uterine contraction in pushing your baby out of the birth canal is the tightening of the abdominal muscles. These muscles often become lax and lose tone during pregnancy. This exercise will help to improve that muscle tone and allow you to work more effectively during the "pushing" stage of labor. Since it straightens the curve in your back, it will also prevent low back pain.

Lying down—Lie on your back on the floor with your hands at your sides and your knees bent. Slowly flatten the curve in your back, pushing your spine down hard against the floor, all the way from your shoulders to your coccyx (tail bone). As you tilt the bones of your pelvic girdle down against the floor, tighten your abdominal muscles inward and upward, so that they become firm to the touch. Then relax your abdominal muscles and pelvis, letting your back return to its natural curve. Remember, the tilting of the pelvis means the bony pelvis; the fatty part of the buttocks must not be raised up but must remain on the floor.

Leg Exercises

Another of the discomforts of the latter months of pregnancy is leg cramps. Maybe you have already had the unpleasant experience of a painful charley horse in your calf. Unfortunately, these often increase, rather than decrease, as the pregnancy progresses.

Leg exercise 1—Do this exercise lying on the floor with your hands at your sides. With legs straight and toes pointed, raise your right leg to as high a vertical position as is possible. Then, with your foot high in the air, tightly flex the ankle so that it is at a 45-degree angle with the leg and slowly lower the leg to the floor. Inhale while raising the leg to the vertical position and exhale as the leg is slowly lowered to the floor. Repeat the exercise with the left leg.

Leg exercise 2—Lie on the floor as before, but this time spread your arms out at right angles to your body. As you inhale, again with the toes pointed, raise the straight right leg to the vertical position as before; flex the ankle as before. But this time, instead of lowering it to the floor as you exhale, let your leg go out to the right side as far as it will go toward your outstretched right hand without raising your left buttock and hip off the floor. When your right foot is out toward your hand as far as possible, you should feel a stretch of the muscles of the inside of the thigh and the right lower quadrant of the abdominal wall. Now point the right toes again, inhaling as you raise the straight right leg back to the vertical position; flex the ankle and exhale as you slowly let your heel go back to the floor. Repeat with the left leg.

Getting Up

As your pregnancy progresses and the size of your abdomen increases, you may feel more and more clumsy when arising from an awkward position. In such instances, you will find it helpful to use your hands and feet as levers.

For example, when lying flat on the floor, turn onto your right side; place your left palm down on the floor in front of your face and push up with it, using it as a lever to raise the top half of your body to a sitting position. Then push with your left hand, with your knees bent, to raise the rest of your body from the floor.

General Movement

In addition to the routine daily practice of the previous exercises, you should now also pay more attention to the way you sit and move.

Posture

As your pregnancy progresses and the uterus enlarges, the weight tends to pull the abdomen forward and the curve in the lower back is sometimes greatly accentuated into a swayback. This is largely responsible for low backaches late in pregnancy, and you should make a conscious effort to "think tall" as you walk or stand, so as to straighten out that hyperaccentuated curve in your back.

Resting

The best rest is achieved by lying down, not by sitting. Never sit when you can lie down. Put a piece of plywood under your mattress. Lie on your back with one pillow under your head and another under your knees. When you wish to get up out of bed, gently roll over on your abdomen and slide out of bed onto your knees. Never jerk or force your back to rotate rapidly or forcibly. When sleeping, do not lie on your stomach. When you lie on your side, draw up both knees. Keep your arms below your shoulders during the night, preferably in a relaxed position along the sides of the body.

Lifting Things

Squat down directly in front of any object you plan to lift, including a baby. Get as close as possible, then stand up slowly while firmly holding the object tightly to your body and letting your legs—not your back—do the work. Never lift while bending forward, as in taking something out of the trunk of a car. Do not lean over furniture to open or close windows. The main point is that you should never lift with your legs straight. In addition, never work or lift with your arms higher than your shoulders or lower than your waist. Do not jerk or force open a drawer.

Sitting

Sit in a straight chair with a firm back. Avoid low, soft chairs or lounges that allow you to sink deep down into the upholstery. You can hurt your back when getting up on your feet. Never sit more than fifteen minutes at a time; get up and move about frequently. Let your feet rest on a low stool so that your knees are higher than your hips. This position relaxes your back.

Standing and Walking

Watch your feet when climbing up and down stairs, stepping over curbs, and walking on rocky or rough ground. You must take care to avoid stumbles and sudden jerks to your back. Open doors wide enough to walk through comfortably. Never stand in the same position for more than a minute. Shift from one foot to the other so that your weight is not on the same leg and foot for longer than a minute. A little footstool or a box that supports one foot or the other, in turn, is comforting to the back.

Driving

Push the car seat forward so that your knees are higher than your hips. Snugly fasten the safety belt and the shoulder harness; they support your body and your back and prevent a sudden twist if there is an emergency stop, turn, or bump.

Doing Household Chores

Get down on your knees to do jobs that otherwise would strain your back to reach. If your back is really hurting, do not vacuum or make beds.

Relaxing Your Back

The simplest and safest way to relax your back is to stand in a hot shower directed against your back, or to soak in a warm tub two or three times every day. Gentle but thorough exercises relax and strengthen back muscles.

NEUROMUSCULAR CONTROL (CONTRACTION-RELAXATION) EXERCISES

This is the most important aspect of the teamwork training of the members of the couple who will be working together in labor. In fact, this entire portion of your training might well be primarily directed toward your partner, since he is the one who will be responsible for your state of relaxation during labor.

The Coach's Role

The coach shares the experience and guides the laboring woman. Giving support in labor requires compassion, skill, patience, and understanding. An awareness of what the laboring woman is thinking and feeling at each moment and complete commitment to the task are essential. It can be hard, exhausting work. But it pays off in the excitement, the deep satisfaction, and the shared joy when a child is born. Your coach can be anyone from a husband or a partner to a friend or a hired nurse.

The Importance of Relaxation

Anyone would probably agree on the importance of being able to relax during labor. Even if you have never had any firsthand contact with someone having a baby, you can imagine how much easier labor can be if you remain completely relaxed.

Research shows that relaxed mothers, who are less anxious during labor and delivery, have shorter labors and deliver babies with high Apgar scores (measures of an infant's respiration, color, heartbeat, and reflexes). Relaxation not only shortens your labor but helps you conserve your energy by preventing the fear-tension-pain cycle, ensures oxygen supply to you and the fetus, decreases your pain, and, above all else, allows your contractions to be effective.

Tensing during childbirth is a natural response to the contractions of the uterus. However, tension not only causes exhaustion, oxygen depletion, and a lower pain threshold, but actually prolongs labor physiologically. The hormone that causes your uterus to contract is oxytocin. Adrenaline, the hormone that accompanies the fear-tension-pain syndrome, actually inhibits the effects of oxytocin and makes your contractions less effective.

Relaxing for labor, however, is different from ordinary relaxation. For example, while working in the office or at home, you may decide to "take ten," sit down, have a cup of coffee, and relax. This is a passive, let-it-happen type of relaxation, which is generally adequate for refreshing you. It is fine—as far as it goes.

During labor, however, one needs more. The laboring woman should be able to employ a controlled type of relaxation. And you can learn to control it by concentrating on the body parts you want to relax, even while other body parts are tight. With daily practice, you can condition yourself to relax this way.

Even the totally untrained woman in labor is admonished by the doctors and nurses in attendance to "just relax," and at the end of each contraction, she may try, but before this let-it-happen type of relaxation can be effective, another contraction begins, and she lets the tightening uterine muscles cause her entire body to become tense.

Anyone who has worked in a labor room can describe some of the mother's reactions to the onset of a uterine contraction. With the beginning tightening of the uterine muscles, she thinks, "Here it comes," and she may clench her fists or squeeze the side rails of the bed, so that her fingernails are digging into the palms of her hands, and her arms become completely rigid. Sometimes her toes will curl tightly downward, as she tightens her ankles and knees until her legs become rigid. Sometimes she will clench her teeth so that her jaws and neck muscles are rigid. She seems to be bracing herself for combat with the uterine contraction, as if to prevent the contraction.

Of course, the uterus must forcibly contract in labor. If it doesn't, something is wrong. This contracting force pushes the baby downward and retracts the cervix from the baby's head. But if other muscle groups and body parts also tighten up when the uterus starts to contract, energy that is needed later on for pushing in the second stage of labor is wasted; oxygen that should be going to oxygenate the baby is wasted; and the end result is nonproductive fatigue.

In contrast, the Lamaze-trained mother who has learned to control relaxation by practicing daily the strengthening of her conditioned response can be relaxed throughout labor—not only between contractions, but during them.

In order for you to realize maximum benefit from your relaxation efforts, you must practice this group of exercises every day (for, as subtle as it is, the process of conditioning does take place daily) and while your husband or other coach is at home to direct you and to check on your progress. Of course, during the day, you may want to do some extra practice to speed up the conditioning. At least once a day, though, be sure to go through all of the steps of relaxing with your coach directing the practice (because without your coach, you can't accurately appraise your own state of relaxation). And during, active labor, your coach will probably first notice any signs of tension before you are aware of them yourself.

At first, the relaxation exercises may seem very time-consuming and difficult as you try to get a feel for the right sensation. Keep in mind that your body is gradually learning to respond to the command to relax, and that the response will continue to increase over time with daily practice, so that when labor begins, you will be able to let your entire body go completely limp on command. This ability will be invaluable.

Practice Exercises for Relaxation

1. Sit, supported by lots of pillows behind the head and the shoulders and under the arms and the knees, or lie on your side supported by pillows. Before your coach begins testing your extremities, make a conscious effort to let your body "go loose." You may have heard of the recommendation given to insomniacs to help them fall asleep: It is said that if you start at the top of the head and, step by step, consciously think of relaxing every part

of your body, you will be asleep by the time you get to your toes.

2. At your coach's command, "Contract your right arm," make a fist, raise the tightened, outstretched arm a few inches off the floor, and keep it up until your coach has time to check successively the relaxation of the joints and the muscles of your left arm and your right and left legs to see that they are perfectly limp before giving the command to release the right arm.

3. Continue this way until you have done all the following exercises, with your coach giving the commands to contract each specific area and then checking the state of relaxation of all other areas before saying, "Release."

Contract left arm; check relaxation. Release.
Contract right leg; check relaxation. Release.
Contract left leg; check relaxation. Release.
Contract right arm and right leg; check relaxation. Release.
Contract both arms; check relaxation. Release.
Contract both legs; check relaxation. Release.
Contract right arm and left leg; check relaxation. Release.
Contract left arm and right leg; check relaxation. Release.

To the coaches: You can help the learning process by your verbal directions "Relax," "Let go," "Let your arm and leg slowly sink downward," "Let me have the weight of the extremity in my hand," and so on. Vocally, you are helping to sharpen your partner's concentration. Begin these verbal directions with the joints — that is, "Relax your shoulder (elbow, knee)" — because they are the easiest for her to relax. She already has voluntary control of joints, which she uses unconsciously when, for example, she bends her knees to walk up steps or bends her elbow to take a bite of food. When you see that the joints are relaxed, then proceed to give her the verbal directions "Let all the muscles in your arm (or leg) go limp in my hand." As she gradually learns to let go, you will feel the weight of the extremity in your hand slowly and gradually increasing, and when you let go of it, the arm or the leg should plop, falling to the floor as a dead weight. When you first start to practice, it may take several minutes to go through the entire process of relaxing all extremities. But as her learning (conditioning) increases, the time spent will grow less and less each day, and by the time labor begins, it will take just one command (without the extra verbal instructions) to have her relax her entire body, even though at the same time the uterine muscles may be tightly contracting.

Again, let us stress how important this ability is in labor, especially when the transition phase arrives, with its strong challenge to the mother's ability to relax.

GENERAL BREATHING TECHNIQUES

One of the most important parts of your Lamaze training is instruction in the method of breathing you use in labor to stay in control of your uterine contractions. Before you start to learn any of the Lamaze breathing techniques, read again the parts of this book that deal with the anatomy and the physiology of labor (chapter 8). Know the signs of the onset of labor and study the course of labor to get a clearer picture of how (and when) your Lamaze techniques are to be employed.

For the sake of brevity here, we'll refer to the longest part of labor, Stage 1, as the "cervical dilatation stage" and the shorter Stage 2 as the "expulsion stage." It is throughout Stage 1 that you will be using your Lamaze breathing methods to control discomfort, changing from one technique to another as your contractions increase in intensity.

At the very onset of labor, contractions are almost always mild, usually occurring at irregular intervals spaced wide apart. Many women describe them as "crampy" in nature, and they probably will not require you to begin any of your special breathing techniques. When asked, "When should I start to use my Lamaze breathing?" most ASPO teachers use the rule of thumb that no Lamaze breathing will be necessary as long as you can comfortably walk and talk throughout a contraction. To start the regime before it's really necessary would only make the period when it *is* necessary seem longer.

When Lamaze breathing becomes necessary, you will first use a slow, rhythmic breathing at a relaxed and quiet pace of approximately six to nine breaths per minute.

When this first technique is no longer effective in controlling your discomfort, you will switch to the second type of paced breathing, which should start slowly but should accelerate as your contraction increases to a peak, then decelerate as the contraction fades away.

You will continue to use this modified paced breathing throughout the cervical dilatation stage of labor, but as the expulsive stage approaches, when the baby's head is lower in the pelvis, most women will feel a sensation of pressure in the rectal area and have an urge to bear down. Then you will need a new type of "transition" breathing — patterned, paced breathing with blowing out — in order to control this urge until the cervix is fully dilated and your doctor has instructed you to start pushing.

When the cervix is fully dilated, the expulsive stage of your labor will begin. Later on in this chapter we will discuss the proper method to use in helping to push your baby through the birth canal.

When you are ready to start your daily practice breathing (approximately eight weeks before your due date), you should incorporate some additional activities into your practice.

1. *Take a deep, cleansing breath,* before and after each minute of practicing each type of breathing. Even though these cleansing breaths may seem the same as the deep-chest breathing you will be doing in the early part of labor, start right at the beginning to establish the habit of taking an extra cleansing breath before and after each minute of practice. These extra "deep, cleansing breaths" will also serve you well when you are further along in labor, using the panting breathing, and during the pushing stage.

2. *Practice effleurage*—gentle abdominal massage—during breathing practice. When the uterine muscles inside your body contract, the muscles and the ligaments that surround and are attached to the uterus also tighten. At the height of a contraction, even the skin over the abdomen is taut. Effleurage, a slow, gentle, light hand massage of the abdomen, feels good when all of these tissues are tightly contracted. Start doing this massage with your first slow breathing, which is done at a rate of about six to nine times a minute. Starting at the lower part of your abdomen, as you inhale, stroke your abdomen gently up toward the top, and as you exhale, slowly let your hands glide back down your abdomen. If you establish this pattern and rate early in your practice, you will not be so inclined to speed up when your coach tells you to accelerate your breathing. It would not feel good—in fact, it would probably be an irritating nuisance—if your hands were to speed up along with your breathing. Effleurage can also be practiced on your thighs or lower back.

3. *Focus your eyes.* Pick one spot or an object on the wall, the ceiling, or the floor and do not let your eyes wander from that one place. At first, you may feel that you look ridiculous staring at one spot as you do your breathing, but this early self-consciousness will soon go away. Focusing your eyes is simply another way to practice concentration. Distractions, visual as well as auditory, are almost

always present when you are in labor. You should condition yourself not to be concerned with the sights and the sounds that do not pertain to your labor, such as traffic in the street outside, a stretcher going down the hall, or people entering and leaving your room. During labor, you should be entirely self-centered. Your sphere should consist only of your contraction, your activities in response to that contraction, and your coach's voice telling you what to do. When you pick out one spot to look at, you are less likely to let your mind wander. In early labor, you may find that an internal focal point is more relaxing.

4. *Develop a conditioned reflex.* Either you or your coach should say out loud "Contraction begins" each time you begin a minute of practice breathing, and "Contraction ends" as the minute ends. Although it may seem a little strange to say words aloud if there is no one but you and the clock present, it is very important that you hear them to establish the conditioned response. You will learn to respond to the sound of the words by starting to do your breathing, beginning your effleurage, focusing your eyes, and so forth.

To the coaches: It is helpful if you call aloud when fifteen seconds have passed, then thirty seconds, then forty-five seconds, and finally one minute, when the contraction ends. For some reason, the minute seems much shorter when it is chopped up into smaller parts. These announcements of the passing seconds are encouraging milestones: the woman knows that she is getting somewhere and this one contraction is not going to last forever. One of the most important functions of the coach in labor is to keep the laboring woman apprised of any and every sign of progress.

Every day, you should practice breathing in each of the four positions you may be in during labor: (1) sitting up in a chair; (2) standing; (3) in a semireclining position, propped up in bed, with pillows supporting your back and shoulders; and (4) on your side. It will give you an added sense of security to have repeatedly practiced your breathing in all four positions. Then, no situation you are in will be strange or unrehearsed when labor begins. If a contraction comes when you are walking from the car into the hospital or standing at the admission desk waiting to go to the labor room, it will not be the first time you have ever done your breathing in a standing position.

Schedule of Breathing Exercises

In the following sections you'll find breathing exercises for each stage of labor — slow-paced breathing for use in early labor, modified-paced breathing with acceleration and deceleration for use as labor progresses, and faster-paced breathing for use in the transition phase to Stage 2. If you are not able to attend classroom instruction or participate in any group sessions, start your daily practice breathing about eight weeks before your due date and establish the following schedule:

1. Eight weeks before due date: Practice the slow-paced breathing with effleurage (see page 208) for one week.
2. Seven weeks before due date: Practice modified-paced breathing with acceleration and deceleration (see pages 209–210) for one week.
3. Six weeks before due date: Practice both slow- and modified-paced breathing, with effleurage, and begin adding practice for transition breathing (see page 212).

Continue practicing the three types of breathing each day until labor begins. By then you'll be a pro.

You may notice a slightly bothersome dryness of the mouth when you start to practice the breathing. After a while, this will diminish somewhat as you become more proficient, because your jaws and facial muscles will become more relaxed and you will salivate more. It may still be something of a problem during labor, however, since this is a slightly open-mouthed breathing. To alleviate the dryness, take with you to the labor room the following articles:

1. A lip balm to keep your lips from feeling dry and cracked.
2. A good supply of sour, tart (lemon or lime, not chocolate) lollipops to suck on between contractions (or a whole lemon, if that suits your taste and your doctor doesn't mind). The tartness will cause you to salivate and the lollipops will also provide some sugar.
3. A small bottle of mouthwash to freshen your mouth.
4. A small paper bag with the edges folded down, the size that will just cover your mouth and nose. Should you feel any light-headedness or signs of hyperventilation during your labor, you can breathe into the bag and, by rebreathing your own exhaled carbon dioxide, end the hyperventilation.

You can bring with you any other small items you think you will need in labor. You should carry those items in a small bag in your hand, rather than putting them in your suitcase, since in most hospitals your suitcase will be taken directly to your postpartum room and you will probably not have it with you in the labor room. You may want to include some talcum powder to sprinkle over your abdomen as you are doing the effleurage. Also, take along a thick washcloth (since many hospitals use disposable washcloths) so that if you feel hot and sweaty during transition, you can wet it with cold water and wash your face and neck to cool off.

BREATHING FOR EARLY LABOR

As mentioned previously, the cramplike, irregular contractions announcing the onset of labor will probably not require any special breathing technique. However, when those contractions have established themselves in a regular, rhythmic pattern and have started to increase in frequency, duration, and intensity (when you can no longer comfortably walk and talk throughout a contraction), you will start to use a rhythmic, slow-paced breathing at a rate of six to nine breaths per minute.

This breathing is easy to do and in no way demanding or exhausting. First breathing is like a sigh. We all sigh without even thinking about it when we are tired or angry or just exasperated by some minor aggravation. The deep, slow inhalation-exhalation of a sigh helps us to relax.

For some women, the slow-paced breathing is adequate for more than half of their labor; for others, it is helpful only during the early part of the first stage, until the cervix is 3 or 4 centimeters dilated. You should use it as long as it is effective for you, whether that is for only two or three contractions, for two or three hours, or much longer.

Practice for Early Labor

1. Take a deep, cleansing breath.
2. At your coach's command, "Contraction begins," start to inhale slowly through your nose, to the full capacity of your lungs, then slowly let the air out through your relaxed lips in a controlled exhalation.
3. Repeat six to nine times per minute. Have your coach count the number of breaths you are taking so that you

can achieve this rate. Your coach should also tell you when fifteen seconds, thirty seconds, forty-five seconds, and sixty seconds have passed, before saying, "Contraction ends."

4. Add the effleurage—bring your cupped hands lightly and slowly up around over the outside of your abdomen as you inhale, and then down the middle of your abdomen as you exhale, or lightly massage your thighs. (Your partner can help here.)

5. Take a deep, cleansing breath at the end of the contraction.

6. Repeat in sitting, standing, semireclining, and side-lying positions.

Let us stress that this, and all the other Lamaze breathing techniques used in the first stage of labor, should be relaxed breathing.

BREATHING AS LABOR PROGRESSES

When the slow-paced breathing is no longer effective (regardless of the amount of time that has passed or the number of centimeters your cervix has dilated), you will switch to a modified-paced breathing. This usually occurs after 5 to 6 centimeters of dilatation but varies from woman to woman.

In labor, you will start slowly, since the beginning of a contraction is mild, and the rate of your breathing will increase as the contraction builds in intensity and reaches a peak. You will use faster, lighter breathing throughout the peak of the contraction and start to decelerate only when the contraction starts to subside.

For your first week of practicing modified-paced breathing, do not concern yourself with speed. That will come more easily later on, when you have mastered the technique of paced breathing evenly, regularly, and without great effort.

For most women, it takes a full week of practice just to learn how to control breathing this way. Practice at a rate that is comfortable for you, approximately twice your normal respiration, achieving a rhythmic, metronomelike quality, rather than trying to increase your speed the first week.

This breathing is done with the mouth slightly open, and it is sometimes helpful to hear the sound of your breathing so that you can regulate the amount of air going in and out with each exhalation. It is imperative that you breathe in the same amount of air that you breathe out. Otherwise, you would not be able to continue for the full minute (much less learn to speed up for the peak).

Two common errors could prevent you from staying comfortable and relaxed during this breathing: (1) If you take in more air when you inhale than you are letting out when you exhale, you may soon start to feel a light-headedness, which is a sign of hyperventilation. If, during a minute of practice, you experience any dizziness or a tingling sensation in your fingers or toes, you will know that you must readjust the amount of air you are inhaling so that it corresponds to the amount you are exhaling. (2) Just the reverse of the previous, if you let out more air with each exhalation than you are taking in with each inhalation, means that you are borrowing some air from the reserve air that always stays in your lungs. Soon your lungs will not let you borrow any more without demanding a repayment, and you will have to make the breathing less shallow and take in a deep breath to replace the air in your lungs before you can continue practicing.

Therefore, if you continue to have difficulty reaching the end of a minute's practice contraction, you (or your coach) should try to identify which of these two errors you are making. You can then correct the problem by carefully listening to your breathing and making a conscious effort to regulate the flow of air in and out.

First Week of Modified-Paced Breathing Practice

1. Take a deep, cleansing breath.
2. At your coach's command, "Contraction begins," start to inhale and exhale in light breaths, keeping your mouth open and your teeth slightly parted, always being aware of equal amounts of air going in and out at about twice the rate of your normal breathing.
3. Continue for one minute (without regard for speed) until your coach says, "Contraction ends." While timing the contraction, your coach should announce when fifteen, thirty, forty-five, and sixty seconds have passed.
4. Take another deep, cleansing breath.
5. Repeat in sitting, standing, semireclining, and side-lying positions.
6. Add effleurage when you are comfortable with the breathing.

Subsequent Weeks of Modified-Paced Breathing Practice

1. Take a deep, cleansing breath.
2. At your coach's command, "Contraction begins," start the paced breathing at a slow rate, and try to imagine that your uterine muscles are just beginning to contract.
3. As your imaginary contraction begins to increase in intensity and your coach says, "Fifteen seconds, accelerate," start to make the breathing lighter and continue to increase your speed as you imagine the contraction rising to a peak and your coach announces, "Thirty seconds." Keep this accelerated speed sustained throughout the imagined peak and then start to slow down when your coach announces, "Forty-five seconds, decelerate." Gradually slow your breathing down to the rate you were breathing when the contraction began, by the time your coach says, "Sixty seconds, contraction ends."
4. Take a deep, cleansing breath.
5. Repeat in sitting, standing, semireclining, and side-lying positions.
6. When you can easily and comfortably accelerate and decelerate at your coach's commands, add the effleurage.

When you first start to practice paced breathing, you will probably have to make a concerted effort to keep relaxed. Your abdomen may move at first, but as you modify the paced breathing, you will see movement at about the level of your breasts.

Modified-paced breathing is usually the most effective Lamaze breathing technique in controlling the discomfort of your contractions, and you will probably use it over a longer period of time than you will any type of breathing. By the same token, it is more exacting and requires greater concentration and more effort than the slow-paced breathing described previously. Therefore, it would be wasteful and tiring for you to begin the modified-paced breathing with your first mild contractions, or when it is not really necessary and the slow breathing is adequate.

On the other hand, do not wait to use this breathing technique until any particular time interval has elapsed or any specific amount of cervical dilatation has occurred; this is not an endurance test. You should begin to modify the breathing whenever the slow-paced breathing is no longer effective in the control of your contractions. Remember, you are the one to determine what breathing is suitable at any given time during your labor. Whatever works for you is what you should be doing.

BREATHING FOR TRANSITION

The change from the end of Stage 1, the dilatation stage, to the beginning of the shorter Stage 2, the expulsion stage, is called the transition phase. This simply means that you are passing from one major stage of labor into another. But to you, in labor, it will probably mean much more, because several new things may start to happen, seemingly all at once.

What Happens in Transition

Contractions. After the onset of active labor, contractions usually maintain a rhythmic, cyclic pattern until transition is reached. Now they usually become longer in duration and stronger in intensity. What is more disconcerting is that they may become erratic, unpredictable in length, strength, or frequency. You may have less time between contractions to rest, and contractions may rise quickly to the peak so that you have to start your acceleration earlier and maintain it longer before the peak starts to wane.

Tremors. At some time in your life, through fatigue or tension, you have probably experienced tremors of your arms or legs. When you tried to hold the extremity still, it would shake even harder. Presumably, by practicing your muscular-control exercises every day and learning how to relax on command, these tremors can be avoided in labor. However, if they do occur, don't be alarmed; tremors are fairly common in transition. You will simply use your relaxation techniques to make them go away, rather than trying to use force to hold the extremity still. With all the activity that is going on inside your body, it is very easy to allow these strong contractions to lead to a state of tension. Therefore, it is most important that the coach be constantly alert during transition and keep you relaxed.

Temperature changes. At transition, you may complain of extreme temperature changes and feel either very hot or very cold. In either case, the treatment is simple. If you are cold, ask the nurse for more cover. If you are uncomfortably warm and sweating, take a large washcloth and wet it with cold water to wipe your face and neck to cool off.

Bloody show. The same type of bloodstained mucous discharge that you saw at the onset of labor will again be present, only now in larger quantities.

Nausea and vomiting. If you tend to feel nauseated during labor, it is usually during transition that this will occur. This is especially true if you ate a heavy meal after labor began.

Irritability. During this period, you may sometimes become very cross and ill-tempered. It is very important for the coach to understand that this reaction is normal and that his or her presence now is even more necessary. You will find comfort in the presence of a reassuring figure and will probably find stronger and more forceful instructions a tremendous help — even if you are insisting on being left alone.

Sometimes in class, women who are in their second or third pregnancy and have returned for a refresher course will try to describe their own mental state during the transition phase of their previous labors. It seems that there is some nebulous quality to it that is hard to verbalize. They use phrases such as: "I would forget what I was supposed to do next," or "Even though I hadn't any medication, I felt kind of like I was drugged." One mother, for lack of a better description, said, "I don't know what it is, you just get a little crazy." This transient loss of perspective and lack of direction and purpose require that the coach take a good firm grip to control the situation until this brief time passes. And it is brief!

Breathing during Transition

These side effects of transition may also appear accentuated because they occur during the most active part of your labor — a period when you are working the hardest to concentrate and stay in complete control of your uterine contractions, when you are tiring, both physically and mentally, and when you would least like to have any extra distractions. It is a time when so much is going on that, alas, *everything* seems grossly exaggerated.

If one (or more) of these annoyances comes along with the transition phase, try to think, "How would I deal with this if I were not in labor?" Such thinking can improve your perspective and may help these minor crisis periods pass quickly.

Even though transition is apt to be the most difficult period of your entire labor, you should not approach this period with fear or dread. Instead, you should think of this as the most welcome milestone you have reached. What a landmark! What a sense of accomplishment when you realize that the long and tedious first stage of your labor will soon be finished. Soon, now, your doctor will examine you and say that your cervix is fully dilated and it is time for you to help push your baby out into the world. It is true that during transition, both you and your coach will have to work very hard to keep you in control, but along with that hard work comes the exciting realization that you will soon give birth.

Throughout your labor, up to now, any sign of progress, any milestone reached was announced by either your doctor or your coach and was dictated by the amount of cervical dilatation you had achieved. To you, it probably was painstakingly slow. But now, when you experience the urge to bear down that comes with transition, you have your own firsthand tangible realization that your baby will soon be born.

It is this urge to bear down, with the feeling of pressure in the rectal area, that gives rise to the need for another change in your Lamaze breathing.

As your uterine muscles have contracted, and as the cervix has retracted, your baby's head has moved farther downward in the pelvis, so that in transition, you will probably feel a sensation of pressure caused by the head pressing on the rectum and a feeling of wanting to move your bowels. This urge can become quite strong, so much so that even heavily medicated women will sometimes be roused by it and insist that they have to go to the bathroom.

As soon as the cervix is fully dilated, and you are in the second stage of labor, that urge will be your signal to start pushing, using your efforts to augment the uterine contractions to help your baby through the birth canal. However, until the cervix is fully dilated, any pushing efforts on your part would be just wasted energy for you cannot push the cervix open. Furthermore, pushing before dilatation is complete may be harmful to the cervix by causing edema (swelling) and possibly even tearing of tissue.

Therefore, the purpose of a different type of breathing for transition is to serve as a more powerful distraction and to counteract the urge to bear down until your doctor tells you it is time to start pushing. The way to accomplish this is to blow out forcibly whenever the urge appears. This blowing of air should not be a slow, long-drawn-out expulsion, but rather a quick, forceful, explosive, staccato blowing accompanied by a tightening of your abdominal muscles. Purse your lips as if you were going to say the letter O, and your cheeks will puff out just as the air is trying to escape your pursed lips. If you are having problems doing this, I suggest that you imagine a large lighted candle situated approximately 2 feet from your face that you have to blow out with one quick expulsion of air.

You can test what effect this blowing out will have on the pressure in the rectal area by sitting in a chair (or on the toilet) with your feet flat on the floor, straining downward as if you were constipated and trying to have a bowel movement, and then quickly blowing out. There is a feeling of release, of "letting go," in the rectal area as soon as the air starts to escape your lips. You will find it is impossible to continue straining downward in the rectal area while you are "straining" with your abdominal muscles and diaphragm to expel the air from your lungs.

When the time comes for you to blow out this way, you will be using your accelerated-decelerated modified-paced breathing to keep control during your contractions. So the next step in your practice will be to learn to incorporate the blowing out into your breathing, without disturbing the rhythm. You can do this by establishing a rhythmic pattern of pant-blow, using six pants and then allowing the blowing out to consume the time that would be required for the next two pants.

After you have practiced this rhythmic patterned breathing for a week, you should easily be able to switch from panting to blowing out and back to panting again without disturbing the rhythm of your panting. Consider the first practice week a learning period, in which you get a sense of how to pant-blow.

When this rhythmic, patterned breathing has become easy for you to do, you should start practicing the transition breathing in a slightly different fashion, in preparation for the way it will probably be used most effectively in labor. Near the end of the first stage, when the urge to bear down becomes strong and persistent, more than one blowing respiration will probably be required to dispel the urge, so that in the midst of your panting, you will start to blow out whenever you feel the urge to bear down. You will repeatedly blow out until the urge goes away, and then you will automatically switch back to your panting rhythm.

In the successive weeks, then, your practice for transition breathing, with your coach calling the commands and timing your contractions, should simulate this sequence of events. The two of you will begin the minute of patterned breathing, the same way that you previously learned it, but at some point (or two or three) in the contraction, your coach will say, "Urge," suggesting the beginning of the rectal pressure. You will now blow out repeatedly until he says, "Stop" or

"Urge ends," whereupon you will immediately return to panting at whatever rate is necessary to control that phase of the contraction. (Note to coaches: This urge does not usually occur in the opening few seconds of the contractions when the uterine muscles are just beginning to tighten up.)

Even though you have progressed to this more sophisticated version of breathing practice for transition, do not abandon your daily practice of this rhythmic pattern of six pants and a blow out. This is a very handy little extra technique to have with you throughout labor, and you may especially want to revert to it when you doctor tells you to stop pushing, just as your baby is being born.

BREATHING FOR THE
SECOND STAGE — EXPULSION

Now that the cervix is fully dilated, you are at last ready for the expulsion of your baby through the birth canal. Even though we refer to this as the second stage of labor, one might just as properly call it birth, since this is what is actually happening — your baby is ready to leave your womb and make its way into the world. Although this stage is, in a sense, a continuation of what has gone before, it is distinctly different. It is true that uterine contractions continue to occur. But they are now performing a different function, and, for you, they take on a different character.

The work you do in the second stage will probably require the greatest physical effort of your entire labor. In contrast to the earlier stage of labor, the second stage requires more brawn than brains. During these contractions, you will use your entire body to augment the efforts of the uterus, and you will assume the proper posture to facilitate the passage of your baby out of the birth canal.

Although it is very important to learn to push correctly, even if the mother is heavily medicated by the time the second stage arrives, the baby will be successfully born. But because the uterus must do all of the work itself, it will take a much longer time. The duration of the second stage is cut approximately in half when the mother is properly trained in the correct posture and techniques of pushing. Here are some reasons why:

- By taking a couple of deep breaths, you can better lean into the contraction.
- You can assume a posture that curves your back, tilts your pelvis, and better utilizes gravity.

- You know to follow up that reflex urge by bearing down with all your might.
- By slowly exhaling, or grunting, you will tighten your abdominal muscles and exert further pressure on the uterus.
- You will relax the perineum (the floor of the pelvis) and be able to visualize the baby's descent and birth.

You can see how much additional help you can give the uterus during each expulsion contraction. Remember, you are trying to help the uterus; it would be counterproductive to try to push between contractions. You cannot push the baby out without the uterus contracting. Instead, use the time between contractions to rest.

This pushing may take place in two different settings. You will still be in the labor room when the second stage begins. In many hospitals, most of the pushing is done in the labor room, so that only a few contractions remain by the time you go to the delivery room. Or you may remain in the labor room or the birthing room throughout delivery.

For the pushing that is done in the labor room, the head of the bed should be elevated to a comfortable position, with two pillows supporting the back and the lower shoulders. During the contraction, you will probably be very grateful for some assistance in positioning, or in supporting your legs. By this time, you may be getting tired and may need extra support and encouragement. Your coach can help by standing near the bed, facing you, and pushing against your knees or feet, or a nurse can stand on one side of the bed and support one leg, while the coach stands on the other side to support the other leg.

You may remain on the birthing bed or move to a birthing chair for the last part of pushing. If the last part of pushing is done in the delivery room, the technique is unchanged, but the position is usually semireclining, with your legs supported at the knees by stirrups so that you do not have to hold them up. Your hands will be resting underneath the sterile drapes, and when the contractions begin and your doctor instructs you to push, you will take hold of the poles that support the stirrups (or the hand grips that are attached to the table) and pull, to help raise your shoulders and lean forward on your diaphragm.

Supplemental Exercises

Before you start to do the practice for pushing, let us pay some attention to the supplemental exercises that will help your actual pushing in labor.

Abdominal Muscle Tone

In the beginning of your training when you started to learn the body-building exercises, we said that one of those—the pelvic rock—would be helpful in getting some tone back in your abdominal muscles, which may have become lax during pregnancy. Continue to do the pelvic rock, but now add on one other abdominal exercise for improving your musculature.

Place your hands on your abdomen; inhale a lungful of air; let the same amount of air out; then blow out, using the residual air left in your lungs. You will feel your abdominal muscles tighten up under your hands and get hard. Do this several times a day.

Perineal Relaxation

The area between the vagina and the anus, which constitutes the floor of the pelvis, is called the perineum, and it is important that these tissues be completely relaxed during the birth of your baby. Perineal relaxation will make for an easier and smoother delivery and will reduce the possibility of lacerations.

You can learn to relax this part of your body, consciously and deliberately, the same way you have used your muscular-control exercises to learn how to relax the other parts of your body when the uterus is contracting. Possibly, in sexual intercourse, you have involuntarily contracted and relaxed these muscles, but before now, there has probably never been a need for you to consciously think, "Now I am going to relax the floor of my pelvis." First, you need to identify where these muscles are and what it feels like when they are relaxed. Then you will learn how to produce this relaxation at will.

The perineum is bounded on the back by the anal orifice (opening) and on the front by the urethral orifice, which leads to the bladder. Knowing the boundaries will help you isolate the area to be relaxed. You can learn to consciously control the area because you already have voluntary control of the sphincters (ringlike muscles) that surround these two openings. In the past, you have deliberately tightened the sphincter around the anus when you did not want to have a bowel movement or tightened the sphincter around the urethra when you did not want to pass urine. Now you will use these sphincters to help you realize the opposite sensation—that of release.

Sit in a chair with your feet flat on the floor and tightly squeeze the muscles around the anus, as if you were trying to prevent a bowel movement. Squeeze tighter and tighter, as tight as you can, hold it for a few seconds, and then release. Now do the same thing in front with the muscle around the urethra. Squeeze tightly, as if you were trying to prevent urination or trying to stop in midstream, hold it for a few seconds, and then release. Now try to tighten both at once; think of the anal orifice and tighten; think of the urethral orifice and tighten; and now tighten the entire area between the two, the whole floor of the pelvis. Squeeze as tight as you can, hold it for a few seconds, and release.

It is this feeling of release that you are pursuing and that you will use during your pushing contractions. The best way to learn it is first to identify and isolate those muscles with your mind, and then to realize the difference in the sensations of *tighten* and *release*.

This exercise, called the Kegel exercise, is very important, not only during the period when you are pushing in labor, but also in the postpartum period (after your baby is born). It helps to eliminate or minimize the discomfort that frequently accompanies the episiotomy repair. Mothers who do these exercises report that they are the single most beneficial exercise for the postpartum period. During the first few days in the hospital after the baby is born, you will see the untrained mothers having trouble with the stitches.

The mere location of the episiotomy probably brings forth anxiety, more so than if the stitches were in some other part of the body. For instance, if you had four or five stitches in your arm, you would probably not be afraid to make a fist or to bend your elbow. But because the stitches are in such a delicate area, new mothers often feel that their stitches must be guarded and protected. This overprotection of the area can increase, rather than decrease, the stitch discomfort, because much of the "stitch pain" begins as edema (accumulation of fluid) between the stitches. With lack of exercise and poor circulation to the area, this is followed by irritation and inflammation, all of which can be a real nuisance in the postpartum period.

You should start to do this exercise at thirty-two weeks so that you will be able to relax the perineum during your labor. You should also start to use this exercise early in the postpartum period to keep the area supple, to improve circulation to the area, and to avoid the collection of fluid between the stitches. By doing so, you can help to avoid stitch discomfort, as well as the nuisance of treatments that go along with it.

Many times, patients who have faithfully done this exercise will comment on the ease with which they passed their urine after their babies were born. At the same time, their postpartum roommates are having difficulty with urination or bowel movements, sometimes to the point of having to be catheterized or requiring laxatives.

It is a simple little exercise that is easy to do, but one that can be very important to you during labor, the postpartum period, and possibly even in later years. Keep it up!

Breathing Exercises for Expulsion

Now, let us go back to the actual exercise for pushing in labor. It may have seemed like an awful lot to learn when we first listed all the parts of your body that are involved in pushing, but it is really not so hard to remember if you will start with your usual deep cleansing breath and then think your way downward from your head to your feet, adding on, one by one, the other parts of the body as you go.

1. Take deep, cleansing breaths: two inhalation-exhalations, and then a third inhalation and hold your breath. These two breaths will allow time for the uterine contraction to build up to the point where your pushing efforts will be most effective.
2. Round your shoulders so that you are leaning on your diaphragm with your lungs full of air.
3. Tighten your abdominal muscles while tilting your pelvis.
4. Bear down, keeping in mind that you are pushing your baby down toward your vaginal opening.
5. Release your perineal muscles.
6. Maintain this pushing effort as long as you can, count to ten, slowly release your breath, then take in another breath, and start all over again.
7. Continue in this fashion until the end of the contraction and then take two or three deep cleansing breaths, and allow yourself to relax all over so that you can rest until the next contraction begins. This rest period, although brief, is very important, because during the contraction, you will be working very hard.
8. Practice pushing (very gentle bearing down in practice) while side-lying, sitting, semireclining, and standing.

You should practice a different position every day and go through the previously outlined steps. If you are afraid that you might rupture membranes when practicing, or if your doctor advises against it, you do not have to bear down as hard as you will in actual labor, since daily conditioning is not important in bearing down. But you do need to practice the pushing posture and procedures so that you will not be embarrassed or ill at ease to assume this posture when your doctor tells you it's time to push, and you will be able to remember all the parts of your body to use.

Earlier, we mentioned that the pushing work you do in the second stage is more brawn than brains. There is, however, one instance — just before the appearance of the baby's head — that requires a great deal of mental effort. That is when you are pushing as hard as you can, bearing down with all your might, and your doctor, right in the middle of a contraction, tells you to stop pushing. The purpose of this directive is to regulate the speed of the delivery and make it a smooth, even procedure. When your doctor gives this instruction to stop pushing, you should let go, lie back on your pillows, and switch immediately to your panting or patterned breathing as you relax your body and let the uterus finish the job. Following this instruction requires some effort, but it is a very welcome sound, because the next instruction from your doctor will probably be the nicest thing you have ever heard: "Now take a look at your new baby."

Your doctor will again ask you to bear down to deliver the placenta after it separates from the uterus. While he or she repairs the episiotomy under local anesthetics, you may lessen any discomfort by relaxing with the breathing techniques used during the first stage of labor and by gazing at your beautiful new infant.

Chapter 10

The Newborn

IN THE HOSPITAL

Often, women remark how quickly attention is shifted toward the newborn baby after delivery. Eyes that were focused on the expectant mother rapidly stare at the new arrival. The entire delivery team will immediately be very busy attending to this new little patient.

The Delivery Room

The birth of your baby will be one of the most exhilarating and rewarding experiences you will ever have. If you are awake during the event itself, which is extremely likely today, you will notice a very odd sequence of events.

Until the moment of birth itself, all eyes will be focused on you in anticipation. After the birth, you will be able to relax for the first time in quite a few hours, while the doctor and the nurses scurry about to accommodate the new citizen of the world.

After the baby is born and lets out its first cry, it is often placed on your abdomen for you to hold while the umbilical cord is clamped and cut. The nose and the mouth will be cleared to facilitate breathing. A bracelet will be put on the baby for identification. The infant's footprint, with your fingerprint, will be placed on a card to register the event officially.

While you are delivering the placenta and having the episiotomy (if necessary) repaired, the baby will be dried off, and the umbilical cord may be further shortened and clamped. He or she may also receive an injection of vitamin K to help with clotting abilities. In some hospitals, routine penicillin injections are also given with the vitamin K to help prevent group B strep infection, the most common cause of newborn meningitis. The nurses will remove the cheesy white

222

material called "vernix," which protected the fetus skin during gestation. Large babies and postmature babies have very little of this coating on their skin at birth. The nurses may also place an antibiotic ointment in the baby's eyes to prevent the effect of maternal gonorrhea on the newborn's eyes. Most hospitals use an antibiotic ophthalmic ointment that is less irritating to the baby's eyes. This treatment can be delayed for an hour or so, until you have held your baby.

You may hear the nurses mentioning numbers. These probably refer to the Apgar score. At birth, most institutions use a general evaluation system to score the physical condition of the infant for purposes of prognosis and treatment. The system is named after Dr. Virginia Apgar, an anesthesiologist who, in the 1950s, was active in newborn medicine and obstetrical anesthesia.

The infant is evaluated on the basis of five signs and given a point score of 0 to 2 for each of these five signs. As seen in table 10.1, the infants can be graded from 0 to 10, with 10 being the highest score.

TABLE 10.1
Apgar Scoring Chart

SIGN	0	1	2
Heart rate	Absent	Slow (below 100)	Over 100
Respiratory effort	Absent	Weak cry	Good strong cry
Muscle tone	Limp	Some flexion of extremities	Well flexed
Reflex response (to catheter in nostril after oropharynx is clear	No response	Grimace	Cough or sneeze
Response to foot slap	No response	Grimace	Cry and withdrawal of foot
Color	Blue, pale	Body pink, extremities blue	Completely pink

Apgar score of	7–10		Healthy infant
	4–6		Moderately depressed infant
	3 or below		Severely depressed infant

Follow-up studies over the past fifteen years have shown that infants with Apgar scores of less than 4 have a higher incidence of neurological problems and defects over the years.

What Else May Happen in the Delivery Room?

Many couples feel a great deal of pressure to save their baby's cord blood. Whether pressure comes from magazine ads, friends, or family, most people understand very little about its true value.

Cord Blood Collection

The fetal blood is pumped by the fetal heart through the umbilical cord to the placenta and then back to the fetal heart. After the baby is delivered, the cord is clamped and cut. A significant amount of fetal blood remains in the clamped cord and the placenta. Traditionally, cord blood has been considered expendable. Usually, after delivery, a sample of cord blood is collected for blood typing and other specialized tests, and then the cord, with its placenta, is discarded.

Fetal blood is quite unique. It contains a very high percentage of special cells called hematopoietic progenitor cells, or stem cells. These cells are usually located in the human bone marrow and, when they mature, become blood cells. These cells are important in treating various blood diseases and cancer. Stem cells are used in a specialized cancer-fighting procedure called a bone marrow transplant.

When a person develops cancer, for example, finding these types of cells may become vital for his or her treatment. The cancer patient must find a donor to supply these cells. The donor's cells must match up with the cancer patient's, or they will be rejected. Finding the right match is often difficult or impossible. If a match is found (often a sibling), the donor must undergo the painful procedure of extracting cells from his or her bone marrow. If the cancer patient had stored his or her own fetal blood, the match would certainly be 100 percent. Not only that, other family members may also be candidates for these cells should the need arise.

In 1988, French investigators were the first to use cord blood stem cells to help treat a rare and fatal blood disease. In that case, fetal stem cells were used on a five-year-old sibling. Since then, many hundreds of such procedures have been performed.

Today, various private companies are available to store collected fetal blood. A list of companies should be available to you at your doctor's office. The cost is usually in the range of $1,000 to $1,500, with a variable yearly storage fee. The decision whether or not to store fetal blood is often difficult. The likelihood that any individual will need a bone marrow transfusion is remote; however, many couples feel that banking fetal blood is like an insurance policy that they cannot do without. If the decision to store fetal blood is made, be sure to discuss it with your doctor and the private company well before your due date.

Attendants at Delivery

At most routine deliveries the doctor and the nurse will be present. Many patients ask, Who will tend to the baby immediately after birth? Will my baby's doctor be there?

Very often, situations arise where the obstetrician recognizes the need for the pediatrician to be at delivery. This is not routine, but the pediatrician is most often summoned as a precaution. The following are possible reasons for having a pediatrician at delivery:

- Amniotic fluid is stained with meconium. Meconium is feces from the fetus, which is usually not released until after birth. If the baby inhales the meconium at birth, it may cause pneumonia. Both your obstetrician and your pediatrician are trained to avoid this occurrence.
- Maternal fever. If there is an elevation of the mother's temperature in labor, the baby should be carefully screened for infection at birth.
- Maternal diabetes. If the mother's sugar is abnormal, the baby's sugar will be affected.
- Untreated or incomplete treatment of maternal group B strep infection (see chapter 12).
- Difficult delivery.
- Fetal distress.

Physical Aspects of the Newborn

At birth, babies appear quite different from the way they do a few weeks later. Television and magazines often use infants who are one to three months old to represent newborns. As a result, many parents are surprised when their baby does not look the way they expected.

A baby who has just emerged into the outside world is often covered with a greasy, whitish coating called vernix. There may also be traces of blood. This is normal. The arms and the legs may be drawn up into the position last assumed in the uterus. Because the head was under pressure in the uterus, the face is likely to appear a bit swollen and the eyes puffy. The skull bones are not fused and are flexible. Therefore, some babies' heads appear elongated or even pointy, due to molding. Babies born by cesarean can have the same appearance if their mothers went through labor before delivery; if labor did not occur, their faces and heads may appear more like those of babies several days old.

In the time just after birth, skin color may not be uniform. In addition to the vernix covering the skin, some newborns may have a bluish or gray appearance, especially of the hands and the feet. This is usually temporary.

After a few days some babies' skin becomes yellow. This condition, jaundice, is caused by a buildup of bilirubin, a substance produced when red blood cells are broken down as a natural process of the body. Normally, the liver removes bilirubin from the body. During pregnancy, the placenta and the mother's liver remove bilirubin from the fetus. The baby's liver cells don't begin to function to remove bilirubin until a few days after birth. It is this lag time that causes temporary jaundice.

Parents should not be overly concerned about jaundice that appears a few days after birth. Although high levels of bilirubin can be toxic to the baby's nervous system, the levels in most babies are not likely to cause problems. Before the liver begins to function naturally, the amount of bilirubin in the blood can be checked and the baby can be placed under fluorescent lights, which lower bilirubin levels.

Everyone wants to know how much a baby weighs at birth. The hospital will give you that figure, usually in pounds and ounces (doctors and nurses express weight in grams; for example, 2.2 pounds = 1,000 grams = 1 kilogram). There is no such thing as a proper or a "good" weight, but there is a range that is considered normal— between 6 and 8 pounds at term.

At the time of birth, the lungs take over the placenta's role as the organ that carries oxygen to the blood. A baby spontaneously takes breaths at the time of birth. Why this occurs is not completely clear, but it appears to result from the stimulation of birth and from changes that take place in the makeup of the baby's blood. Many babies will cry loudly and often at birth, but some don't cry at all. Some babies even begin to breathe without crying. Once the lungs are working, however, most babies cry. In addition to the first cry, babies will often respond to handling with cries.

Blood moves to and from the placenta through vessels in the umbilical cord. At the time of birth, the placenta comes loose from the inside of the uterus and is expelled. Thus, a major flow of blood to the fetus stops suddenly. At the same time, blood flow to the lungs increases dramatically.

Just after birth, when the baby's lungs are filling with air and receiving more blood, doctors and nurses often listen to the chest carefully with a stethoscope. In addition to the sound of air entering the lungs, they can often hear sounds or murmurs associated with the changes in blood flow that are a normal part of the baby's adjustment.

The healthy fetus gives off heat through the placenta to its mother, and it is protected from heat loss by the surrounding warmth of the mother. At birth, the baby enters an environment that is much cooler than the mother's uterus. Being wet, the baby is at risk for serious heat loss through evaporation. This loss can be kept to a minimum by drying and wrapping the baby just after birth.

Newborns have controls to maintain their body temperature, but these systems are not as efficient as those in older children. Environments that are too hot or too cool can overwhelm the newborn.

A newborn baby's basic reflexes, such as those that control breathing, function well. The baby is able to interact with people and respond to sound and light. Parents may notice a complex reflex action, such as the startle, or Moro, reaction, in which a newborn extends the arms, the legs, and the head and then draws the arms back to the chest in response to a strong stimulus such as a sound. Sight, hearing, and pain sensation are present from birth but are more easily recognized as the baby matures.

The placenta was the main source of food for the fetus before birth. After birth, the baby is able to feed by sucking and swallowing milk through the mouth and moving it into and through the intestinal tract. Although unable to handle an adult diet, a baby can digest carbohydrates, proteins, and fat soon after birth. Feeding can take place early the first day. The fetal intestine contains a dark, tarry greenish substance called meconium that is usually seen within twenty-four hours, when the first bowel movement occurs.

Behavior of the Newborn

All newborns have similar biological needs and respond with limited reactions. Beyond this, however, each baby expresses a unique personality. There are wide variations in how each baby behaves and interacts with people. Some seem quiet and subdued and indeed may have seemed quiet in the uterus; others exhibit lusty crying and vigorous kicking.

After the stress and the physical adjustments of birth, the baby often has a brief period (an hour or so) of being alert and may suckle if put to the mother's breast. The baby may then fall asleep or be drowsy for the next several hours or even a few days.

At first, babies spend most of their time sleeping (in short intervals that total fourteen to eighteen hours per day) with only brief periods of alertness. Some babies spend more time awake from the beginning and are fussy, rather than quiet and alert. Others will spend long stretches sleeping and will gradually awaken to a quiet state. Parents can alter sleep/wake patterns to help babies adapt to a fixed schedule. For example, by encouraging the baby to stay awake during the day and by ignoring fussiness and avoiding anything that keeps the baby awake at night, parents may be able to alter cycles. The need to feed during the night may continue for two to three months after birth and sometimes longer.

Bonding is the magic feeling that a mother has toward her infant shortly after birth. Not all mothers feel this way immediately. The baby may not look as she expected, or a difficult birth may prevent bonding. In a short time, a few days at most, interaction will become closer as mother and baby adapt to each other. Attachment is the gradual process of developing a loving relationship between a baby and his or her parents over time.

The Nursery

After you have held or breast-fed your baby, the baby is taken to the nursery, where most of its needs will be met for the next few days. Nurses will check its bowel movements (the brownish-green meconium) for the first few days after birth. Failure to void feces and urine may indicate some congenital problem in need of correction. They will check for jaundice, which occurs in about a third of all newborns (caused by immaturity of the baby's liver, with a resulting increase in bile pigment). The nurses will change and bathe the baby and help you with feeding and learning about being a mother.

A pediatrician or a general practitioner will usually take over the care of the infant after birth. Most hospitals give the baby to the mother for feedings, whether the baby is breast- or bottle-fed. All babies lose weight immediately after birth. Most are too sleepy to eat the first few days. But when they are ready, they will let you know. No baby starves quietly.

Rooming-In

In some hospitals, babies can stay in the rooms with their mothers. This arrangement, called rooming-in, has advantages and disadvantages.

Proponents say it is good for several reasons. Since the baby is in the room with the mother, to be fed on demand, rooming-in encourages bonding and promotes lactation for breast-feeding. They say the mother's attention will be focused on baby care immediately, reducing her worry about what will happen at home. Then, once she gets home, caring for the baby won't seem so strange to her. She will also learn that the demands of most newborns are not so great—some may sleep as much as twenty out of twenty-four hours a day. Fathers can also spend more time with their newborns when they room-in.

Opponents say rooming-in is not necessary, especially for a mother who does not feel well after delivery. They feel that two days are not going to make that much difference in learning to be a mother, since the mother and the baby have the rest of their lives to become acquainted in the comfort of their home. Some opponents are against the idea of paying for the high cost of postpartum care and then doing all the work themselves.

Newborn Intensive-Care Unit

Most babies born today are healthy, with an almost certain chance for survival. However, about 10 percent of babies are born with some risk of medical problems. They may be premature or have some condition that requires special attention or very special care. These higher-risk babies require the minute-to-minute care of doctors, nurses, and other trained personnel. Therefore, in every part of the country, hospitals have established intensive-care nurseries, called either newborn intensive-care units or perinatal centers, to which babies who need this kind of care are sent as soon as the baby's doctor is aware of the need. Most hospitals have a staff able to care for most babies; however, babies requiring special care are either brought to the special unit or transferred to a center that has one. Babies who have to be transferred are transported in a specially equipped ambulance that contains all the necessary equipment to keep their condition stable en route.

The most common cause for intensive care is prematurity. Premature birth and the other illnesses and conditions that put babies at greater risk are quirks of nature and have many causes. Your doctor will talk with you about your baby's condition and try to relieve any anxiety you may have. It is important for you to have all your questions answered.

In intensive care, your baby will be placed in a warmer bed or an incubator, providing an enclosed environment. Here, heat and moisture can be controlled, and extra oxygen, if needed, can be supplied. An incubator also provides protection against infection. The entire nursery and the incubator are designed to enable caregivers to observe your baby for any signs of distress. Special wires are taped to your baby's skin to keep a constant check on body temperature. The heart and the breathing rates are continuously monitored. Many of these small babies will require feeding, initially by intravenous techniques and then perhaps by a tube entering the stomach. But as the baby gains weight, he or she may nurse from a bottle or eventually breast-feed. After a while, your baby will be well enough to move out of the intensive-care nursery and, eventually, be ready to go home. Before your baby is discharged, you may want to spend several days in the nursery to make sure you know you can begin to provide for your baby's care. It is important that you feel secure in starting to take care of your baby at home; therefore, don't hesitate to ask questions. You can then be ready to enjoy caring for your baby and watching him or her grow.

Circumcision

Circumcision—cutting away the foreskin that covers the end of the penis—is controversial. In the United States, circumcision of male infants became more common after World War I, and today, most newborn baby boys in the United States are circumcised. Jewish and Muslim people still practice circumcision as a religious rite.

Circumcision is one of the oldest surgical procedures known. This surgery is usually done before your baby leaves the hospital and has very few risks involved. In 2001, both the American Academy of Pediatrics and the American College of Obstetrics and Gynecology stated that the existing evidence is insufficient to recommend routine neonatal circumcision.

The choice of circumcision is completely up to you. Discuss it with your doctor. Some doctors routinely recommend circumcision, often for reasons of hygiene or traditional values. In uncircumcised males, a substance called smegma, made up of cells shed from the outer layer of skin, gathers under the foreskin. This can lead to odor or infection if the penis is not cleaned regularly. In circumcised males, the foreskin is gone, so smegma cannot build up. It is important for parents of uncircumcised boys to clean the penis during the child's bath until he learns to do this on his own. Some parents choose circumcision because they want their son to look like his circumcised father or older brothers.

Many people believe that circumcision prevents cancer of the penis in old age. Circumcision could be considered an effective means of preventing cancer of the penis, but good hygiene—liberal use of soap and water—can be just as effective a preventive measure. When the penis is not cleaned regularly and properly, large quantities of smegma, which may contain a cancer-causing agent, can build up. High rates of penile cancer have been found in circumcised males who have very poor hygiene, yet uncircumcised men who have very good hygiene have very low rates of this cancer.

Although a male can be circumcised at any time in his life, it is usually done soon after birth—before you and your baby leave the hospital. A circumcision can be performed with or without analgesia. Currently, surveys have shown that most are performed without analgesia. Many studies have confirmed that newborns who are circumcised without analgesia experience pain and stress. A study done in 1999, using various stress indicators such as heart rate and crying during the circumcision procedure, found a significant decrease in stress for those babies who received analgesia.

Types of analgesia in use today include topical EMLA cream, dorsal penile nerve block, and subcutaneous ring block. Most commonly, EMLA cream is used. EMLA is a cream consisting of two local anesthetics. The penile tip is covered with EMLA cream. After approximately one hour, the cream is removed and the foreskin will be appropriately anesthetized for the procedure. The medicine acts topically so there is little, if no, absorption into the baby's system. Both dorsal penile nerve block and subcutaneous ring block require injection and therefore have a higher potential for complications. Studies seem to indicate similar stress reduction with each method. We prefer topical EMLA application if analgesia is used. As with any surgery, there are possible complications. But when the circumcision is performed by a doctor in a hospital, complications are rare. When complications do occur, the most frequent are hemorrhage, infection, and trauma. After a circumcision, diapers should be changed frequently so that urine and feces do not irritate the skin and cause infection. Wash the penis with soap and water daily. The circumcision should heal in about ten to fourteen days.

It is your choice as parents whether your child should or should not be circumcised. Talk with your doctor about your questions or concerns.

The Role of the Pediatrician

At the hospital, your baby will be checked thoroughly by a staff pediatrician. In most instances you can have the pediatrician of your choice come to the hospital and check your baby. Many mothers find this practice tremendously helpful. The doctor will look at the baby from stem to stern and alert you to little birthmarks and rashes that might frighten you when you discover them at home. Since most mothers are lying in high, narrow beds when the baby is given to them for feeding, they never unwrap the baby until they get home.

The doctor will also give feeding instructions and answer any questions you may have. He or she will tell you certain things to look for: Girl babies, for example, often have a slightly bloody vaginal discharge soon after birth. A mother seeing this in a week-old baby, without expecting it, could be quite upset.

The doctor will also set up an office appointment for you to bring in the baby for a weigh-in, a checkup, and immunization after the first two weeks and every month thereafter until the baby is about eight months old, when visits become less frequent.

THE NEWBORN AT HOME

Common Concerns about Infant Care

The most common issues that arise concerning newborn care include the following.

Crying

Some women are afraid they will have a baby who cries insistently and inconsolably. Actually, newborn babies usually cry for only a few reasons: They are hungry or thirsty, too cold or too hot, or sleepy. Whereas the adult human is ruled by the brain, the infant is ruled by the stomach. Most chronically unhappy babies have some kind of digestive disturbance, and most of these have some medical remedy. Often, the baby just needs more to eat or may need solid foods. (Some doctors will prescribe cereal as early as the second or third week of life.) Colic, the early indigestion, is often caused by intolerance to cow's milk. Breast milk or soy milk is often used as a substitute.

It has been pretty well established that a newborn does not have the cerebral capacity to be spoiled. Being spoiled requires some memory, which is not yet developed. The current thinking among child psychologists is that crying should be viewed as a signal of a physical need that must be tended to. The thinking here is that by answering the need, you show the infant that the world is a friendly place that will take care of him or her.

Newborns want to be as warm and snug as they were inside the womb. This is why a baby might cry when its clothes are taken off. It's also the reason that babies are usually wrapped snugly in little cotton flannel receiving blankets—even in summer—until they get used to being on the outside. Normal infants in the first week after birth need some clothing, such as a cotton shirt or a gown, in addition to a diaper and perhaps a light blanket. The room should be draft free and not too warm or too cool (70° to 75°F) or too dry (35 to 60 percent humidity).

Scheduling

In past generations, a good deal of effort went into putting the baby on a regular schedule. Mothers sat waiting for the minute hand to hit the hour before they fed a baby who had been crying for a half-hour. Or they woke up a perfectly contented sleeping baby because it was "time to eat," only to find that the infant was not really hungry, refused to eat on command, and then woke up demanding food before the next scheduled feeding.

Modern mothers are much more relaxed and more likely to feed babies when they let mothers know that they are hungry. Actually, most mothers find that, if left to regulate themselves, most babies want to eat about every four hours. Some eat more often, some less often. Larger babies who have bigger stomachs that can accommodate more food will probably eat less frequently. As a rule of thumb, a baby who eats everything at every meal is probably not getting enough to eat. Most of the baby-care books have tables to use as informal guides to the amount a child should be eating, according to the child's size.

Sleeping

A newborn baby usually sleeps more than he or she is awake. For most mothers, this sleeptime is a welcome opportunity to rest. But many mothers who are eager to interact with their baby find it difficult to feed, clothe, bathe, cuddle, and immediately put the sleepy one down. Eventually, however, the sleeping beauty does awaken. That's when you may long for the return of the angelic little child you once wished would wake up.

Care of the Cord

There will be a scab on the baby's belly where the umbilical cord attached the baby to the mother. About ten days following birth, this drying remnant of a cord will fall off, leaving in its place the navel, or belly button. Until this happens, however, the cord should be cleaned off daily with an alcohol-soaked pad. If possible, the baby's diaper should not cover the cord. You should refrain from bathing the baby in a tub until the cord falls off.

Bathing the Baby

For the first few days, the baby should be given sponge baths. If possible, only a little part of the baby should be exposed and washed at a time, so that the baby remains comfortable and warm. Most hospitals provide instructions for bathing the baby in prenatal classes or in mothers' classes after birth.

Fresh Air

Fresh air is usually recommended for new babies, weather permitting. In the summer, fresh air is no problem. When you should take the baby out in the winter is another matter. Your doctor will give you specific instructions, usually based on your baby's size. There is a tremendous tendency for new mothers to overdress babies when they take them out. Remember, they require no more clothing in any weather than you do.

Feeding

The decision to breast-feed or bottle-feed is a mother's personal preference. Just as many mothers were attracted to general anesthesia for delivery when it became widely used in the 1940s, so were many mothers attracted to bottle-feeding when prepared formulas became more widely available, reducing the need to make formula. Bottle-feeding today can be as easy as screwing a sterilized nipple onto a bottle of prepared formula that requires no refrigeration until it is opened. But the pendulum of maternal and medical preferences seems to be swinging back to the more "natural" way of child caring, and the number of mothers nursing is on the rise.

Breast milk has special properties that make it superior to even the most carefully made home or commercial preparations. It not only provides substances (antibodies) that protect against common illnesses, such as colds and respiratory disease, but also helps produce a protective environment against infection in the intestinal tract. It contains the complete range of nutrients necessary to the young infant and is easier to digest than substitutes. Breast milk as a food contains protein, carbohydrates, and fat in sufficient quantities to make it a complete food. Except for iron and vitamins B and D, breast milk contains all the nutrients a growing baby needs. These other substances will probably be prescribed as a supplement by the pediatrician. In 1997, the American Academy of Pediatrics released a statement that research in the United States, Canada, Europe, and other developed countries has provided strong evidence that human breast milk decreased the chances of diarrhea, lung infections, ear infections, various bacterial infections, urinary tract infections, and a severe and often deadly condition of the intestinal tract called necrotizing enterocolitis (NEC). In addition, breast milk may protect against sudden infant death syndrome (SIDS), diabetes, Crohn's disease, ulcerative colitis, lymphoma, allergic disease, and digestive problems. Finally, breast-fed babies may have superior intelligence.

Breast-feeding costs less (it's free!) than feeding with substitutes. While nursing eliminates formula and bottle preparation, it requires a more careful maternal diet and a little more privacy at mealtime, unless you feel comfortable enough with the process to nurse the baby in public. Women who have generally busy schedules or who return to work when the baby is very young often compromise and nurse for some meals and bottle-feed for others.

Besides being the best form of nutrition for the infant, breast-feeding may be an important means of spacing births and preventing pregnancy, especially in religious groups that cannot use artificial methods of contraception. Breast-feeding postpones ovulation and is somewhat of a contraceptive—albeit not a good one.

For those who do decide to nurse, some background will be useful. Throughout pregnancy, the breasts are sensitive to the hormonal changes in the body. Very early, the breast becomes enlarged and the nipples grow larger and darker in color. By the end of the third month, a premilk, called colostrum, is formed and may ooze from the nipples throughout pregnancy. The amount of colostrum increases just after delivery. Until the milk comes in, the baby will drink colostrum.

When the milk does come in, your breasts may be painful and engorged. For up to ten days after birth, colostrum and milk are both secreted. The supply of milk is determined by the amount of sucking your baby does, which is why it is suggested that you start the baby on both breasts at each feeding to get the milk to flow.

Several factors determine how satisfying nursing will be for the baby. Besides the baby's demand, the amount of milk available also depends on a satisfactory schedule; an adequate diet for the mother, including a good deal of liquids; an emotionally relaxing environment; general good health; and good care of the breasts to prevent cracking of the nipples. This last condition can be prevented by using a good cream on the breasts and by letting them dry off after a feeding. A breast shield can also be used to protect tender nipples. Breasts should be supported by a firm brassiere for comfort and to eliminate sagging after you stop nursing.

Successful Breast-Feeding

Here are some suggestions that have proved helpful to many mothers who continue to breast-feed after they have left the hospital. Your doctor may feel that some points should be modified for you or your baby. Your doctor's advice is based on your individual baby, and the doctor will be happy to explain the reasoning behind each recommendation; ask as many questions as you need to.

Bowel Movements

The bowel movements of the breast-fed baby are typically soft, even liquid, in consistency, yellowish-brown or greenish-brown in color, and may contain curds or mucus. Your baby may have bowel movements as seldom as once every other day or even once in three days, but most often at every feeding. What would certainly be called diarrhea in an adult is the normal bowel movement of the breast-fed baby. If anything else seems unusual, have your baby checked by a doctor.

Frequency of Feeding

The newborn breast-fed baby typically demands and needs to eat every two to four hours in the daytime after first leaving the hospital. (Formula-fed infants eat less frequently at first.) The breast-fed baby may also gain weight at a slower rate than the formula-fed baby, but this is fine so long as the gain is sufficient and the baby is well. If, during the first month, your baby does not demand at least six feedings a day, try to nurse more often than demanded, since some babies are not as efficient at making their needs known as are others. At your baby's first checkup, you might want to check with the doctor if you wish to feed less often.

Milk Supply

If at any time you or your doctor feels that your supply of breast milk is not fully meeting the baby's needs, you can usually build it up to the required level by nursing as often as possible for forty-eight hours (as often as every two hours during the day and every three at night), while trying to rest and take fluids. Most babies have times when they suddenly seem hungry, but this need not mean your supply has dwindled; the baby may suddenly need more because he or she is entering a growth spurt. If you nurse more often for a few days, you will probably find that your baby will return to a more stable schedule and seem happy with it again.

Nighttime Bottles

Mothers who breast-feed often like to leave a nighttime bottle so that the father or a helper can tend to the 4 A.M. feeding. While the nighttime bottle does sometimes work out, often the mother finds that her supply is scanty by the time the baby is a few weeks old because she isn't nursing frequently enough. If you do have help at home, the bottle is best used for housekeeping, shopping, preparation of meals, and perhaps some care of the baby between feedings, rather than for feedings themselves. But it is likely to work best if you do not use it at all during the first month. Once the baby is about a month old, however, leaving a bottle for one to three feedings a week will not interfere with continued breast-feeding. After several months, even a daily bottle will not interfere.

Duration of Feeding

When you first get home, continue to limit the time on each breast at each feeding to ten to twelve minutes (not counting time when the baby dozes). Prolonged feedings may lead to soreness, while frequent short feedings should not. Remember that the baby takes the largest portion of the milk present in the breast in about five to seven minutes of sucking time. Of course, there is no harm in letting the baby nurse longer at some or all feedings if you and the baby both wish to and if you are still comfortable. If the baby wants additional sucking time, it's usually because many babies have a need to suck, but it is not necessary for the baby's nutrition. Some mothers supply this need to suck by allowing additional time on the breast, some by using pacifiers or empty bottles with blind nipples, and some by giving water (boiled to sterilize, then cooled) between feedings. The healthy breast-fed baby does not need extra water unless the weather is very hot or the temperature of your home is high.

Introducing Solid Foods

Your doctor or clinic will recommend when to introduce your baby to juice and to solid foods. Your breast milk contains everything the baby needs for nutrition, except for some vitamins and iron. Since a vitamin supplement will probably be prescribed for your baby, and the healthy infant does not need iron until four to six months, solid foods will not be nutritionally necessary for quite a while. The baby who has started solids is naturally less eager to nurse and may slacken nursing enough to lower your milk supply even below what he or she still needs. Also, the younger the baby, the greater the chance that introduction of a food other than breast milk will elicit an allergic response. The later you start solids, the less likely they will interfere with an adequate milk supply. If your doctor suggests solid foods earlier, you may wish to discuss postponing them.

Pacifying the Baby

Remember that your baby may cry for many reasons besides hunger. In order to soothe the crying baby, you might try swaddling (wrapping the baby with the arms at his or her sides in a light blanket), burping, changing diapers, adding or removing a layer of clothing or blanketing (in case the temperature is uncomfortable), rocking, and offering a pacifier. Trying to determine whether the baby is hungry by offering a bottle is inadvisable, since many breast-fed babies will drink from a bottle even when they have been well fed. In general, offering a bottle because of *possible* hunger only makes the baby wait longer before nursing again, and this will decrease your milk supply.

Breast Size

It is perfectly normal for your breasts to lose their initial hardness and gradually return to normal size even while you continue breast-feeding. This does not mean you are losing your milk. In about six months, you should be back to your nonpregnant size, even if the baby is fed only from the breast and is, of course, taking much more milk than at six days.

Breast-Feeding and Menstruation

You may not menstruate for quite a while if you continue to breast-feed. This is normal and no cause for concern. When your periods do resume, they may be irregular for a while, and the baby may appear to be fussy for a day or two. Your milk is just as good at this time, however, and the baby should continue to be breast-fed. It is possible to ovulate while you are breast-feeding, even if you have not yet menstruated since the baby was born; you can become pregnant again without ever menstruating. Although certain birth-control pills are inadvisable while breast-feeding, since they do tend to dry up the milk, your doctor or clinic can suggest other means of family planning if you wish. If you should become pregnant, you should wean the baby who is breast-feeding, but make sure this is done gradually, rather than suddenly.

Weaning

The best time to wean the baby is when you want to. If you wish to breast-feed for a relatively short time and then stop, that is fine. In fact, most authorities feel it is better to stop than to continue reluctantly. However, if you wish to continue for a relatively long time, that is fine, too, for there is no point at which your milk becomes a poor food for your baby. At about six months, though, it is no longer adequate as the only food. Our hope is not that you will breast-feed for any specified length of time, but that you will stop because you are ready and wish to, rather than because of poor information or lack of support. Weaning should be done gradually for your own comfort and the easiest transition for the baby. This means that you substitute the bottle (or the cup, with an older baby) for the breast at one feeding a day for several days, until you find that your breasts no longer feel full at that feeding. Then eliminate a second breast-feeding for a few days, and so forth.

Breast-Feeding When the Mother Is Ill

Mothers often ask if it is all right to breast-feed the baby when they themselves are ill. It is perfectly all right, providing you have checked with your doctor, are not taking medication that would harm the baby by passing through the milk, and do not have an illness that precludes contact with the baby. For example, you are not protecting a breast-fed baby from catching your cold by giving a bottle instead of the breast, since germs don't pass through breast milk and the baby is equally exposed to your germs while being bottle-fed. However, any medications you take should be checked with the baby's doctor, since you want to be very careful about what substances reach the baby through the milk.

Antihistamines temporarily decrease your milk supply and should be avoided unless essential to your health.

The Mother's Diet

You may hear many dos and don'ts of diet while breast-feeding, most of which you can ignore. In general, you can eat what you wish, as far as your milk and the baby's health are concerned, but a good sound diet is naturally preferable to a poor one for your own health, just as at any other time. Make sure that you get enough calcium by drinking several glasses of milk a day or eating cheese, ice cream, yogurt, puddings, and other foods containing milk (skim milk is just as good as whole milk in providing calcium and is much lower in calories). Since you do not need to eat fatty foods and will need only about 600 to 1,000 calories more a day than if you were not breast-feeding, you certainly need not gain weight or remain heavy in order to breast-feed. In fact, this is a good time for the really overweight woman to lose some weight or for the underweight woman to gain weight for her own sake during the nursing period. Since few babies react with any appearance of digestive upset to any one food, you can probably eat as you wish. Then, if your baby seems upset several times after you have eaten a specific food, try eliminating it. There is no particular food or beverage that helps to make milk or improve its quality, but it is important to drink enough fluids (water is as good for this purpose as any other beverage), since lack of fluids can decrease your milk supply. Drink whenever you are thirsty and try to drink something at each nursing, but you need not drink to the point of discomfort. Alcoholic beverages and coffee and tea will not affect the milk in a manner harmful to the baby unless taken in large quantities.

The Mother's Attitude

You may hear that a woman must be calm and relaxed in order to breast-feed successfully. Although anxiety, tension, and fatigue do not lessen the mother's supply of milk, they may make it difficult for her to release or "let down" milk that is present in her breasts. Therefore, it is best to arrange for circumstances that will permit you to be as calm and comfortable as possible before and during each nursing.

Milk Supply

The biggest question in the minds of most women who are breast-feeding is whether their baby is getting enough milk. It is hard for many women to believe that they can produce enough milk for their babies, and they may envy the ability of the woman who bottle-feeds to count the ounces that the baby takes. Weighing the baby often, and especially before and after feeding, creates unnecessary anxiety in most mothers. It is advisable only for the small minority of cases where a doctor feels the baby has not been gaining well enough and wants to see if more frequent feedings may improve matters.

Manual Expression of Breast Milk

Manual expression of breast milk—removing breast milk with your hands—is useful to stimulate and increase your supply of milk; to relieve a full, uncomfortable breast; to maintain your supply of milk if the baby is temporarily unable to feed at the breast; and to give the infant breast milk in a relief bottle.

The technique for manual expression consists of the following:

- Wash your hands.
- Expose the breast.
- Gently wash your breasts with a soft cloth and plain water; pat dry with a soft towel.
- Assume a comfortable position.
- Place a towel or a cloth under the breast to protect your clothing if the milk should drip.
- Hold the pitcher or the container beneath the nipple. (The container should be sterile if the milk is to be given to the infant.)
- Grasp the breast gently just back of the areola (the brown part surrounding the nipple) with the ball of the thumb on the upper surface of the breast and the forefinger beneath the lower surface.
- Press the thumb and the forefinger together gently but firmly, squeezing that part of the breast between them.
- With a forward pull and downward pressure, the milk is forced out in a stream without your fingers touching the nipple.
- If the milk is to be discarded, it can be expressed directly into the sink.
- Breast milk is sterile and does not have to be sterilized for use.

Bottle-Feeding

If you have decided to bottle-feed your baby, you must allow your body to stop producing breast milk. You can help this by wearing a snug bra (one cup size smaller than you usually wear) during the first week after delivery. At first, your breasts will be engorged with colostrum. You may need to apply ice packs to both breasts and take analgesics for discomfort. Heat and manual expression will only stimulate them to produce *more* milk. Without the stimulation of breast-feeding, your body will begin to reabsorb the colostrum, and swelling will go down. The complete reabsorption process can take as long as four weeks. Some limpness may remain in your breasts until then, or your nipples may leak during this time.

Infant formula preparations today try to imitate breast milk as closely as possible. Since they are derived from cow's milk, the milk curds take longer to digest, and bottle-fed babies will usually sleep longer between feedings. Nutrition in formula is basically the same as that of breast milk.

Discuss sterilization processes and choices of formula with your pediatrician. Formula powder or concentrate is substantially less expensive than ready-to-use formula. Make enough formula to last twenty-four hours, but never reuse formula left over from a prior feeding.

After each feeding, wash the bottle immediately. If formula sits overnight, a ring will form in the bottle that is difficult to scrub out.

Bottle-feeding can be a happy experience. It's important that your infant be held and cuddled while he or she eats, nourishing stomach and soul. Burp your baby halfway through bottle feeding and at the end of each feeding.

Some babies will develop an allergic reaction to cow's milk, usually apparent as a rash or gastric distress, in which case your pediatrician may recommend a change to a soy-based formula.

One of the advantages of bottle-feeding is that everyone can help out. It's nice for you to be able to step back and let fathers, grandparents, other children, and friends feed the baby and share this enjoyable experience.

Car Safety

Motor vehicle crashes are the leading cause of death for Americans from birth to thirty-four years of age. Many of these fatalities and serious injuries are preventable through the proper use of safety belts and child restraints. Most states have passed laws requiring drivers and adult passengers to wear safety belts and all child passengers to be placed in safety seats.

Seat Belts and Pregnancy

For the best protection, you should wear a lap-shoulder belt throughout your pregnancy every time you travel in a motor vehicle, including during your ride to the hospital for the birth of your baby. In the event of a crash, the lap-shoulder belt will keep you in the vehicle and prevent your head and chest from striking the steering wheel, the dashboard, or the windshield. About 40 percent of injuries in motor vehicle crashes occur when a person hits the steering wheel or the windshield. A lap belt will protect your lower torso and will keep you from being thrown from the car. Some motor vehicles have only lap belts in the backseat. If a lap belt is all that is available, use it.

Place the lower part of the lap-shoulder belt under your abdominal bulge, as low on your hips as possible, and against your upper thighs. Never place the belt above your abdomen, since this could cause major injuries in a crash. Position the upper part of the belt between the breasts. Adjust both the upper and the lower parts of the lap-shoulder belt as snugly as possible.

You should adjust your position in the seat so that the belt crosses your shoulder without chafing your neck. Never slip the upper part of the belt off your shoulder. Safety belts worn too loose or too high on the abdomen can cause broken ribs or injuries to your abdomen. But more damage is caused when they aren't used at all.

Child Safety Seats

In 1987, child safety seats saved the lives of about 200 children under age four. If child safety seats had been correctly used on all child passengers that year, an additional 300 lives could have been saved.

When your child is traveling in a motor vehicle, the safest place for him or her is in a child safety seat correctly installed on the rear seat of the vehicle. The most dangerous place is in someone's arms—even yours or a loving grandparent's. During a crash, an unbelted person holding an infant or a child is thrown forward with enough force to crush the child against the unyielding, hard surface of the dashboard or the windshield. Even if the adult holding the child is wearing a safety belt, the adult will not be able to hold on to the child during an accident. Sometimes the force of a collision is so great that the child is thrown from the person's arms and out of the vehicle.

Each child should have his or her own safety seat. A child should never share a safety belt with an adult.

All fifty states and the District of Columbia now have child passenger protection laws requiring the use of child safety seats. Before giving birth, make plans to bring your newborn baby home from the hospital in an infant safety seat. Many hospitals require parents of newborns to have an infant safety seat before they leave the hospital with their new baby. Often a safety seat can be rented from the hospital. A plastic infant carrier is *not* a safety seat, even if a seat belt is placed around it—it can shatter in an accident.

Various models of car seats are designed for infants and small children. The seats can be rented or purchased. Check with your doctor, hospital, baby stores, car dealers, or local consumer safety council about purchase or rental.

It is important that the safety seat you choose is safe and simple to use. Some seats are harder to use than others, with an elaborate system of straps and buckles. The most important aspect is safety, but the simpler the seat is to use, the more likely you'll be to use it *every* time you travel with your baby. The best safety seats are equipped with restraints that hold the baby's body at each shoulder and hip and between the legs. This design reduces the impact during a crash by spreading the force over more of the baby's body, much as a lap-shoulder belt does for an adult.

The four basic types of safety seats are

1. Infant—birth to about 20 pounds
2. Convertible—birth to about 40 pounds
3. Toddler—twenty to 40 pounds
4. Booster (for older children)—about 40 pounds

For younger infants, the safety seat should be installed on the backseat of the car, with the baby facing the rear of the car. In a head-on collision, the baby will then be pressed backward into the safety seat, with less risk of injury, and in a rear-end collision, the backseat of the car acts as a buffer to hold the safety seat more securely.

If your newborn is premature or very small, consult with the doctor about the type of seat to use. An infant seat will need to be replaced as your baby nears 20 pounds. Many parents prefer to use a convertible seat right from the start. These seats are usually designed to hold newborns and also have restraints that can be adjusted for a larger baby or child. If your vehicle is equipped with automatic safety belts or air bags, refer to your owner's manual for information on how the child safety seat should be installed and used.

Chapter 11

Postpartum Care

———— ∞ ————

THERE IS PROBABLY no more neglected stage of childbirth for the mother than the period immediately following the birth of the baby. So much energy and interest are directed to the event itself that often there is less preparation for the period following delivery. Your doctor, who paid very close attention to you those last few weeks, relaxes more about your condition once he or she is certain you are fine.

For one thing, you will be tired. Labor requires an expenditure of energy equal to that needed for a 12-mile hike, and while this is more than compensated for by the exhilaration of birth itself, the postpartum period can be a little anticlimactic.

Most women do not anticipate or are not prepared for the pain that may be present in the episiotomy: The stitches that close it hurt. This is temporary, usually lasting four to five days, and can be greatly alleviated by analgesics, local preparations, and sitz baths.

Hemorrhoids can also develop after birth, especially after prolonged pushing in the second stage of labor. These painful engorged veins in the rectal area are also temporary and can be relieved by various medications.

Uterine cramps are bothersome after delivery, especially when breast-feeding. Uterine cramps are a manifestation of the body getting back to its normal state. They usually last for less than a week and are worse after having a previous baby. Analgesics help lessen the discomfort.

A few days following delivery, you may become very depressed for no apparent reason. This postpartum depression—the "baby blues"—is not clearly understood but is rather common and should be no cause for concern.

The discomforts of the episiotomy, hemorrhoids, or uterine cramps may add to your blues. But remember, those are temporary discomforts that can be greatly alleviated by medications. It won't be long

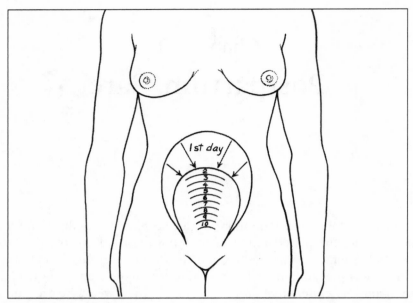

The speed with which the uterus returns to normal depends on many factors.
In women who do not nurse, the shrinkage is slower than shown above.

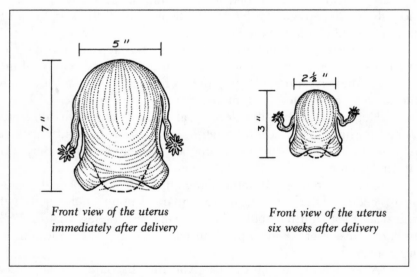

Front view of the uterus
immediately after delivery

Front view of the uterus
six weeks after delivery

INVOLUTION OF THE UTERUS POSTPARTUM

before you are feeling great and strolling with your new infant in the park for all to admire.

Basically, you must remember to prepare for the period following birth as actively as you prepared for birth itself. This may include hiring a nurse or inviting a family member to come help with cleaning, cooking, caring for other children, or showing you how to take care of the baby when you come home from the hospital.

GENERAL INSTRUCTIONS

After delivery, you will be taken to your room to rest. The baby may not be brought to you for the first eight to twelve hours, to allow you both time to get acclimated. If you have chosen rooming-in as an option, your newborn will be with you right after birth, so that you can begin bonding immediately.

You will be encouraged to urinate so that a tube will not have to be passed into the bladder to help you void. This procedure, called catheterization, is often required when you have not been able to void because prolonged labor has weakened your bladder muscles.

You will probably be given pain relievers for the stitches and heat-lamp treatments or sitz baths for the episiotomy and the hemorrhoids. A cream will be supplied to put on the stitches to keep them moist—they have a tendency to pull when they dry out. The nurses will show you how to change your sanitary pads and clean off after you go to the bathroom, to prevent infected stitches.

You should move your bowels within four days following delivery. If you do not, a mild laxative or a gentle enema or suppositories are often required.

A nonnursing mother requires no special breast care except a good support bra. In the past, nonnursing mothers were sometimes given pills to prevent lactation; however, those medications have been removed from the market for this purpose due to dangerous side effects. Mothers who have breast engorgement can use ice packs and pain relievers and should restrict fluid intake for about two days, allowing the problem to solve itself. Nursing mothers suffering from engorgement can squeeze some of the fluid out, either by hand or by using the hospital's breast pump.

If you are Rh negative and your baby is Rh positive, you should receive your immunization with Rh immunoglobin within seventy-two hours after delivery.

Upon returning home, you should rest for the first few weeks, and, as tolerance permits, resume normal activity slowly. Keep socializing to a minimum. You will be tired enough receiving family and friends who come to see the baby.

You should bathe daily. Baths will help the episiotomy, and primping a little will make you feel better.

Begin exercising slowly. Walking with the baby is probably as much as you will need to do for a little while. Many women like to do exercises to firm up stomach muscles. Ask your doctor when you can start these.

You should refrain from intercourse for the first six weeks following delivery to give your body a chance to return to normal, allow the stitches to heal, and avoid the possibility of infection. Upon resumption of sexual relations, you may experience some discomfort for a while. Pain of some sort is common. With patience, relaxation, lubricants if necessary, and tender loving care, this, too, will soon end, and sexual relations will be normal again.

If the vagina feels relaxed and open upon resuming sexual activity, the so-called Kegel exercises can help (see page 219). As you practice these isometric exercises more frequently, you will increase vaginal tone.

While pregnancy and postpartum care are states of health and not illness, a little conservative management does not hurt. Rest will affect the milk production in a nursing mother and will therefore influence the satisfaction of the baby's needs. Try to take a nap each day.

PHYSICAL CHANGES AND EXERCISES

Although everything appears to return to normal very quickly, physical changes occur in the body for a long time following delivery.

The organs of reproduction begin returning to their prepregnant state almost immediately in a process known as *involution*. The uterus slowly shrinks in size, going from 1½ pounds the first week following delivery to its normal weight of 2 ounces in six weeks.

The vagina and the external genitalia, which stretched tremendously for delivery, gradually regain their muscle tone over an eight-week period. The vaginal opening also becomes smaller as muscles firm up.

The uterus continues to shed the lining it used to support pregnancy. This discharge is called lochia. It is bloody at first and then becomes white in color and creamy in consistency. It has a characteristic odor, which some women find unpleasant. Lochia usually stops three to six weeks following delivery.

When ovulation and menstruation return depends on whether or not you are nursing. Ovulation resumes in the first three months following delivery for 90 percent of nonnursing mothers. The hormonal changes caused by lactation generally delay the return of menstruation, although most nursing women will have a period long before nursing is ended.

The delay of ovarian function in nursing has led many women to think that nursing is a good method of contraception. It is not.

Many women find that muscle tone in the abdomen returns very slowly. The rate at which this occurs is determined by several factors, including the individual mother's muscle constitution and the amount of stretching the abdomen has undergone. Exercises to remedy this are outlined in the following section.

Postpartum Exercises

You should check with your physician before instituting an exercise program. The following exercises are helpful to most healthy women after they give birth.

First Week

Leg raises. Lie flat on your back, legs straight out. Raise your legs alternately 6 inches, keeping them straight. Repeat four to five times.

Tighten abdominal muscles. Lie on your back. Contract your abdominal muscles, arch your back, and push your buttocks against the floor, then push your back against the floor and raise your pelvic area. Repeat four to five times.

Second Week

Increase the number of times you do the previous exercises and add a *pelvic twist:* Lying flat on your back, bring your knees to your chest, arms straight to your sides. Keep your shoulders flat and twist your pelvic area so that your left knee touches the floor. Rest, then do a right pelvic twist. Work up slowly to ten twists.

Third Week

In addition to the previous exercise, you can start *sit-ups:* Lying flat on your back, with your knees bent and your arms in front, raise yourself slowly at the waist. It will help if your toes are placed under a couch or a ledge for countertraction. This exercise will be difficult at first, but in the long run, it will get your abdominal muscles back into shape. Slowly work up to ten to twenty per day.

Fourth to Sixth Week

Walking, jogging, tennis, swimming, and other aerobic exercises can be restarted and prepregnancy activity levels gradually resumed.

DISCOMFORTS

After delivery, you may find that you are physically uncomfortable at times. Most of these discomforts don't last and can be relieved. Some common problems are discussed as follows:

Afterbirth pains. Afterbirth pains are caused by the uterus contracting and relaxing as it returns to its normal state. With first babies, the pain is usually mild. The contractions get stronger with subsequent babies and with nursing, but in all cases they last only a few days. Try changing your position or lying on your stomach with a pillow under your abdomen. Keep your bladder empty. Medication to help you feel more comfortable is available.

Painful episiotomy. Cold packs applied immediately after delivery often lessen the discomfort of an episiotomy. Later on, cold packs or a warm sitz bath (sitting for a short time in warm water) can also make you more comfortable and help the healing process. In the hospital, you will be taught how to clean the area to prevent infection.

Hemorrhoids. Hemorrhoids can protrude or become swollen and painful during pregnancy, labor, and delivery. Sprays, ointments, or dry or moist heat can provide some relief. Cold witch hazel compresses are also very soothing. The hemorrhoids will gradually decrease in size and may even disappear.

Constipation. Reduced movement through the intestines and relaxed abdominal muscles often contribute to postdelivery constipation. Fear of having a bowel movement because of the pain from an episiotomy or hemorrhoids may add to the problem. A high fiber diet, plenty of fluids and juices, dried fruit, or mild laxatives can help.

Breast engorgement. You may have fullness and discomfort in your breasts two to four days after delivery. A well-fitting support bra will help. Ice packs may be applied to relieve the discomfort. If you are not nursing, you should not empty, stimulate, or pump your breasts; this will only cause more milk to be produced. The discomfort should disappear in about thirty-six hours and can be relieved by pain medications.

Postpartum warning signs. After delivery, you should continue to watch for any abnormal changes in your health. Call your doctor if you notice any of the following symptoms:

- Fever over 100.4°F (38°C)
- Nausea and vomiting
- Painful urination, burning, and urgency (a sudden, strong desire to urinate)
- Bleeding heavier than your normal period
- Pain, swelling, and tenderness in the legs
- Chest pain and cough
- Hot, tender breast
- Persistent perineal pain with increasing tenderness

BABY BLUES AND POSTPARTUM DEPRESSION

About 75 percent of women have the baby blues after childbirth, due to extreme changes hormonally and emotionally (after all, their lives will change forever!). Feelings of depression, anxiety, and anger can begin about three days after birth. New mothers may feel sad, anxious, and moody. For no clear reason, they may feel angry at the new baby, at their partner, or at their other children. They may cry and have trouble sleeping, eating, and making decisions. They almost always question whether they are able to handle caring for a baby. Many new mothers are surprised at how fragile, alone, and overwhelmed they feel after the birth of a child. Their feelings don't seem to match their expectations. They fear that these feelings somehow mean that they are bad mothers.

As bewildering and frightening as these thoughts and feelings seem at the time, the baby blues usually last only for a short time— a few hours to a week or so—and go away without the need for treatment.

Some women develop a postpartum depression, which is marked by more intense feelings of sadness, anxiety, or despair that disrupt their ability to function. This true psychiatric illness is estimated to occur in 10 to 20 percent of all women after delivery. Known risk factors for this condition are a history of manic depression (bipolar depression) and schizophrenia or a family history of those illnesses. A 2002 study looked at pregnancy-related risk factors and found that sick leave and an increased number of office visits during pregnancy were risk factors for developing postpartum depression. In addition, women who had hyperemesis gravidarum, premature contractions, and psychological disorders were more likely to develop this condition. Interestingly, there was no relationship between the type of delivery, whether natural or cesarean, or economic status and postpartum depression. If not recognized and treated, postpartum depression may become worse or may last longer than it needs to. If you have any of the following signs of postpartum depression, you should discuss this with your doctor and take steps right away to get the support and the help you need.

- Baby blues that don't go away after two weeks, or strong feelings of depression and anger that begin a month or two after delivery
- Sleep disorders: being unable to sleep even when exhausted, or sleeping most of the time
- Feelings of sadness, doubt, guilt, helplessness, or hopelessness that seem to increase with each week
- Extremes in concern and worry about the baby, or lack of interest in or feelings for the baby
- Anxiety or panic attacks
- Fear of harming the baby or thoughts of harming yourself
- Marked changes in appetite

Periods of sadness, fear, anger, and anxiety after childbirth are quite common and do not mean that you are a failure as a mother or that you are mentally ill. They do mean that you and your body are adjusting to the hormonal and other changes that follow the birth of a child.

THE SIX-WEEK CHECKUP

You will probably see your doctor for a checkup six weeks after delivery. The doctor will weigh you, check your breasts, do a pelvic exam, and take a Pap smear. If you have any questions about sexual hygiene, contraception, or minor physical concerns, ask them now.

At this time, you can be refitted for a diaphragm, or you can start on birth-control pills if you are not breast-feeding. And you'll probably be given the go-ahead for sexual relations at this time.

You should continue to see your doctor on a regular basis—twice a year if you are taking birth-control pills, once per year otherwise—for a general checkup.

NUTRITION AND DIET

You will lose about 10 to 20 pounds within ten days after delivery. You might be disappointed that you're not losing more so that you can get back to your old self, but be patient. If you continue to eat the well-balanced diet that you began in pregnancy, in an amount appropriate for your body weight, you will return to your normal weight within two months of delivery. Coupling this diet with exercise will keep your muscles in tone.

If you are breast-feeding, you need extra fluid, calories, calcium, and protein. A nursing mother needs the foods normally required for her own body, plus extra food to produce milk for her baby—about 600 to 1,000 more calories a day than she needed before pregnancy. It is easy to add the extra food needed for nursing if you are already eating a well-balanced diet made up of a variety of foods.

WORK

There are a number of factors to consider in deciding whether and when to resume working after the birth of your baby. Your doctor may recommend that you remain at home for a certain period of time to recover your strength before returning to work.

Finances should be considered, of course, as well as the cost and the availability of child care. If you are breast-feeding, you may have to wean your baby or cut down the number of feedings before you return to work full time. Breast milk can be saved to be given to the baby later, if you can't be there.

Employers are becoming more flexible and offering more options to working mothers. Many women work part time or even share one full-time job with someone else. With home computers, copiers, and fax machines, some women find that they can work comfortably at home.

SEX

Before having sexual intercourse, you should wait until the healing process is complete to avoid hurting delicate tissues. Sexual intercourse can usually be resumed when your pelvic structures and the episiotomy are healed and you feel comfortable. This usually takes about four to six weeks. It is important for you and your partner to discuss this beforehand with your doctor and with each other.

When you think you are ready to resume sexual relations, proceed slowly and gently. Try to choose a time when you are not rushed. You may notice a dryness of the vagina. This decreased lubrication is a normal response of your body. It may last as long as you breast-feed or until your first menstrual period. Use a water-soluble cream or jelly or saliva to provide extra lubrication during this time. For your comfort, try different sexual positions.

Sometimes you may not be as interested in sex as you were before you gave birth. Fatigue is often the main cause of a lack of interest in sex at this time for both men and women. The emotional stress caused by the changing roles of both new parents and the constant demands of the baby may decrease your desire. You just may be too tired. You may also be afraid that intercourse will be painful because you have had an episiotomy or you may fear becoming pregnant again. If there are difficulties, it is important to talk about them. Spend time together without the baby.

ON BECOMING A PARENT

After waiting nine long months, you suddenly are a parent. The bonding process, whereby parents and their baby become closely attached to each other through touching, eye contact, and face-to-face relationship, will help you be relaxed about handling and caring for a tiny baby. This process is the first step toward becoming a closely knit family. It will help your newborn begin to develop emotional and social attachments.

Take every opportunity to become acquainted with your new baby as soon as possible after birth. Every time you pick up your baby, you increase the feeling of belonging to each other. Hold your baby close, talk, sing, cuddle, and look into his or her eyes. The newborn can detect a warm, friendly presence and will respond in many ways.

Through the close contact you and your baby have in the hospital, you get to know a great deal about each other. At home, your mutual interests will grow stronger every day, although your baby will be mostly self-centered during the first few months. When your baby cries, don't hesitate to show your love by holding, patting, and kissing. We don't believe that parents spoil babies by loving them.

As time goes by, your infant will become more familiar with the sound of your voice. Talk to your baby while you bathe, diaper, play with, and feed him or her. Eventually, the infant will respond to the rhythm and the tone of your voice with smiles, sounds, and gestures long before what you are saying becomes intelligible. Communication systems will gradually develop. They are unique to the two of you, and your baby will learn to make you aware of likes and dislikes in a private way.

Your baby's daily life will consist of many feedings, naps, baths, and, eventually, daytime walks. Establishing a predictable daily routine will make the baby feel more secure and more relaxed. It may even help develop memory skills. An orderly routine will also help you to be more organized and efficient in baby care. As the weeks go by, your baby will grow and learn. Remember, no two babies are exactly alike, and your baby won't develop according to a precise schedule in a book. The individual pace is what makes your baby unique. It allows him or her to develop a personality and achieve new accomplishments. Development takes time. Encourage your baby but do not push. Physical and emotional growth occur together. In addition to rapid growth in weight and length, development will occur in the coordination of the muscles, the recognition of objects and people, and an increasing ability to perform little tasks. Don't forget that your baby is an individual who is different from any other. Your doctor will evaluate his or her individual physical and emotional progress during periodic checks.

Being a Father

A good opportunity for the baby and the father to be alone together is during night feedings. If the baby is not being breast-fed or if supplemental bottles are occasionally used, this private time together while the rest of the family is asleep helps a father and his baby form a special closeness. A close relationship with the new baby starts during the pregnancy and continues in the hospital and at home. Many fathers feel a little insecure about handling a baby because of little experience in doing so, but your baby won't mind if you are awkward. Giving love is much more important than changing a diaper expertly or holding a baby just right.

Since the advent of the prepared childbirth classes and Lamaze deliveries, fathers have become a very vital part of the birth process. This should continue at home.

Being a Mother

Delivery is a strenuous physical experience. Your body will need rest. In order to get that rest, you cannot permit the baby to demand your attention every minute. Child rearing should not become exhausting. Other members of the family should share in child care and household tasks. This will enable you to overcome your tiredness, to rest, and to feel better about yourself and your baby.

Becoming a mother should not interfere with your being a person in your own right. Some depression or blueness is common during the first few months, but soon afterward you will be able to resume your normal activities. The demands of continued baby care may be exhausting, so it's important for you to concentrate on looking and feeling your best. If you can, have a grandparent, a friend, or a sitter take care of the baby for an afternoon or an evening so that you can get out, visit a friend, have dinner, go to the movies, or do whatever else you enjoy. Your baby will be there when you return, and you will be ready to spend some solid time with him or her.

Many professional women will go back to work six to eight weeks after delivery. You may have ambivalent feelings about leaving your baby. But remember that in the long run, the most successful mother is one who is happy and satisfied with her own life; her baby will reflect this.

You may have many mixed emotions about becoming a parent. You may find yourself resenting the baby and then feeling guilty, and you may have fears about your ability to become a parent. These feelings are not unusual. Most parents experience them at some point. Don't aim to be perfect—no parent is. But if you do your best, you probably will be a better parent than you think you are.

Remember to find time for yourself. It is important to you as an individual to keep the interests you have developed after the baby comes and as your family grows. You may not have as much time for them, but there is no reason for you to give them up completely.

Part IV

GENERAL CONSIDERATIONS

Chapter 12

Conditions Associated with Pregnancy

——∞∞∞——

THE PURPOSE OF prenatal care is to watch for certain conditions of pregnancy that can prove harmful to both mother and baby. Knowing what they are and their danger signs will help you understand the nature of pregnancy and what can be done to ensure a successful outcome for both patients.

PRETERM LABOR

Labor that begins after twenty weeks but before the end of thirty-six weeks is called preterm labor. Approximately 40 to 50 percent of the time, preterm labor accounts for preterm deliveries. The remainder of preterm deliveries results from preterm premature rupture of the membranes. Being born too early—before a baby is fully ready for life on its own—is a major cause of problems in infants. Most of the preterm deliveries in the United States are close to term. Even though only 1 to 2 percent of births are less than thirty-two weeks' gestation, they account for almost 50 percent of the babies who are brain damaged and around 60 percent of the babies who die. In the United States, the preterm delivery rate is approximately 11 percent, while in Europe the rate varies between 5 and 7 percent. Despite all the improvements in medical care, the rate of preterm delivery has actually increased slightly over the last forty years. For about two-thirds of women who begin labor before the end of thirty-six weeks, the exact cause of preterm labor is never known.

Preterm labor seems to be linked to a number of risk factors:

- Nonwhite race
- Age younger than seventeen or older than thirty-five

- Low socioeconomic status
- Previous preterm labor or history of preterm birth
- Pregnancy with twins or multiple fetuses
- A history of several induced abortions
- Abnormalities of the cervix (e.g., incompetent cervix) or the uterus (e.g., malformations or fibroids)
- Abdominal surgery during the late second and the third trimester of the current pregnancy
- Presence of serious infection in the mother
- Bleeding in the second trimester of the current pregnancy
- Poor maternal weight gain or weight of less than 100 pounds
- Diabetes
- Hypertension
- DES exposure of mother in utero
- Placenta previa or placental separation
- Increased or decreased volume of amniotic fluid
- Maternal smoking

Women who have little or no prenatal care seem to be at increased risk for preterm labor. A number of other factors have to do with the mother's medical history, as well as her previous and current pregnancies. Having one or more of these factors does not mean that you will have preterm labor, only that you are at increased risk of giving birth to a preterm baby during this pregnancy.

Preterm labor is of serious concern because premature infants often have problems outside the uterus. Depending on how early they are born, preterm babies often need special medical care in order to breathe, eat, and keep warm. The medical problems are most common and most severe for infants born before thirty-two weeks of pregnancy, but they may affect all preterm infants to some extent. Despite the rise in the incidence of preterm deliveries over the years, the survival rate has improved dramatically, thanks to major improvements in the special care nurseries around the United States. It is possible these days to see normal survival of a 1- to 2-pound baby born extremely premature.

Table 12.1 shows the chances an infant has of surviving when delivered at various weeks of pregnancy in the best centers and its chances of having major problems after birth.

Major advances in neonatal facilities and improvements in treatments for the preterm laboring patient have clearly improved infant survival. The extremely premature babies (twenty-five weeks and less)

TABLE 12.1
Chance of Survival Based on Mean Birth Weight

GESTATIONAL AGE (WEEKS)	MEAN BIRTH WEIGHT (G)	CHANCE OF SURVIVAL (%)	CHANCE OF SURVIVAL FREE OF MAJOR PROBLEMS
22	500	rare	0
24	650	25	9
26	900	80	41
28	1,150	91	67
30	1,400	95	81
32	1,750	97	90
34	2,200	99	95
36	2,600	99+	98

that do survive, however, have about a 50 percent chance of having disabilities, and 25 percent have major disabilities. Because preterm babies are usually of low birth weight (weighing less than 5 ½ pounds at birth), their health and survival may be threatened. Babies born too early often have organs that are not developed enough to function properly. For instance, the lungs of a preterm infant are often not fully developed, and the newborn may have trouble getting enough air. This condition is called *respiratory distress syndrome (RDS)*. Recently, it was discovered that giving injections of corticosteroids (steroids) to the mother threatening to deliver at between twenty-four and thirty-four weeks' gestation improves survival and reduces the risk of RDS. This is now considered to be the standard of care. Apnea, or interrupted breathing, often occurs in preterm and low-birth-weight babies in the first days or weeks of life. A preterm baby may also have problems with swallowing, making it necessary for him or her to be fed through a tube. Sometimes the very premature infant may have undeveloped intestines, and a fatal intestinal infection called necrotizing enterocolitis (NEC) can develop simply from feeding the baby. Since the skull is very soft, there can be bleeding in the brain, called intraventricular hemorrhage. Since preterm babies often don't have enough body fat, they may have trouble maintaining body temperature.

The first signs of preterm labor are often subtle and painless and may begin slowly. If preterm labor is discovered early enough, preterm delivery can often be prevented or postponed. Sometimes the signs that preterm labor may be starting are fairly easy to detect—for example, when the membranes rupture (your water breaks). Other times, though, the signs of preterm labor are very mild and may be very hard to detect. The following is a list of the early signs of preterm labor. If you experience any of these signs, call your doctor.

- Abdominal cramps, with or without diarrhea
- Regular contractions or uterine tightening
- Low, dull backache
- Pelvic or lower abdominal pressure
- Vaginal discharge: change in type (watery, mucous, or bloody) or increase in amount

Finding out whether you are actually in labor is often quite difficult, as many women throughout pregnancy will have occasional uterine contractions without being in preterm labor. Traditionally, the doctor would examine you to see whether your cervix has begun to change. Fetal monitoring tests are usually used to record the heartbeat of the fetus and contractions of the uterus. Ultrasound is used to estimate the size and the age of the fetus and to determine its position in the uterus. You may be watched for a time and then examined again to see whether your cervix continues to change, which confirms preterm labor. Often, if you wait to see changes in the cervix, it may be too late to stop labor. New methods have recently been developed and are available to your doctor to check whether labor has started. Scientists have discovered a biochemical marker that is released into the cervix and the vagina at the very early stages of labor. This marker is called fetal fibronectin, and it can easily be detected with a special kit. This test can be reassuring to women who are not sure if they are truly in labor, because if the test fails to detect fetal fibronectin (negative test), there is less than a 1 percent chance of delivery in the next one to two weeks. In addition, advances in ultrasound have enabled the obstetrician to evaluate more subtle changes in the cervix and the surrounding tissues to detect really early evidence of preterm labor.

If labor is detected at its earliest stages, and there are no apparent signs that you and your baby are in danger from infection, bleeding, or other complications, your doctor may try to stop the labor. Sometimes bed rest and hydration—extra fluids given by mouth or through a tube inserted into a vein—are enough to stop contractions.

Your doctor may treat preterm labor by giving you drugs that can stop or suppress contractions. These drugs are usually given by injection but can also be taken orally or rectally. The following is a list of currently prescribed drugs, known as *tocolytics*, used to reduce contractions:

Magnesium sulfate. This drug must be given intravenously. It can have dangerous side effects, so the preterm labor patient must be monitored closely in the hospital while on this drug. With proper monitoring, magnesium sulfate can be safe and effective in halting delivery for at least twenty-four to forty-eight hours.

Terbutaline (Brethine). This medication was originally known as a treatment for asthma, as it relaxes the muscles in the lungs and helps with breathing. In addition, it helps to relax the muscles of the uterus. Usually, terbutaline is given by injection under the skin. A newer delivery method for terbutaline has been designed. It is given through a special pump that releases the drug continuously. Additional amounts of the drug can be given when uterine contractions increase. The terbutaline pump can be used both in the hospital and at home. Common side effects include heart palpitations.

Nifedipine (Procardia). Also used for high blood pressure and other heart problems, this drug is effective in decreasing contractions. Nifedipine is given by mouth every six to eight hours. Side effects include low blood pressure in the mother.

Indomethacin (Indocin). Also used to treat generalized pain and fever, this drug can be effective for preterm labor. It can be given orally, vaginally, or rectally. It may cause intestinal side effects in the mother, and it cannot be used for more than forty-eight hours, because it can affect the production of amniotic fluid.

If you have had signs of preterm labor, your doctor may advise you to make changes in your lifestyle, including learning how to monitor your contractions or taking drugs.

If you are at risk for preterm labor, you should take special care of yourself during pregnancy. A healthy pregnancy—including early prenatal care, good nutrition, and adequate rest—is the best prevention. Your doctor may ask you to come in more often for exams and tests. Avoid lifting and other strenuous or tiring tasks during pregnancy. Women at risk may also be advised to cut down on travel. And they should avoid nipple preparation for breast-feeding, since stimulating the nipples can sometimes lead to uterine contractions. Your doctor may advise you to restrict sexual activity or to monitor yourself for contractions after intercourse and may suggest that your partner use a condom during sex, since this may help decrease the chance of infection.

If you are at increased risk for preterm labor, your doctor may advise you to monitor yourself for signs of uterine activity or tightening. Monitoring may be done with a machine that you use at home or by palpation by hand. If you monitor yourself by hand, it is best done at the same time each day so that you will be sensitive to any changes in uterine activity.

If you detect contractions, turn onto your side and continue monitoring for an hour. Keep track of when each contraction starts and ends and the total number of contractions per hour. Having some uterine activity before thirty-seven weeks of pregnancy is normal. But if your contractions occur more than once every ten minutes (six or more per hour) call your doctor. Remember, a diagnosis of preterm labor can be made only if changes of the cervix have been detected.

If you have had preterm labor or birth, bed rest may be prescribed. The kind of bed rest advised can vary from partial bed rest, where you can get up, go to the bathroom, and have limited activity, to staying off your feet and restricting certain activities, such as climbing stairs. It may mean that you will have to stop working. Or total bed rest may be required.

Sometimes preterm labor may be too advanced to be stopped. Or there may be reasons, such as infection, bleeding, or signs that the fetus may be having problems, that the baby is better off being born, even if it is early.

Home uterine activity monitoring (HUAM) has been in existence for almost two decades. A machine connects to a woman's abdomen over the uterus and to a telephone line. A signal is transmitted to a service to look for uterine contractions. In addition, there is daily contact between the patient and an obstetrical nurse. It was hoped that this system would help to detect preterm labor earlier than traditional means. To date, many studies have been done to test the benefits of HUAM. The largest study, which looked at approximately 2,500 women, failed to show any benefit. In fact, the U.S. Preventative Task Force in 1995 concluded that the HUAM device was not effective. The U.S. Food and Drug Administration has approved this device only for use in women with a history of preterm birth. Ask your doctor about it if you are in a high-risk category or are experiencing problems.

Your preterm baby may not look like what you expected. Most preterm babies appear quite red and skinny, because they have little fat under their skin and their blood vessels are close to the surface. After a few days, your preterm baby may develop jaundice, causing the skin to appear yellow. This condition is usually temporary.

Many preterm babies are tiny and fragile and are not ready to live on their own. They may be cared for in a neonatal intensive-care unit (NICU) for weeks and sometimes months. Your baby may be placed in an incubator to keep warm, fed through a tube, helped to breathe with a respirator, and monitored by specially trained nurses and complicated equipment. Today, with this special care, even very early, low-birth-weight babies have a much better chance of survival than they did in past years.

Your baby needs you in order to thrive. It needs to hear your voice and to feel your touch. Contact with the baby is important for the parents, too. As soon as possible, talk to your baby. Stroke him or her in the incubator. After a time, you may be able to hold and cuddle your baby for longer periods of time and help with the baby's care, and before long, you can bring the baby home with you.

POSTDATE PREGNANCY

Only 5 percent of babies are actually born on their due dates. Eighty percent of women give birth between thirty-eight and forty-two weeks of pregnancy; these are so-called full-term pregnancies. While 10 percent of women will deliver before thirty-eight weeks, the remaining 10 percent will deliver after forty-two weeks and are referred to as postterm or postdate pregnancies.

Knowing the gestational age of the fetus is the most important factor in diagnosing postdate pregnancy. Inaccurate menstrual histories, irregular menstrual periods, and other causes may make it difficult to predict the exact due date. As discussed in chapter 2, we use more than one method to cross-check the gestational age of the fetus.

About 95 percent of babies born between forty-two and forty-four weeks are delivered safely. However, if gestation extends beyond forty-two weeks, there are increased risks to the health of the fetus. It is important to remember that risks to the fetus, although real, occur in only a small number of postdate pregnancies.

The postdate fetus may be in danger because the normal functioning of the placenta may begin to decline. Also, the volume of amniotic fluid in the sac surrounding the fetus may begin to decrease. Decreased amounts of amniotic fluid may cause the umbilical cord to become pinched.

As pregnancy continues past forty-two weeks, a fetus has an increased risk of the following problems:

- *Macrosomia*—A condition in which the baby is too large to pass safely through the birth canal during delivery
- *Dysmaturity syndrome*—A condition characterized by a long and lean body, alert facial expression, abundant hair growth, long fingernails, and thickened skin

- *Fetal distress*—A sign that the baby may be having problems before delivery
- *Meconium aspiration*—Inhalation of meconium, a greenish substance that builds up in the fetus's bowels and is normally discharged shortly after birth

If a postdate pregnancy is suspected, a number of tests can help us monitor the well-being of the fetus. Generally, tests are begun at around 41 weeks of pregnancy.

- A *fetal movement chart* is simply a record of how often you feel your baby move. Healthy babies tend to move about the same amount each day. If you notice decreased movement, you should perform *kick counts*. This is done by lying on your side and recording specific fetal movements. Once you have counted ten discrete movements, you may stop counting. If more than two hours pass without ten movements noted, this is considered five standard deviations below the mean, and you should report this to your doctor immediately.
- In *electronic fetal monitoring*, electronic instruments are placed on your abdomen to record the fetus's heart rate in response to its own movements or to contractions of your uterus. The two types of tests that can provide reliable information on the fetus's health are the nonstress test (NST) and the contraction stress test (CST).
- *Ultrasound* can be used to measure the amount of amniotic fluid and to reveal important information about the placenta.
- *Amniocentesis* can sometimes provide further information about the amniotic fluid. Examination of the fluid can detect the presence of meconium and can determine whether the fetus's lungs are mature enough for it to be born.

If the fetus appears to be active and healthy and the amniotic fluid appears to be normal, your pregnancy may continue to be monitored at regular intervals until labor begins on its own. If the fetus appears to be in danger, it should be delivered, either by inducing labor or by cesarean birth. (See chapter 8.) Labor can also be induced electively. Recent studies have evaluated elective induction versus waiting and performing testing on the fetus. There have been various results with regard to costs and cesarean section rates. As far as outcome data (the health of the newborn), there appears to be no difference in either group. We feel that if the cervical exam is favorable, induction of labor should be performed after 41 weeks, and it should be performed after forty-two weeks in almost all circumstances.

With postdate pregnancies, continuous electronic fetal monitoring is usually recommended during labor. If problems occur during labor, the baby may be delivered by cesarean birth. Once born, a postdate baby may need special care and monitoring.

Remember, most postdate babies are born healthy and delivered safely. Tests and careful monitoring during the last weeks of pregnancy and during labor will help ensure this outcome.

IF YOUR BABY IS BREECH

If an infant delivers with its feet or buttocks first, this is called breech presentation. It occurs in about 3 out of every 100 full-term births. Although most breech babies are born healthy, they do have a higher risk for certain problems than do babies in the head-first position.

By the last month of pregnancy, most babies move into the head-down, or vertex, presentation. Most of the babies who don't turn by then will be in a breech presentation when it's time for delivery. The baby will be sitting in the uterus, with its head up and its buttocks, feet, or both down.

The doctor makes the diagnosis of a breech presentation by carefully feeling the baby through your abdomen and uterus. By placing his or her hands at certain points on your lower abdomen, the doctor can try to make out the general position of the baby's head, back, and buttocks. Ultrasound may be used to confirm the diagnosis. Because your baby may keep moving around until the end of pregnancy, the diagnosis of a breech is sometimes made when labor begins.

Breech presentations are more common when certain other factors are present:

- The mother has had more than one previous pregnancy.
- There is more than one fetus (twins or more) in the uterus.
- The uterus is not normal in shape or has abnormal growths, such as fibroids.
- The uterus has too much (polyhydramnios) or too little (oligohydramnios) amniotic fluid.

- The placenta partly or fully covers the opening of the uterus—a condition known as placenta previa.
- The baby is premature.

What Makes a Breech Delivery More Difficult?

At the time of birth a baby's head is the largest part of its body, as well as the firmest. When the baby is in the normal head-down position, the largest part of the body is born first, after a long period of molding to fit the birth canal, and the rest usually follows easily. In a breech birth, though, the baby's head is the last part to emerge, and it may be harder to ease it through the birth canal, especially without the benefit of molding.

Breech presentation can pose serious risks for premature babies. Because they are so small and fragile, and because their heads are relatively larger, their bodies don't stretch the cervix as wide as full-term babies do during birth. This means that there may be less room for the head to emerge. For this and other reasons, breech babies who are premature are often delivered by cesarean birth.

Another problem associated with breeches is called cord prolapse. This means that the umbilical cord slides to the bottom of the uterus, toward the birth canal, during delivery. As the baby's buttocks and legs move down into the birth canal, the cord can get squeezed, slowing the baby's supply of oxygen and blood.

According to the National Center for Health Statistics, in 1999 approximately 85 percent of women whose babies were not head down (i.e., they were breech presentation) at term went on to have a cesarean section. In 2000, a large well-respected study was released that compared a planned vaginal breech delivery to an elective cesarean section. The researchers found unequivocally that although there was no difference in the maternal outcome, the babies who had planned vaginal deliveries had a significantly higher rate of problems. Therefore, the current recommendation for women with breech babies is to have cesarean section.

External Cephalic Version (ECV)

By the completion of your thirty-seventh week of pregnancy, the position of the fetus should be known. If your doctor diagnoses a breech position, a lengthy discussion of options should be presented. If the baby stays in the breech position, a cesarean section is extremely likely. Because it is unlikely that the fetus will spontaneously turn to the head-down position by this time, your doctor may offer an external cephalic version (ECV). This procedure involves applying pressure to the mother's abdomen to turn the fetus in either a forward or a backward somersault to achieve a head-down position. The procedure is somewhat painful but is usually well tolerated. In rare cases, ECV can lead to fetal distress, so it is important to be close to a facility equipped to perform an immediate cesarean section. The success rate of ECV varies but averages around 60 percent. This rate generally increases in women who have had more than one baby, have a larger volume of amniotic fluid, are thinner, and whose placenta is behind the fetus. Although ECV is easier before thirty-seven weeks, this is generally not recommended, as there is risk of fetal distress, and many fetuses will turn on their own.

Remember, most breech babies are born healthy and normal. When you know about the problems and possible solutions, you will be in the best position to work with your doctor to ensure the best possible outcome.

PREMATURE RUPTURE OF MEMBRANES

Premature rupture of membranes (PROM) is the rupture of the membranes prior to the onset of labor. The interval from the rupture of the membranes to the onset of regular contractions of labor is called the latent period.

The cause of PROM is not well understood. At term, membranes undergo changes that cause them to weaken. Therefore, the rupture of the membranes at term is normal. Overall, PROM occurs in approximately 10 percent of patients and is associated with at least 30 percent of preterm deliveries. PROM, like preterm labor, is more common among those of poor socioeconomic groups, teenagers, and smokers. It is more likely to occur with the presence of sexually transmitted diseases. Many cases of PROM are caused by infection.

When PROM occurs, the next likely event is labor. Generally, the closer you are to term, the sooner labor is likely to begin. Over 90 percent of term patients and 50 percent of preterm patients will be in labor within twenty-four hours after PROM; more than 85 percent of preterm patients will be in labor within one week.

In the patient who does not go into labor immediately after the membrane's rupture, there is an increasing likelihood of infections in both the mother and the fetus as time passes before labor sets in. Depending on the degree of prematurity, the most significant fetal risks with preterm PROM are from complications related to immaturity.

Sometimes leakage of urine or a vaginal discharge is mistaken for PROM. Making the correct diagnosis of PROM depends on assessing a combination of the patient's history, a physical examination, and laboratory information.

It is important that you be examined when symptoms suggestive of rupture of membranes occur, in order to confirm the diagnosis. Examination is performed carefully to avoid introducing infection. Your doctor may confirm the diagnosis by identifying a pool of fluid in the vagina. The next step is generally to confirm the presence of amniotic fluid by testing for an alkaline environment with special paper indicators. (The environment of the vagina in pregnancy is usually acid and that of amniotic fluid is alkaline.)

The management of PROM will depend on many factors, including the age of the pregnancy, the presence of infection, the presence of labor, and evidence of fetal distress.

If your pregnancy is thirty-six weeks or older, the general course is delivery. If you are a known carrier of Group B streptococcal infection or if the status is unknown, an antibiotic should be given. (This information is covered later in this chapter.) In the absence of fetal distress or infection, you can be observed for signs of labor. However, some physicians actively induce labor with PROM after thirty-six weeks. Both methods are currently acceptable.

Between thirty-two and thirty-six weeks, many factors can determine management. Often, the amniotic fluid can be collected either through a vaginal pool of fluid or through amniocentesis. The fluid can then be tested for a chemical that provides evidence that the lungs of the baby are mature and that the baby is therefore ready to be delivered. In this case, waiting may increase the risk of infection and poor outcome. If the amniotic fluid test fails to demonstrate lung maturity, the doctor will try to prolong the pregnancy, provided there is no evidence of infection, fetal distress, or active labor, because the main risk to the baby is prematurity. The patient will most likely be hospitalized for continuous monitoring for infection, fetal distress, and labor. Occasionally, a patient will stop leaking and can go home. If infection does occur after PROM, delivery should be hastened. The use of an antibiotic prophylaxis at this stage is recommended because it has been shown to improve outcome. As mentioned earlier, the use of steroids in the mother can help accelerate maturity. With PROM, their use is controversial at this fetal age. Steroids can not only make it more difficult to diagnose infection, they may weaken the mother's immune system, thereby increasing the risk of infection.

If the gestation is less than thirty-two weeks—unless there is infection, fetal distress, or active labor—the doctor will attempt to prolong the pregnancy. Studies have shown that both prophylactic antibiotics and steroids should be used at this stage, as they improve outcome. Even at this early gestational age, any evidence of infection requires delivery.

Your doctor may want to consider using drugs (tocolytics) to stop contractions if labor begins. Currently, no studies in the literature have shown that these medications prolong pregnancies more than forty-eight hours. This may prevent labor long enough to administer steroids and antibiotics.

PROM at less than twenty-four weeks is associated with poor fetal outcome. The overall survival rate is approximately 30 percent. About half of the babies who survive have severe disabilities. Because of these data, parents may want to consider pregnancy termination. The only exception to this is when the membranes rupture following a genetic amniocentesis (see chapter 7). In this case, if amniocentesis causes rupture of the membranes, the hole created will often seal on its own, without any treatment.

PROM is one of the more common complications of pregnancy, but modern obstetrical and neonatal care can often ensure a happy ending.

TOXEMIA OF PREGNANCY

Preeclampsia is probably the best-documented but least understood condition of pregnancy. It is seen only in pregnant human beings and is thought to be caused by a toxic agent that originates in the placenta, the kidneys, or both, although doctors are not certain of this. We still do not know the cause of toxemia.

The condition is characterized by high blood pressure, fluid retention, and the presence of protein in the urine, usually during the third trimester. There are varying degrees of severity of this disease, though most cases are mild. General treatment requires early recognition. During prenatal examinations, doctors look for the predisposing factors of high blood pressure, kidney disease, multiple pregnancy, poor nutrition, and obesity. The incidence is higher among poor women.

Toxemia is a problem because it can cause a chemical environment in the mother's body that prevents the placenta from properly doing its job. Early detection and treatment of mild toxemia are the best ways to keep severe problems from occurring. Precautions include ensuring a well-balanced diet to minimize weight gain. Early prenatal care is important to prevent toxemia. A good deal of rest is required for the toxemic mother, especially if she also has high blood pressure. If the latter condition persists, the doctor may prescribe some of the new blood pressure–reducing drugs that have been so successful lately. Many doctors admit toxemic women, especially those with severe cases, into the hospital before their due date to monitor them and to prepare for early delivery, so that the toxic agents in the mother's system do not interfere with the continued growth of the baby. Six decades ago, toxemia was a real problem. Today, however, with good prenatal care, the seriousness of toxemia has been reduced tremendously.

The use of nonstress tests, fetal monitoring, serial sonograms, and amniocentesis for lung maturity has helped a great deal in our management of this pregnancy complication. Much research has been devoted to finding ways to prevent preeclampsia. Treatment with low-dose aspirin and calcium supplementation was thought to help prevent the development of this condition. Unfortunately, studies have failed to show any benefit. Recently, treatment with 1,000 mg of vitamin C and 400 mg of vitamin E daily has shown some promise in reducing preeclampsia.

DIABETES

Medical science has made it possible for a diabetic mother to go through pregnancy safely and have a healthy baby. Yet diabetes, a disorder in the body's use of sugars, should be closely monitored in pregnancy.

All pregnant women between the twenty-fourth and the twenty-eighth week of pregnancy should be screened for diabetes. In fact, more than 94 percent of obstetricians surveyed in the United States recommend universal screening. Your doctor will give you 50 grams of sugar orally, usually supplied in one bottle of flavored soda. After one hour, your blood will be tested for sugar levels. If the test shows elevated sugar levels, a formal glucose tolerance test should be performed. This test is performed after a fast with a fasting sugar blood level, a large glucose load, then one-, two-, and three-hour blood sugar levels. If two out of four sugars are elevated, the diagnosis of diabetes is made. Approximately 2 to 5 percent of women will have diabetes in pregnancy. Almost all women diagnosed with diabetes in pregnancy will no longer be diabetic after pregnancy is over.

Once the diagnosis of pregnancy-induced diabetes, or gestational diabetes, has been made, the patient should receive nutritional counseling to reduce the sugar in her diet, and she should learn to periodically check her blood sugar levels. Most often, diabetes can be well controlled through diet alone. Sometimes it is necessary to use oral medications and insulin to help with sugar control. If a woman is able to achieve good sugar control, fetal outcome is expected to be excellent.

If the sugar control is poor, pregnancies can be complicated. Babies of diabetic mothers can get very large, and this can increase the risk of birth trauma. Diabetics also have an increased risk for high blood pressure, preeclampsia, and unexplained fetal demise. The use of fetal monitoring, ultrasound, and amniocentesis is especially valuable in the care of these pregnancies. Often, induction of labor is recommended early in these patients.

RH DISEASE

Rh incompatibility, in which the mother has Rh-negative blood and the father and the baby have Rh-positive blood, occurs in 13 percent of all pregnancies. The Rh factor is named for the rhesus monkey, a species of animal in whose blood it is always found. Humans who have the factor are Rh positive. Those who do not have it are Rh negative. Fifteen percent of women are Rh negative.

Rh disease can occur because, following the delivery of the placenta, a small amount of the baby's red blood cells spills into the mother's circulatory system. If the baby is Rh positive and the mother is not, the mother will begin to build up permanent antibodies to the Rh factor. If a subsequent pregnancy produces a baby who is also Rh positive, the mother's new antibodies will cross the placental barrier and systematically destroy the baby's blood. To eliminate some of the toxic by-products of this blood destruction, the baby must be given an exchange transfusion at birth.

Through the development of a vaccine called Rh immunoglobulin, however, Rh disease is on the way to eradication. Given within seventy-two hours of delivery, the vaccine prevents the mother from developing antibodies, so that a second Rh-positive baby would not be growing in a hostile maternal environment. Rh immunoglobulin is almost 98 percent effective, as long as it is also given after every spontaneous or elective abortion. It also should be given to Rh-negative women who have an amniocentesis, ectopic pregnancies, and bleeding in the third trimester. Your physician will advise you on this great advance in obstetrics. Many centers use Rh immunoglobin routinely at twenty-eight weeks in normal Rh-negative women. This use is safe and does not hurt the fetus. It decreases the chances of Rh disease from 2 percent to 0.2 percent. A second dose is then also given after delivery if your baby is Rh positive.

The vaccine is not helpful to any mothers who became sensitized prior to the development of the vaccine. Those women must still rely on developments such as amniocentesis and intrauterine transfusions. In intrauterine fetal transfusions, a needle is passed through the maternal abdomen into the uterus and into the baby's umbilical cord, where blood is placed for transfusion.

ABRUPTIO PLACENTAE

Abruptio placentae is the partial detachment of the placenta from the uterus before the baby is delivered. The condition is a problem because detachment interferes with the nutrition and the respiration of the fetus. If detachment is complete, the baby has no source of food and oxygen, and the baby dies. The condition can by mild, moderate, or severe. It occurs in around 1 in 86 to 1 in 200 pregnancies. Approximately 85 percent of the time, abruptio placentae is mild or moderate, and the remainder are severe.

Abruptio placentae usually makes itself known first by bleeding, followed by sudden severe pain over the uterus.

A slight amount of premature separation is usually treated only by waiting. Often, a slight amount of separation is not diagnosed until after delivery, when a small blood clot is seen attached to the outer surface of the placenta.

Advanced separation is treated by early delivery, sometimes even by cesarean section, if there is heavy bleeding. The rate of placental separation increases with age and the number of previous pregnancies. Maternal smoking, poor nutrition, cocaine use, and infection all increase the risk. High blood pressure seems to be the most common predisposing factor. Blunt trauma is another common cause of placental separation and should always be ruled out after any injury involving the abdomen.

PLACENTA PREVIA

Sometimes the fertilized egg implants itself too low in the uterus and partially blocks the cervical opening. This condition is known as placenta previa. It usually becomes a problem late in pregnancy when the cervix begins to shorten, causing a partial separation of the placenta from the uterus, or abruptio placentae. This condition occurs in about 1 in 200 pregnancies, and its biggest risk factor is a history of having had a cesarean section.

Coverage of the cervical opening may be partial or complete. It is characterized by painless vaginal bleeding in the last trimester but can be positively diagnosed by vaginal examination in the operating room. At that point, cesarean section may be required. In general, physicians try to delay treatment for this condition until after thirty-seven weeks of gestation. Sonograms can be very helpful in the diagnosis and the management of placenta previa.

Any significant vaginal bleeding in the third trimester of pregnancy should be immediately reported to your doctor.

HERPES INFECTIONS

Herpes simplex is a virus that causes infections in men and women. It is usually transmitted by sexual contact, especially the type 2 herpes virus, which is almost exclusively in the genital tract. The virus causes painful and recurrent lesions on the external genitalia. The newborn can be infected with the virus as it travels through the birth canal, which is infected with herpes virus. Infection is more likely when there is an increasing amount of virus, such as when there is an active herpes blister in or around the birth canal. The newborn who is infected most commonly develops blisters on the skin around the eyes and the mouth. This is mild and there is no risk for serious illness or death. Less likely, the condition can affect the central nervous system (CNS). In cases of CNS disease, there is a 15 percent chance of death. Rarely, the infection can spread throughout the entire body. Here, the risk of death is around 60 percent. Considering the potential seriousness of a newborn's herpes infection, the following course of management has been suggested.

If the mother's genitalia have active herpes lesions during labor, the infant should be delivered by cesarean section to prevent infection. If the blister is completely healed or is in another location away from the genitalia, the mother can have a vaginal delivery without fearing infection to the newborn. Rupturing membranes are no longer considered to increase the likelihood of newborn infection; however, if this occurs at term and a woman has the active herpes virus in the birth canal, a cesarean section should be performed as soon as possible. If membranes rupture preterm, delivery should be considered only if indicated as outlined in the previous section under PROM.

If the mother has a known history of a recurring herpes virus, she can be given antiviral herpes medication, starting in the last four weeks of pregnancy. Although these medications have, to date, not been approved by the U.S. Food and Drug Administration for use in pregnancy, they have been used for many years now and have demonstrated no ill effects on the newborn. The newer antiherpetic drugs are much more active against the virus and therefore require less frequent dosing to cause similar effects. They are categorized as class-B medications, which indicates absence of human risk but with the caveat of limited data. Using these drugs has decreased the need for a cesarean delivery when the mother has the herpes virus. Despite the increasing incidence of genital herpes, the need for delivery by cesarean because of infection is rare and decreasing.

INTRAUTERINE GROWTH RETARDATION

Any infant born small for his or her gestational age—that is, an infant whose birth weight is in the bottom tenth percentile for his or her particular gestational age—is termed a growth-retarded baby. The risk of fetal death and possible neurological and intellectual impairments goes up with growth retardation. The causes of fetal growth retardation are many: poor maternal weight gain; diseases of the blood vessels, such as preeclampsia and high blood pressure; chronic kidney disease; severe anemia; smoking; the use of drugs and alcohol during pregnancy; multiple births; and fetal intrauterine infections, such as rubella. The diagnosis of intrauterine growth retardation depends on taking a careful history and on careful monitoring in the presence of any of the previous situations. A series of sonograms of the fetus can aid in the diagnosis. Nonstress test antepartum fetal monitoring is also of value in determining when to deliver. With good obstetrical care, intrauterine growth retardation can be prevented or appropriately managed.

MULTIPLE BIRTHS

Between 1 and 2 percent of pregnancies in the United States result in multiple births. The most common kind of multiple pregnancy is twins, but three or more fetuses can also develop. The introduction of fertility drugs (which help a woman become pregnant by stimulating multiple ovulations) has caused an increase in the number of multiple birth pregnancies.

Twins occur naturally in about 1 of every 90 births. When two separate eggs are fertilized, fraternal twins result; when a single fertilized egg divides into two fetuses, identical twins result.

Less frequently than twins, three or more fetuses can be produced in a single pregnancy. The risk in these pregnancies is even greater than in pregnancies with twins. Triplets occur naturally in only 1 of every 10,000 births, although they are more common with the use of fertility drugs.

Naturally occurring fraternal twins are the most common type of twins. Certain families have a higher incidence of fraternal twins. Identical twins are fairly rare. Their incidence is not related to a history of twins in the family.

With multiple births, the mother and the fetuses are all at increased risk for certain problems. Women carrying more than one fetus will need more frequent visits to the doctor and will be watched more closely to prevent problems that may occur. The most important factor in preventing problems in a multiple pregnancy is early diagnosis. Several signals may alert your doctor to the possibility of a multiple pregnancy.

- A genetic history of twins in your family
- A larger-than-expected uterus for your length of pregnancy
- A history of taking fertility drugs
- Excessive nausea and vomiting in the first three months of pregnancy
- More fetal movements than you felt in any previous pregnancies
- The detection of more than one heartbeat

Ultrasound offers the most accurate diagnosis of multiple fetuses and, in fact, often reveals twins incidentally during an exam done for other reasons.

Once multiple pregnancy is diagnosed, you will schedule more frequent visits with your doctor and may have ultrasound exams more often to monitor the growth of the fetuses. You will need to eat more and may gain 35 to 45 pounds during pregnancy. You should take iron and vitamin supplements because of the increase in nutritional needs. Your physician may reduce your physical activity.

Preterm labor and delivery are more common in a multiple pregnancy. The choice of method at delivery is often complex. Doctors consider the positions and the number of fetuses, their condition during labor, and whether they are preterm. Depending on the positions of the fetuses in the uterus, a cesarean birth may be needed. In pregnancies with more than two fetuses, cesarean birth is performed. Even though multiple pregnancy often involves greater problems and risks than a pregnancy with one fetus, with early diagnosis, frequent visits to your doctor, and testing, you should have few problems. And you get a premium for your efforts: two—or more—happy, healthy babies.

GROUP B STREPTOCOCCAL INFECTION

Group B streptococcus (GBS) is a type of bacteria that inhabits the vagina and the rectum. It is quite common and is present in up to 30 percent of all pregnant women. This bacterium also happens to be the most common cause of early onset infection, pneumonia, and meningitis in newborn babies. There are approximately 1,600 cases of early onset GBS infections and 80 deaths annually in the United States. Until recently, obstetricians have adopted several guidelines for GBS infection prevention in newborns. Currently, the Centers for Disease Control and Prevention (CDC) has released data indicating that the best preventative means of reducing newborn GBS infection is by testing all pregnant women between thirty-five and thirty-seven weeks for GBS, and, if present, the women will receive intravenous (IV) antibiotics in labor. Your doctor will test you by taking a culture swab of the vagina and around the rectum. Unless you are allergic, the antibiotic used is either penicillin G or ampicillin. There is no value in treating women prior to labor because the bacteria will almost always come right back after therapy is completed. Women with a history of GBS infection or who have had a urine infection with GBS should receive treatment during labor, regardless of their culture status.

DEPRESSION IN PREGNANCY

Depression is one of the most common health disorders in women. It occurs in 25 percent of women at some point during their lifetimes and affects almost 10 percent of women during pregnancy. Because depression is so common, especially during the childbearing years, two important points must be recognized with regard to pregnancy. First, many women go undiagnosed. This may have very serious consequences for both the mother and the fetus. Second, many women are currently being treated for depression and may become pregnant while on potentially dangerous medications.

Since depression occurs in around one in ten pregnancies, it is often not recognized by either the woman or her doctor. Left untreated, depression has a negative impact in the overall health of the pregnant mother and her fetus. Frequent tearfulness, irritability, insomnia, or any combination of these, may be clues that you are suffering from depression. Symptoms must persist for longer than two weeks to make the diagnosis. Mild illness may respond to nonmedication therapies. They can include diet changes, improving sleep time, stress management, and exercise. Support from your family and your doctor is essential and may help with the symptoms. In more severe cases of depression, medication may be necessary. As a general rule, when the risk of a disease is greater than the potential risk of a drug, the drug is used. This is especially true when the disease has a serious risk to the mother, her fetus, or both. Depression has been associated with poor fetal growth and negative newborn outcome. More dramatic pregnancy outcomes from untreated depression include risk-taking behavior, fetal abuse, and maternal suicide. Certain medications used under supervision of your obstetrician and your psychiatrist may alleviate symptoms and improve outcome.

Some women who are maintained on medications for depression become pregnant. Since some medications cause fetal malformations, a careful evaluation of your depression and its treatment should be performed by your doctors prior to conception. If you discover you are pregnant and are on depression medication, don't panic. Many of these medications are perfectly safe, and those that are known to cause birth defects are likely to have no effects if stopped and changed to a safer medication.

Chapter 13

Preventing Pregnancy

❦

DESPITE MAJOR ADVANCES in medical science, preventing pregnancy still remains a considerable challenge for both fertile people and their doctor. This chapter discusses what is currently available.

CONTRACEPTION

Not until the baby is born and settled in the household does an old problem pop up—contraception. There are several effective contraceptive methods to choose from, until you decide to have another baby.

The choice of contraception is something every woman, and every couple, has to grapple with. As soon as you decide to have sex, you must also decide what method of birth control to use. The choice of contraception varies from couple to couple and changes as each person's life changes. A single person not currently involved in a long-term relationship has very different needs from a newly married couple looking forward to starting a family. And the woman who plans to establish her career before having children faces yet another set of options. A woman who hopes to have children in the future needs a method that is as safe and effective as possible, and one that will not jeopardize her ability to have children when she decides to do so. A woman who has completed her family has a somewhat different contraceptive outlook. She and her partner may, for example, want to consider one of the forms of sterilization. A birth-control method must also be considered from an aesthetic viewpoint: It must be as pleasant to use as possible—or it *won't* be used consistently and correctly. And using any method carefully, every time, is the key to effectiveness.

Unfortunately, there is no perfect method of birth control. World population exceeded 6 billion in the year 2000 and is expected to reach 9 billion by the year 2050. Currently, 50 percent of the pregnancies in the United States are accidental. Family planning is therefore a critical health-care concern today.

Every birth control technique has its side effects, drawbacks, or limitations, as well as its advantages. Some methods—the IUD, for example—may be distinctly hazardous to women who want no risks to their subsequent fertility. Others, such as the diaphragm, may be extremely safe but not as effective as other options. Together, you, your partner, and your physician can make the best decision about the method that works for you right now without causing problems in the future. Try to be open and clear about your needs, likes, and dislikes and take the time to do a little homework about various methods so that you can talk to your doctor about them.

Most reversible methods of contraception fall into one of three general categories: barrier, hormonal, and intrauterine devices. But there are other, less effective techniques, such as withdrawal and rhythm, as well as permanent birth-control options, such as sterilization.

Barrier Methods of Contraception

The barrier methods—so called because they work by physically keeping sperm away from the egg—are among the oldest forms of birth control. In Egypt, medicated vaginal inserts are mentioned as early as 1500 B.C. Condoms have also been used since ancient times. The original models were fashioned from the intestines of animals. Modern-day barrier contraceptives—primitive diaphragms, cervical caps, and condoms—began to appear toward the end of the nineteenth century. For many years, these were the only birth-control methods available.

In addition to preventing pregnancy, the barrier methods have an added bonus. The spermicidal jellies, creams, and foams used in conjunction with them inhibit the growth of some of the organisms associated with sexually transmitted diseases: gonorrhea, syphilis, trichomonas, and even herpes. These infections are thought to cause infertility.

There has been a recent increase in the use of barrier methods because of their safety and their availability (often without a doctor's prescription). They appeal to women who are postponing the start of their families until their late twenties or thirties and who are concerned about the effects of exposure to the pill's hormones or the IUD's risk of infection. Barrier methods are also attractive to women who have sex infrequently or sporadically. "I don't have to take a pill every day or live with a foreign object in my uterus. I just use birth control when I need it" was how a young single woman put it.

The fact that barrier methods must be used every time you have sex, however, deters many potential users. Couples may find it inconvenient and distracting to pause in their lovemaking or to prepare in advance for sex (some vaginal spermicides require a specific length of time for a suppository to melt or foam). Some women find spermicides too greasy and messy or are disturbed by the sensation of heat and itching that they sometimes produce; and men complain that "it just doesn't *feel* the same" with condoms. As with all methods of contraception, the effectiveness of the method depends on two things: First, how effective is the item being used? Second, how well does one use the item? With the barrier methods, the main problem seems to be mistakes made with using the item, its so-called *use effectiveness*. It is therefore important to discuss in detail any contraceptive method with your health-care provider.

The Diaphragm

Prior to the introduction of the pill and the intrauterine device (IUD), the diaphragm was the most frequently used form of contraception in the United States. Diaphragms are shallow rubber cups with flexible metal rims that fold or bend for insertion, then pop open and slide into place, covering the cervix. They have two roles: first, to provide a physical barrier that keeps sperm from getting into the cervix; and second, to hold spermicidal gels and creams that increase effectiveness by immobilizing sperm that try to sneak in around the rim.

Many types of diaphragms are currently in use, but the design of all of them is basically similar. The effectiveness of the diaphragm at preventing pregnancy depends on two factors: getting the right type and fit, and using it correctly and consistently. The correct type and size of diaphragm depend on your pelvic anatomy and your vaginal tone. Since only your doctor can determine this for you, diaphragms cannot be obtained without a prescription. The vagina expands during sexual excitement, so the largest diaphragm that fits and is comfortable is the one that should be used. If it is too small, it may slip out of place. If it is too big, it may rotate and not cover the cervix completely. Therefore, it is essential that an experienced person fit a diaphragm. Childbirth may change the size and the shape of the vagina, so after pregnancy a new fitting is required before sex is resumed. Some physicians also recommend a new fitting with a weight change of 15 to 20 pounds.

You should be taught how to use and care for the diaphragm when you are first fitted for it. The diaphragm must be inserted before sexual intercourse. Many couples find stopping to do this an interruption and prefer to insert the diaphragm up to an hour or so before sex begins. You may choose to incorporate insertion into foreplay. Before inserting the diaphragm, place a teaspoonful (or applicatorful) of spermicidal jelly or cream inside the dome, which will cover the cervix, and spread a little bit more around the entire rim. After insertion, you or your partner should slide a finger into the vagina to check that the diaphragm is, in fact, covering the cervix. The front rim should be tucked up behind the pubic bone. If a diaphragm is correctly in place, you should be able to walk around, go to work, or bathe without feeling it, and your partner should not be able to feel it during sex. Let your doctor know if this is not the case.

Leave the diaphragm in place for at least six, preferably eight, hours after the last time you have sex. If you have intercourse more than once while the diaphragm is in place, each time you should insert another applicatorful of spermicidal jelly or cream *without removing the diaphragm*. A diaphragm can be used during menstruation but should be removed as soon as possible after the required time because of the slight risk of toxic shock syndrome (TSS).

Six or more hours after the last time you have sex, the diaphragm can be carefully removed. (Although diaphragms are quite sturdy, a fingernail can tear them.) Wash the diaphragm with warm water and a mild soap and dry with a towel. Some women dust it lightly with cornstarch before storing (talcum powder should *not* be used because of its possible relationship to cancer of the ovary). Before storing it, inspect your diaphragm for small holes or rips by holding it up to the light. With careful handling, a diaphragm generally lasts about two years.

When the diaphragm fails, it may be due to a poor fit, a hole or a tear in the device, failure to add spermicide for repeated intercourse, removal too soon, or failure to use it at all. Theoretically, if it is used correctly every time, its effectiveness should be about 98 percent. However, since we are human and occasionally impatient, careless, or forgetful, its actual effectiveness is quite a bit less—about 92 percent. The cost of the diaphragm is about $20, plus the cost of spermicide and the initial visit to your physician.

The Cervical Cap

The cervical cap was developed in the mid-nineteenth century by a German gynecologist. A thimble-shaped rubber device that was fitted over a woman's cervix, the cap was custom-made from a wax impression of each user's cervix. The cervical cap of today is smaller than a diaphragm, fits directly over the cervix (instead of blocking the entire upper part of the vaginal canal, as a diaphragm does), and is made out of a more rigid plastic or rubber.

Although cervical caps have always been popular in Europe, they never achieved widespread acceptance in the States. Their use was minimal because they were much more difficult to insert properly and to remove than the diaphragm. Recently, however, the cap has achieved a resurgence in popularity and interest. New research efforts have made it easier to insert and remove, and it can be left in place for longer time periods. Currently, the cap is used much like the diaphragm, being filled with spermicide prior to use and left in place six to eight hours following intercourse. The cervical cap was approved for general use in this country by the Food and Drug Administration (FDA) in May 1988. The most recent FDA-approved study rated its effectiveness in preventing pregnancy at around 89 percent. If used correctly, the cervical cap should be around 97 percent effective, but because of its reported difficulties with use, no studies report this number.

Vaginal Spermicides

A very old method of birth control is placing sperm-killing (spermicidal) agents inside the vagina before sex. Over the ages, many different preparations have been used. Today vaginal spermicides come in five general forms: jellies, creams, suppositories, aerosol foams, and foaming tablets. While the form may vary, almost all of them contain the same spermicide, nonoxynol-9.

It is essential that spermicides be used in the proper manner and before *each* act of intercourse. They must be placed where they will cover the cervix completely. If intercourse does not take place within one hour, a new application should be used. If foaming tablets or suppositories, which must first melt, are used, you *must* wait the stated length of time after putting them in before having intercourse. Avoid douching for at least six hours after the last act of intercourse, since it can take that long for all the sperm to be killed.

An advantage of spermicides is that they are available over the counter, without a prescription. But the tradeoff is their relatively high failure rate. A study released in 1999 compared pregnancy rates among very fertile couples using various nonoxynol-9 preparations versus no contraception. With no method of contraception, around 60 percent of couples became pregnant within six months. When couples used spermicides alone, around 25 percent became pregnant in that same time period. Although spermicides reduce pregnancy rates, women who strongly desire contraception should use other methods.

The Sponge

The sponge is a synthetic spongelike material saturated with the same spermicide, nonoxynol-9, used in other vaginal contraceptives. It is inserted prior to intercourse and is as effective as most barrier methods of contraception. The sponge was withdrawn from the market for a time because of allegations of unsafe production processes, leading to increased risk of infection. It was reintroduced in 2003.

Male Condoms

These are the only main established form of male barrier contraception used today. The newest condoms, usually made of latex, are thinner than ever and are available prelubricated, often with spermicide. This is the method most often used in Japan, Sweden, and the United Kingdom and is, in fact, the most widely used form of contraception in the world.

Although the condom's theoretical effectiveness is an impressive 97 to 98 percent, its actual in-use effectiveness varies from population to population. Most failures are due to ripping or tearing but also occur from insertion of the penis in the vagina before slipping on the condom, failure to unroll the condom completely on the shaft of the penis, and failure to leave enough space for the ejaculation at the tip of the condom. If used with a vaginal spemicide, the condom's effectiveness is a remarkable 99 percent. The condom-plus-spermicide combination is probably the most underrated form of birth control in the United States today.

In addition to being a highly effective contraceptive, condoms offer very good protection against many types of sexually transmitted diseases and AIDS. They are inexpensive and available over the counter, without prescription. The main drawback for women, however, is that they must rely on their male partners to use this method. Many men are reluctant to do so.

Female Condoms

The female condom is a thin plastic pouch that lines the vagina. Two rings are attached on each end of the pouch: a larger ring that lies outside the vagina and a smaller closed ring that lies on top of the cervix like a diaphragm. Insertion is similar to inserting the diaphragm, where the inner ring is pushed into the vagina, while the outer ring stays about 1 to 2 inches outside the vagina. Right after ejaculation, squeeze and twist the outer ring and then gently pull out the pouch and discard. Like the male condom, this can be used only once. Many women like this method because they feel that it gives them more control over the situation than does the male condom.

Hormonal Contraceptive Methods

Various types of hormones can be prescribed that can be used through different routes to offer very reliable methods of contraception. Hormones can be taken orally, they can be given by injection, and currently, they are available in preparations such as a patch or a vaginal insertion or released in an IUD. Hormonal contraception is used by over 100 million women worldwide and over 12 million women in the United States.

Oral Contraceptives

The development of the oral contraceptive, or the pill, as it is commonly known, is one of the great scientific achievements of the last four decades. In many ways the pill is the closest thing available to an ideal contraceptive. It is almost 100 percent effective when taken as instructed. It is easily reversible when children are desired, and it is inexpensive.

In 1960, the FDA authorized the marketing of the birth-control pill called Enovid. A whole generation of women has used it and its successors effectively. It has produced quite an impact on our society.

Oral contraceptives are made from synthetic hormones in various combinations. They are taken every day for twenty-one days of the menstrual cycle. Basically, all pills contain a combination of the hormones estrogen and progesterone, in varying quantities. Developments over the last twenty years have made possible a pill that contains minute amounts of these agents. When taken for twenty-one days, the hormones in the pill produce an inhibition of ovulation. Without ovulation, pregnancy cannot occur. These hormones also cause other changes that inhibit pregnancy. Progesterone makes the cervical mucus thick and impenetrable to sperm, thereby preventing them from entering the uterus. The hormones also alter the lining of the uterus, making it unreceptive to a possible fertilized egg.

Despite its relative safety, no woman should take the birth-control pill without a gynecological checkup, a breast examination, and a Pap smear. A complete history must also be taken before the pill is prescribed. Women with a history of blood clots or embolism, strokes, heart disease, serious liver disease, or unexplained bleeding from the vagina should not take the pill. Also, if she has a history of high blood pressure, diabetes, epilepsy, migraine headaches, serious mental disturbances, visual problems, or kidney disease, a woman should not take the pill. Your doctor is the best person to advise you about the safety of the pill in your individual case. You can then better arrive at the decision by balancing the risks against the benefits.

If a woman should decide to become pregnant, stopping the pill will easily reverse the contraceptive effect. She simply finishes her pill series and does not start another series. The pregnancy rate after the cessation of oral contraceptives is the same as the rate in women who have never taken the birth-control pill. That is, 90 percent of women will become pregnant within one year of trying to do so. Babies born to women who have used oral contraceptives show no aftereffects from the medication. A few women experience a delay in ovulation and menstruation for a number of months after stopping the pill. This condition is called post-pill amenorrhea, or lack of menstruation, and usually occurs in women who had irregular menstrual cycles before taking the pill. It can be treated, however, by the use of other medications, which can bring on ovulation, menstruation, and pregnancy.

There are common side effects in women taking the pill. Most women, however, take the low-dose contraceptives and do not experience any side effects at all or are bothered by only mild, transient effects. Psychological factors seem to play some part in the incidence of these effects. Nausea is common during the first couple of cycles and usually can be avoided by changing the time of day that the pill is taken from morning to midday. Fluid retention may be a problem, as may bloating, swelling of the legs, and weight gain. This can be treated by a low-salt diet or by diuretics, if necessary. Other occasional, minor changes are an increase in vaginal discharge and an increase in facial pigmentation, especially when exposed to strong sunlight. This pigmentation change is reversible on stopping the pill.

Some women experience mild mood changes, including depression, as well as increased appetite and weight gain. Breast enlargement is also common during the early cycles of taking the pill. Breakthrough bleeding or spotting between menstrual periods is another common side effect, which usually disappears after the third cycle. If this is persistent, a higher dose of medication can be prescribed. Recurring vaginitis, or vaginal infection, is common among women on the pill, especially infections caused by an organism called yeast fungus. This condition should be treated by your doctor.

There are occasionally serious complications associated with pill usage, such as blood clots in veins and possibly an embolus or traveling blood clot in the lungs. Even though there is a greater risk of a blood clot in women taking the pill, the death rate from clots caused by the pill is very low. The new low-dose pills are even safer than previous ones. There is no conclusive evidence of cancer resulting from the use of the birth-control pill. Some recent studies have suggested that there is a lower risk of ovarian cancer occurring in women who were on the birth control pill in past years.

For women who are breast-feeding who would like the convenience of the pill, the combination oral contraceptive, as described previously, may have the effect of decreasing the quantity of milk produced. Although breast-feeding women have decreased fertility, they can become pregnant. This is especially true if the baby is older than three months or the mother is supplementing breast milk with formula. For these women, there is a special type of pill that contains only one type of hormone, progestin. The progestin-only pill must be taken all twenty-eight days of the month, and it will not affect milk production. With this preparation, women rarely see menstrual flow and may have more "bloating"-type side effects.

The Patch

A new form of hormonal contraception is now available in a transdermal (patch) delivery system. In 1995, the National Survey of Family Growth estimated that the pill had a failure rate of approximately 8.3 percent in its first year of use. When used correctly, the pill should have a failure rate of well below 1 percent. There is likely a serious problem with its use effectiveness. The patch form of contraception was therefore developed to improve use effectiveness. This new system called "Ortho-Evra," consists of a series of patches that is applied, one at a time, to the skin. A fertile woman sticks a patch on the skin. After a week, the patch is removed and a new patch is put on. This continues for three consecutive weeks, and then no patch is worn for one week. A woman will likely bleed during this week. Because a woman does not have to remember to take a pill every day, this method of contraception is expected to improve compliance and therefore decrease pregnancy rates. The medication delivered by this system is similar to that in the pill and therefore has the same side effects and may also interfere with milk production in breast-feeding women. A 2001 study rated its overall failure at about 0.7 percent and its side effects to be minimal.

The Vaginal Ring

Recently, a new hormonal contraceptive method has been developed, in which a small, transparent, flexible ring is inserted into the vagina. It is inserted for three weeks and then removed for one week. During the no-ring week, the menstrual flow will occur. The ring releases a low level of hormone that is similar to that of the pill and the patch, thereby preventing pregnancy. This product became available in July 2002, so its success is still questionable. A study just released, however, showed very low pregnancy rates and few side effects.

Depo-Provera

For those women who are not afraid of injections, Depo-Provera offers an excellent method of contraception. An injection of this medication is given into a muscle every three months. The medication is nearly 100 percent effective in preventing pregnancy and has few side effects. The most common complaints are abnormal bleeding and weight gain. Because this method contains no estrogen, there is no effect on breast-milk production, and it can be used as an alternative to the pill if the woman has a history of blood clots (thrombosis).

Intrauterine Devices

The effectiveness of the intrauterine device to prevent conception has been known for more than 2,000 years. Turkish camel drivers inserted small round pebbles into the uteri of their camels centuries ago before going into the desert to prevent the camels from becoming pregnant during the long journey. Hippocrates, the ancient Greek doctor, even placed an intrauterine device into the womb of a woman to prevent pregnancy.

During the last thirty-five years, doctors have devoted serious attention to perfecting intrauterine devices that are placed inside the uterus and left there. Worldwide, 12 percent of married women use the IUD for contraception, whereas in the United States only 0.7 percent of married women seeking contraception use the IUD. This is likely due to fear that an IUD leads to pelvic infection. In fact, pelvic infection is very unlikely in the married population using an IUD.

There are many conflicting theories as to how the IUD works. Its exact mode of action is still not understood. The three main theories are that it (1) changes the muscle balance of the uterus and the fallopian tubes; (2) changes the lining of the uterus, called the endometrium, which prevents the implantation of the fertilized egg into the lining; and (3) alters the chemical environment of the uterus, preventing fertilization and implantation.

New synthetic plastics are now being used for intrauterine devices. These flexible and moldable devices do not react with body chemicals, and, because they are malleable, they are easy to insert.

One type of IUD contains small amounts of pure copper added to the plastic devices to improve effectiveness.

Another type of IUD uses the hormone progesterone to decrease side effects. This IUD, Progestasert, must be replaced each year since it contains a small amount of progesterone, which is released slowly into the uterus. Recently, a new progesterone IUD, called Mirena, has become available, which is effective for five years.

In order to evaluate an IUD, its expulsion rate, failure rate, and side effects must be considered. Most of the IUDs are 98 or 99 percent effective over a year's use. But it appears that the IUD is successful or tolerated by only about 80 percent of women, for 10 percent of women spontaneously expel the IUD, and another 10 percent have the device removed because of troublesome side effects.

Insertion of an IUD is usually a simple, quick, and more or less painless procedure. It is inserted following a complete examination, usually during or immediately following a menstrual period. Your doctor will insert the IUD into the uterus, leaving some nylon threads protruding into the upper vagina. These strings are left so that you may check to make certain it has not been expelled and so your doctor can remove it without difficulty. The IUD is effective immediately following insertion, and neither you nor your partner should be aware of its presence after insertion. Women who have never been pregnant do not tolerate the IUD as well as women who have had children. They tend to experience a greater degree of pain on insertion and immediately after insertion of the IUD. Women who have had children have a greater expulsion rate and a higher incidence of cramps during the first couple of menstrual cycles after insertion. Some side effects of the IUD are common but not serious. These side effects will often disappear after a few months' use. They include increased menstrual cramps, irregular bleeding during the month (spotting), and occasionally very heavy menstrual flow.

The intrauterine device should be checked periodically by your physician, at least every six months. Serious complications are possible with the IUD; they include pelvic infection and possible uterine perforation. The risk of serious pelvic infection is 1 to 2 percent. These infections can lead to sterility. Uterine perforation most often occurs upon insertion; once the IUD is properly inserted, its passage into the abdominal cavity would be quite unusual. These factors should be considered in your choice of IUD.

The IUD is less efficient than the pill, since the pregnancy rate is 1 to 2 percent during a full year's use. For unknown reasons, the IUD appears to be most effective in women who have had several children and are over thirty years of age.

The IUD is still one of the best contraceptive methods available. It is safe, easy to use, and inexpensive. It requires only an initial insertion, and is therefore indefinitely effective (the Copper T can be left in place for ten years), and it does not interfere with the enjoyment of sexual intercourse. Its contraceptive effect is completely reversible when it is removed.

The Rhythm Method

The rhythm method of birth control consists of abstaining from sexual intercourse on those days of the menstrual cycle when you are most likely to become pregnant. This is not an effective birth-control method, but it may be the only method available to some women because of religious beliefs. Women who, for medical reasons, must not become pregnant should not rely on this method. It cannot be used by any woman who has irregular cycles.

The method depends on the fact that conception occurs near the time of ovulation, and ovulation usually occurs fourteen days before the onset of the next menstrual flow (or in the middle of a twenty-eight day cycle). Therefore, conception is most likely in mid-cycle and least likely at the beginning and the end of the menstrual cycle. In order to use the rhythm method, a woman should keep a record of her menstrual cycles for eight months. When a regular pattern becomes clear, the first day of menstrual flow is designated day one. To calculate the unsafe period, she subtracts eighteen from the length of the shortest cycle to find the first unsafe day, and then subtracts eleven from the longest menstrual cycle for the last unsafe day. A woman must not have intercourse from the first unsafe day through the last unsafe day. Suppose, for example, your longest cycle over eight months is thirty days and your shortest is twenty-six days. To determine your first unsafe day, subtract eighteen from twenty-six to get eight. To determine your last unsafe day, subtract eleven from thirty to get nineteen. Now abstain from sex between days eight and nineteen of your menstrual cycle. You should also continue to record the length of each cycle and revise your calculations monthly so that they are based on the last eight cycles.

Another rhythm method of birth control combines calendar calculations with basal temperature readings. It relies on the fact that a woman's body temperature is higher during the second part of her menstrual cycle. This increase in temperature is caused by the release of the hormone progesterone following ovulation. To use this method, you take your temperature before getting out of bed each morning. This temperature is known as the basal body temperature, or BBT. Special thermometers with fine gradations are available to determine basal body temperature accurately. By recording basal body temperature daily, you can assume that three days after the rise in basal body temperature, ovulation is completed and the safe period has begun. The unsafe period cannot be determined except by the calendar method. The first unsafe day is calculated from the shortest cycle, as outlined previously. The last unsafe day is the third day after the rise in basal body temperature.

Coitus Interruptus or Withdrawal

Withdrawal is one of the oldest methods of birth control known, but it is difficult to use properly and has a very high failure rate. When this method is used, sexual intercourse continues until just before male orgasm. When the male feels ejaculation coming, he withdraws his penis from the vagina, preventing the emission of the sperm into the vagina.

As a contraception technique, it has several problems. It relies purely on willpower. And even if withdrawal is completed, the method may not work because some sperm is often ejaculated in small amounts prior to orgasm. With the existence of cheap, easily available mechanical and hormonal contraceptives, this method should not be considered a valuable birth-control technique.

The Morning-After Pill

Scientists have developed a pill to prevent the implantation of a fertilized egg following contraceptive failure. The pill is commonly called the "morning-after pill." This form of emergency oral contraception is now available by prescription. The U.S. Food and Drug Administration has approved two specific prescription methods. They are the Preven Emergency Contraceptive Kit and the Plan B method: Preven consists of four pills that are taken two at a time twelve hours apart, and Plan B consists of 2 pills that are taken twelve hours apart. Patients seem to prefer Plan B because Preven is more likely to cause nausea.

As soon as possible after unprotected sex occurs, emergency oral contraception should be taken. Although it can be effective up to seventy-two hours after sex, it is more reliable if taken within the first twenty-four hours. Once it is taken, the risk of pregnancy should be reduced but not eliminated. Therefore, if there is no menses within twenty-one days following emergency oral contraception, a pregnancy test should be performed.

ABORTION

Elective abortion is becoming an increasingly available alternative to contraceptive failure. In January 1973, the Supreme Court legalized abortion in the United States. In states where the decision resulted in changed laws, the maternal death rate dropped, as did the illegitimacy rate and the infant mortality rate. The decision to have an abortion rests between a woman and her doctor. In 1997, 1.18 million legal abortions were performed in the United States.

There are several kinds of abortion techniques, the use of which is usually determined by the stage of pregnancy.

D&C (Dilation and Curettage)

The D&C is probably the oldest of the abortion techniques used today. It consists of dilating the cervix and scraping the uterus clean. It is performed under local or general anesthesia up to the twelfth week of pregnancy. The D&C is also used to clean out the uterus following a spontaneous abortion or miscarriage.

Vacuum Aspiration

The most common technique used today is vacuum suction. All but 1 percent of abortions performed today use this technique. It, too, requires a slight dilation of the cervix, after which an instrument called a suction cannula is held in the uterus. The cannula is attached to a pump, which suctions out the contents of the uterus like a vacuum cleaner. This method is also confined to the first twelve weeks of pregnancy. It is widely used because it results in only a small loss of blood and it is less likely to damage the uterus. It is the quickest and the simplest of the abortion techniques. It can be performed using local anesthetics in an office or an outpatient operating room.

Late Abortion Techniques

After fourteen weeks of pregnancy, different abortion techniques are used. Generally, two methods are available. One is called a D&E

(dilatation and evacuation). It involves dilating the cervix sufficiently to allow special instruments to be inserted to evacuate the uterine contents manually. Suction is also used in this method.

The other technique involves the injection of certain substances into the uterine cavity to produce labor. Amniotic fluid is usually removed and substances, such as salt solutions, urea, or a chemical called prostaglandin, are instilled. Labor usually occurs within eight to twelve hours, and the fetus and the placenta are passed spontaneously. Some states allow this type of abortion up to twenty-four weeks of gestation.

Medical Abortion

In 1988, France became the first country to license specific medications used for abortion. The drug known as RU-486, or mifepristone, was originally banned in the United States, and that led to the development of other less-effective drugs to induce abortion. Finally, in September 2000, the U.S. Food and Drug Administration approved RU-486.

Currently, several methods use medication to induce abortion. The process usually involves several visits to the doctor and requires follow-up. The treatment is more successful if used earlier in the pregnancy, prior to forty-nine days after the last menstrual period. The most effective method involves taking an RU-486 (mifepristone) tablet and then forty-eight hours later taking another medication called misoprostol. Within four hours, the pregnancy is usually expelled with little or no discomfort. A follow-up exam is usually scheduled for ten to fifteen days later to make sure all is well. If the pregnancy fails to expel or does not expel completely, a surgical abortion should be performed. After forty-nine days past the last menstrual period, the success rate drops to 85 percent. As the gestational age increases, it maybe better to consider a surgical abortion.

Hysterotomy

This method is the least commonly used of all. It requires surgical incision into the uterus, the same approach used for a cesarean section. This method is usually reserved for a second-trimester abortion, in which the other methods have failed, or for an abortion accompanied by a sterilization procedure, such as a severing of the fallopian tubes.

Considerations in Abortion

Although moral and theological considerations may delay a decision to seek an abortion, abortions are safer from a medical standpoint when performed between the sixth and the tenth weeks of pregnancy.

The woman seeking an abortion needs certain basic information. First of all, she should be certain she is pregnant. One abortionist who recently summarized his experience of a twenty-five-year period said that 10 percent of the women who came to him were not pregnant. Many women seek abortion when they are only two days late with their menstrual flow, unaware that several factors other than pregnancy can delay the onset of the period, such as weight change, anxiety, illness, travel, and normal variation in the cycle. The new blood pregnancy tests are very accurate in early detection and should be used if a woman suspects she's pregnant.

The patient's physician is the best one to determine the diagnosis of pregnancy and recommend the best type of procedure. Moreover, an examination by a competent physician may reveal that other problems need treatment, in addition to or prior to an abortion. Occasionally, pregnancy may be in the fallopian tube or there may be ovarian cysts or vaginal infections present. Women who are Rh negative and have either a spontaneous or an induced abortion should also get Rh immunoglobulin.

Often, after an abortion, women feel that there is no reason to see a doctor again, especially if they feel normal and are not experiencing excessive bleeding and infection. Occasionally, however, we see a woman who may still be pregnant despite an attempted abortion. It is important that a postoperative examination be performed approximately one to two weeks following the operation. At the initial visit, after a medical checkup is performed, contraception can also be discussed. Following an abortion, a woman should think about developing a contraceptive plan.

The emotional aftereffects of an abortion should not be forgotten. Some women will have an immediate response of relief, while others suffer periods of depression with crying, fatigue, and insomnia. However, these are usually short-lived and not serious, and they do pass.

STERILIZATION

Sterilization is a permanent surgical means of preventing pregnancy. It is often advised when another pregnancy would endanger the life of the mother or when there are already children with genetic birth defects and the possibility of their recurring is strong. Increasingly, however, couples are turning to sterilization once their family has reached optimal size.

Abdominal Tubal Ligation

Female sterilization leaves the main organs of reproduction untouched. The most common method, tubal ligation, consists of cutting the fallopian tubes and sewing them shut so that the egg never meets with sperm or reaches the uterus. The unfertilized egg disintegrates. The woman continues her normal menstrual cycle.

The operation is fairly simple and can be performed vaginally or through a small incision in the abdomen. If performed immediately following delivery, tubal ligation requires only a 1½-inch incision and a few days' stay in the hospital. In fact, the operation can be performed immediately following delivery under the same anesthesia used for delivery. Performed at other times, the procedure is a little more of an operation.

Sterilization by tubal ligation does not affect the woman's menstrual or hormonal cycle. Ovulation will occur in the usual fashion, and the uterus will react normally to the cyclic ovarian hormones. Menstruation will take place, but the pathway for the egg and the sperm combination has been interrupted and therefore pregnancy does not occur. Sexual responsiveness and orgasm are not affected by these techniques.

Laparoscopic Tubal Ligation

Currently, almost all tubal ligations are done using a procedure called laparoscopy, which was developed for sterilization purposes. A laparoscope is a long, tubelike instrument fitted with lights and mirrors that is inserted through a small incision, usually in the navel area of the abdomen. Through this instrument, the pelvic organs can be seen, including the tubes. The tubes are then cauterized—that is, burned closed with a plastic band. Usually, general anesthesia is required for this procedure. The risks of the procedure are minimal. The main risks seem to be those related to the general anesthetic, plus the rare complication of injury to the bowel or the tissues by the cauterization. Current experience with laparoscopic tubal ligation has proven it to be safe and successful. Laparoscopic technique requires a shorter hospital stay than the abdominal operation, usually only one day, and is most often less expensive.

Other Sterilization Techniques

Research is currently being carried out in many institutions on an even more simple outpatient sterilization procedure. One procedure uses an instrument called the hysteroscope to look inside the endometrial cavity of the uterus. Techniques that close the entrance to the fallopian tubes from the endometrial cavity, either permanently or temporarily, are being evaluated. However, at this time, these procedures are still experimental.

Vasectomy

Some men equate male sterilization with castration. This is not the case at all. The most common form of male sterilization used today is called vasectomy.

Vasectomy involves cutting the sperm ducts in the testicles, thus preventing the passage of sperm to the penis. Sexual desire and activity should remain the same. The only observable difference will be a 10 percent decrease in the volume of ejaculate.

Vasectomy is easy to perform and can be done as an outpatient procedure under local anesthesia. A small incision is made in the scrotum over the sperm duct (the vas deferens), which is then cut. It will then take about three weeks for all the sperm to leave the tract, completing the procedure. A semen sample should be examined under a microscope for sperm before the operation can be called completely successful.

Vasectomy carries with it a 1 percent failure rate, since every once in a while the two ends of the sperm duct rejoin and allow the flow of sperm through the penis. Attempts to reverse the procedure and restore fertility, however, are less than 50 percent successful.

Chapter 14

Infertility

——◦◦◦——

ANY BOOK ON pregnancy and childbirth should include a chapter on infertility. Because reproduction is an essential aspect of many marriages, the inability to conceive often ranks high among the causes of marital unhappiness. Whether true or not, many people believe that a child is necessary for a strong family relationship.

The exact incidence of infertility is difficult to compute. It is estimated that infertility affects 6.1 million American women and their partners, which is around 10 percent of the reproductive population. Approximately 1.25 million women will seek infertility treatment each year. We may define sterility or infertility as the inability to conceive after a year of trying. The primary form of sterility is that in which conception has never occurred. The secondary variety is one in which previous conception has taken place, but a repeat attempt at conception has been unsuccessful. We may say a couple is absolutely sterile when it is clear that conception is impossible. This would be true if a woman has had a hysterectomy or if the man has no sperm in his semen. Many couples experience a relative sterility where factors are present that make conception difficult, although not impossible. It is estimated that 10 to 15 percent of couples have problems with conception.

The one-year definition outlined previously is not an arbitrary one. Many analyses have shown that two-thirds of pregnancies occur within three months of initiation of unprotected intercourse. Within six months of trying to conceive, 75 to 80 percent of couples are successful, and by the end of one year, 80 to 90 percent have conceived. At least 5 percent of normal women will conceive during the second year of trying. But partners who have been unsuccessful after trying for one year should seek medical help and should be regarded as candidates for a full-scale investigation to determine the cause of their

298

trouble. Couples in their thirties or forties should wait somewhat less than one year before seeking medical advice.

ESSENTIAL FACTORS IN INFERTILITY

Before discussing the causes of infertility, let's review the mechanisms involved in normal reproduction. In every case of infertility, one or more of these mechanisms is altered:

- The testicles must produce healthy sperm that are able to propel themselves to meet the female egg.
- The ovaries must produce healthy eggs that must be discharged at ovulation at regular intervals.
- The semen must be deposited at or near the cervix so the sperm can make their way toward the ovum, and, of course, this occurs by the male's satisfactory completion of orgasm during sexual intercourse.
- The ovum, after ovulation, must meet with no obstruction as it passes through the tube toward the sperm.
- The sperm, likewise, must meet no physical or chemical obstruction as it passes through the cervix, into the uterus, and toward the tube, where it will meet with the egg.
- The fertilized egg must arrive in the uterus at the time when there is a ready site of implantation in the uterine wall.

The causes of infertility can be either male or female in origin; partners with a problem should seek medical advice and treatment together.

The doctor you choose will organize a diagnostic search and a survey. This investigation begins with the first office visit, when a thorough family history is taken. Information concerning previous marriages, previous pregnancies, menstrual cycle, and sexual habits will be explored, and a general physical examination and some laboratory studies will be performed.

The doctor will probably investigate five major areas:

1. *Pelvic conditions.* Tumors, infections, and anatomical variations should be ruled out. These abnormalities are uncovered in fewer than 5 percent of women.
2. *The process of insemination.* The doctor will explore impotence problems, how close to the cervix the semen is

deposited, and failure of sperm to pass through the cervix because of a hostile chemical makeup of cervical mucus. This latter reaction can be detected by performing a Heuhner or postcoital test on cervical secretions after intercourse. Surprisingly, this condition may be remedied by the use of condoms for a short period of time to remove the allergic reaction.

3. *The condition of the tubes.* Partial or complete closure of the fallopian tubes is determined by an X-ray examination of the uterus and the tubes, called hysterosalpingography. Laparoscopy has become a very useful tool in the evaluation of tubal and pelvic conditions. Direct visualization of the pelvis can document such problems as chronic infection, adhesions, endometriosis, and ovarian disease.

4. *Hormone problems.* An endocrine problem in the female reproductive system may cause alterations in menstruation and ovulation, or inadequate preparation of the endometrium (the uterine wall) for implantation of the fertilized egg. Problems can be diagnosed by performing endometrial biopsies, by taking the basal body temperature, and by hormonal studies of various types.

5. *The male reproductive tract.* Problems here account for infertility among 40 percent of couples studied. Examination of the semen, usually performed by a urologist, can reveal problems.

If a problem in two or more of these five areas exists, the probability of successful conception is reduced. Multiple problems are found in more than 60 percent of infertile couples. The investigation and the treatment of these five major problems are the main objectives in the management of infertility.

Another aim of the infertility investigation, besides enabling a couple to bear children, is to determine the chances of eventual pregnancy. This permits the couple to have an intelligent outlook on the problem and to adjust and make plans concerning the possibility of adoption or artificial donor insemination.

The chance of successful pregnancy following infertility evaluations and therapy is estimated to be between 20 and 50 percent. In general, one out of every three couples that seeks medical help following one year of inability to conceive will be successful in having a baby. This can be compared to the one out of twenty couples that will conceive during the second year of trying without seeking medical help. Medical evaluation and therapy for the infertile couple can obviously be worthwhile.

THE CAUSES OF INFERTILITY

There are many reasons why couples fail to conceive. Most problems are quite simple to correct and require very little intervention. Occasionally, problems exist that require more advanced reproductive technologies. Working with your doctor to determine the problem may be less stressful if you have some understanding of the main causes of infertility.

Sexual Problems and Infertility

Minor physical problems can interfere with satisfactory sex. If a woman has a tight hymen (the piece of tissue around the vaginal opening), it may be painful or impossible for her partner to push his penis completely into her vagina. Incomplete penetration means sperm will not be deposited as close to the cervix as possible, and the discomfort involved may discourage the couple from wanting to have sex at all. Yet this situation can be quickly and easily remedied, often right in the doctor's office, by a small surgical incision in the too-tight hymen.

Sometimes the man is unable to achieve sufficient rigidity of his penis to penetrate his sex partner. Or the woman may involuntarily constrict the muscles of her vagina so that penetration is impossible, a situation called vaginismus. In either event, the result—unsatisfactory sex—is the same. This may in itself decrease a couple's chances of enjoying sex in the future. Sex therapy and sometimes medications such as Viagra can bring about excellent improvement when problems like these exist.

Certain social and cultural traditions can interfere with conception. For example, very orthodox Jews do not have sex during menstruation or for one full week after bleeding ceases. If a woman menstruates for eight days and then must wait another seven, ovulation may have already occured by the time she next has sex.

And, finally, the infertility workup itself may prompt sexual difficulties that hamper conception. A couple told to have sex on a regular schedule may lose the desire to have sex at all. What should be a great spontaneous pleasure may now seem mechanical, empty of meaning. Not surprisingly, such feelings may leave a man unable to achieve erection, a woman dry and tight, and both partners unable to reach orgasm. In addition, some specialists feel that stress may affect the ovulatory mechanism so that periods become irregular; and if ovulation does occur, stress may diminish the coordinated functioning of the fallopian tubes so that the egg and the sperm can't be properly transported through them.

Male Factors in Infertility

Inadequate Sperm

Only strong, healthy sperm in adequate numbers are capable of producing a pregnancy. A look at a sample of sperm under a microscope, a semen analysis, may reveal that a man is producing too few sperm, that the sperm are not moving vigorously enough to wend their way to an egg, or that the sperm are abnormally shaped. Or it may reveal no sperm in the semen.

Male infertility problems may be a result of several types of defect. The structure of some part of the reproductive organs may have been askew from birth or been damaged by infection, drugs, or accidents.

A *varicocele* is an example of a structural problem. This is a cluster of enlarged veins surrounding the tubes that lead from the testicles to the penis. Its presence may raise the temperature in this area, which would result in infertility. Even a small varicocele can be associated with infertility, although many men with a varicocele have completely normal semen production and sperm counts and no fertility problems at all. The enlarged veins can be felt if a man's scrotum and testicles are gently examined while he bears down, such as he would during a bowel movement. Varicoceles have been described as feeling like "a bag of worms." The enlarged veins can be removed by surgery, which sometimes results in an improvement in fertility.

Another structural problem is a *blockage* in the tubes that sperm pass through on the way from the testes to the penis. In this case, even though sperm are being produced by the testes, they can't get out to fertilize an egg. Some men are born with such a blockage. Others opt for it surgically—as in the case of a vasectomy, in which the tubes are severed. To check for obstruction of the tubes, the doctor will test a semen sample for the presence of fructose. This sperm-nourishing sugar is added by the epididymis, a structure through which the sperm pass on their journey from testicle to penis. If testing the semen reveals no sperm and no fructose, chances are the problem is an obstruction of the tubes. If, on the other hand, no sperm are present but fructose is detected, then the problem probably lies in an inability of the testicles to manufacture sperm.

Cryptorchidism

Another structural problem leading to male infertility is called cryptorchidism. In a male fetus, the testes are found in the lower abdomen—much like a female's ovaries—but they normally migrate down into the scrotum (the sac of skin behind the penis) by the time a male baby is born. When the testes don't descend into the scrotum, the condition that results is cryptorchidism. It severely affects the development of the testes and, if not surgically corrected soon enough, can prevent normal sperm development entirely. A baby may also be born without testicles at all. This condition, called anorchia, results in untreatable sterility.

Hypospadias

Another structural abnormality of the male, called hypospadias, occurs when the opening of the penis is somewhere along the underside of the shaft, back from the tip. This means that at ejaculation, sperm are not deposited at the top of the vagina next to the cervix, and the chances of conception are reduced. Pregnancy can often be achieved if a semen sample, collected after masturbation, is deposited next to the cervix, a process called artificial insemination.

Retrograde Ejaculation

Retrograde ejaculation is a condition in which the sperm are pushed backward into the bladder instead of being projected out of the penis at ejaculation. It can be caused by drugs or various types of pelvic surgery and is diagnosed by finding sperm in the urine instead of in the ejaculate. Infertility from retrograde ejaculation can be treated by threading a tube through the penis into the bladder after ejaculation, and using this sperm sample for artificial insemination.

Infection

Infection can also cause male infertility, either temporary or permanent. For example, any significant inflammation of the testes after puberty (as can happen with mumps) may damage the testicles so that they can't produce normal sperm. Common infections like gonorrhea, chlamydia, or mycoplasma bacteria have also been implicated in male infertility. Until they are treated with antibiotics, these infections can adversely affect both the production of sperm and the fluid portion of semen.

Genetic Problems

Men can also be born with genetic infertility problems. A normal male has forty-six chromosomes—twenty-two pairs, plus one X and one Y chromosome that determine his sex. (Normal women also have forty-six—the same twenty-two pairs, plus two Xs.) Any variation from this normal chromosome composition often hampers that person's ability to reproduce. In a syndrome called Kleinfelter's, a man has an extra X chromosome—so his cells have twenty-two chromosome pairs, plus two Xs and a Y—and he is generally unable to father children. Chromosomal studies will quickly determine this problem and aid in treatment.

Hormonal Imbalances

Hormonal imbalances in any of the glands of the complex hormone system can cause infertility. The pituitary gland is a kind of master gland that sends signals to other glands throughout the body. If it malfunctions, it can make the testicles poor sperm producers and can cause thyroid and adrenal gland upsets. A hormonal workup, which involves checking the levels of various hormones in the blood, is usually done on men with abnormal sperm counts.

Drugs

Certain drugs and medications can also affect sperm production. Narcotics, alcohol, tranquilizers, some antidepressants, and blood pressure medications may leave a man unable to become erect or ejaculate properly. Other drugs, such as methotrexate (used to fight cancer and other disorders), antimalaria drugs, nitrofurantoin (an antibiotic), and marijuana, can cause abnormally low sperm production.

Pressure on the Testicles

Even something as simple as having a job that requires a lot of time sitting—like truck or taxi driving—or wearing tight pants or underwear can lower a man's sperm count. For optimal sperm production, the testicles need to be at a relatively low temperature, but in these situations they are pressed close to the body for long periods of time, causing their temperature to be raised higher than is optimal. Sometimes simply changing from close-fitting jockey shorts to loose, airy boxer shorts that let the testicles fall farther from the body will bring the sperm count back to normal.

Even this partial listing of the types of reproductive problems a man can have should start to make one thing clear: It takes time, patience, determination, and a true detective's nose to zero in on important clues—while not getting bogged down in the mass of potential false leads. And these qualities are called upon from each member of the search party—not only the doctor, but the couple, too.

Female Factors in Infertility

Earlier in this book, we described the complex process of ovulation. As with male fertility problems, things can go awry in almost any step of a woman's cycle and can cause problems with her fertility.

Hormonal Problems

Hormonal factors can keep a woman's ovaries from releasing an egg (ovulating) or can fail to prepare the lining of the uterus to accept an egg once it's fertilized. Approximately 20 percent of infertile women have ovulatory problems. Once a problem with ovulation has been diagnosed, the cause must be determined. Approximately 70 percent of women who have ovulatory dysfunction have a condition known as polycystic ovarian syndrome, or PCOS. This condition is seen in approximately 5 percent of the reproductive-age population. It is characterized by symptoms such as absent or infrequent periods and higher than normal levels of male hormones, leading to increases in facial and body hair and acne. About 10 percent of women with ovulatory dysfunction have a condition known as hypothalamic anovulation. In this condition, an area of the brain called the hypothalamus is not functioning properly. This is common in women who are very thin, who exercise too vigorously, or who are under excessive stress. Women suffering from anorexia nervosa usually have associated hypothalamic anovulation. Another 10 percent of women with ovulation issues have a condition known as hyperprolactinemia. This condition prevents ovulation by the overproduction of the hormone prolactin, produced in the pituitary gland. The remaining 10 percent of women with ovulation issues have a failure of the ovaries called premature ovarian failure, or POF.

Although that doesn't normally happen until a woman is about fifty to fifty-five years old, premature ovarian failure occasionally occurs between the ages of thirty and forty, often for unknown reasons. Surgical damage to both ovaries and radiation therapy aimed at cancer in the pelvic organs may also produce premature ovarian failure. There is, unfortunately, no treatment that can make the ovaries start up again. However, recent advances in *in vitro fertilization* (so-called test tube babies) may make it possible for a woman with nonfunctioning ovaries to carry and deliver a baby. A donor egg, fertilized with her partner's sperm, can be implanted in a woman's uterus and, as long as the uterus itself is healthy, the embryo can develop from then on exactly as her own egg would.

Hormone problems can also prevent a fertilized egg from implanting properly once it reaches the uterus. If the ovaries do not produce enough progesterone after ovulation, the endometrium will not build up and develop properly. This situation is called inadequate luteal phase or luteal phase defect, since the luteal or after-ovulation half of the cycle is when the problem occurs. Luteal-phase defects can also cause early miscarriage if the endometrium is developed enough to accept implantation of a fertilized egg but not to support the growing embryo.

Fallopian Tube Problems

Fallopian tube problems are most likely to be caused by scar tissue. The tubes must be lined with healthy hairlike cilia and be capable of coordinated contractions so they can move the sperm in one direction and the egg, both before and after fertilization, in the other. The fingerlike projections, called fimbria, at the end of the tubes must also be able to sweep over the ovary and guide a just-released egg into the tube. The fimbria's ability to move freely is an important factor in this process. The inflammation that accompanies infections like gonorrhea and chlamydia can cause scar tissue to form around a tube, in its walls, or inside the channel, leaving it either squeezed from without and unable to move properly or blocked off from within. Scar tissue can clump fimbria into a solid immobile mass. Inflammation and infection can also cause a related process, called adhesion formation, in which tough, thin strands of fibrous tissue, like stringy cobwebs, bind internal organs together. Adhesions can twist the fallopian tube into such contorted positions that the pickup of an egg is impossible.

Any irritating process in the pelvis, from appendicitis to endometriosis, may produce inflammation and scarring in the reproductive organs. Endometriosis is a condition in which bits of uterine lining stick to pelvic structures instead of being expelled during menstruation. The intrauterine (IUD) contraceptive device, as previously discussed, can cause tubal infection and produce tubal scarring, and pelvic surgery or sterilization procedures can affect the functioning of the tubes as well. More recent data, however, seem to indicate that the modern-day IUD does not lead to an increase in the risk of pelvic infections.

Cervical Mucus

The role of the cervix in conception is to serve as a gateway through which sperm pass in their search for an egg. The cervix also produces a mucus that fills the canal. Healthy cervical mucus is specially formulated to speed sperm through as quickly and easily as possible. This mucus is vital to the process of conception. Some women, however, produce too little mucus, while others produce mucus so thick it stops sperm like a barricade. In some, the cervical mucus contains antibodies that attack and immobilize the sperm as if they were unwanted invaders like bacteria.

Uterine Structure

Due to other structural abnormalities, the uterus may be unable to accept pregnancy. In the most common of these, called a bicornuate uterus, there is a wall dividing the uterine cavity into two halves, each usually having one fallopian tube connected to it. This type of problem can interfere with conception and with the process of pregnancy itself, causing miscarriages and premature delivery.

Fibroids

Another common uterine problem is fibroids. These noncancerous growths in the walls of the uterus may distort the uterine lining and compress or twist the fallopian tubes, making implantation or sperm-and-egg travel impossible.

Infertility from No Known Cause

One of the most difficult challenges of all occurs with a small number of infertile couples: All studies are completed and still no reason is found for their inability to conceive. Medical science is simply not advanced enough to completely understand all of the subtle complexities of the process of creating a new human being. As science advances, however, this happens less often. We will probably never know the reasons in every case. Sometimes couples are able to have a child after months or years of trying, without ever knowing the reason for their previous infertility. As we will see later, extraordinary new treatments, such as in vitro fertilization, have started to make this once-impossible dream a reality.

INFERTILITY TESTS

When a couple goes to a gynecologist or a fertility specialist, the partners usually have two pressing questions: First, Why have we been unable to conceive? And, second, What are our chances of being able to have a baby in the future? In spite of their understandable impatience, it usually takes two to six months to be able to answer even the first question completely: The success of the treatment and how long it will take depend, of course, on the causes.

Step one of a fertility workup includes a careful medical history and a thorough physical examination of both partners. The sperm count is the first basic test for the man. The number, the ability to move, and the types of sperm in a sample obtained through masturbation are evaluated under a microscope. A count of over 20 million sperm, with 80 percent moving normally and less than 10 percent oddly shaped, is considered normal for one ejaculation. As discussed in the section on causes of male infertility, if certain indications exist in the history, the physical exam, or the sperm count, your doctor may also request a genetic workup and various hormone tests.

For the woman, some basic tests are performed during different stages of the menstrual cycle. A postcoital test will be performed to see if your cervical mucus is normal. Your doctor will instruct you to have intercourse at the time ovulation is anticipated. Then, four to eight hours after intercourse, he or she will quickly and painlessly remove mucus from the cervix for study under the microscope. This will be done in your doctor's office. The number of sperm the mucus contains and their movements will be studied, and the mucus itself will be examined for signs of infection. Poor postcoital test results reveal a low number of sperm or sperm that are unable to move correctly. In this case, the cervical mucus may actually be killing the sperm because a cervical infection, a hormone imbalance, or an immune response has changed its chemical composition.

The health of a woman's uterus may be checked with an endometrial biopsy done during the second half of the menstrual cycle. This test involves slipping a narrow instrument through the vagina and the cervix and into the uterus, where it snips a tiny chunk of the uterine lining, or endometrium. This tissue may reveal that the endometrium has not become thick and ready to receive a fertilized egg. This may be due to infection, or a condition called inadequate luteal phase. The latter is usually due to a deficiency of progesterone.

Another technique discussed earlier, called hysteroscopy, lets the physician actually see the interior of the uterus by inserting a tiny viewing instrument through the cervix. This technique can reveal a number of abnormalities and irregularities of the endometrium, as well as

structural abnormalities of the uterus. A hysterosalpingogram, in which
dye is injected through the cervix and x-rayed as it coats the inside of
the uterus and flows out the fallopian tubes, can spotlight many uterine and tubal abnormalities as well. Finally, your gynecologist may perform a test called a saline sonohystogram. Here, salt water is injected
into the uterus while a vaginal ultrasound is performed. Any abnormalities in the uterine cavity can usually be spotted.

The last major test for evaluation of the tubes and the pelvic
organs in general uses laparoscopy. This test most often requires the
use of general anesthesia. Carbon dioxide is pumped directly into the
abdomen through a small incision made at the edge of the navel, to
separate the internal organs enough so that individual parts of them
can be seen. Next, the laparoscope, the viewing instrument for which
the procedure is named, is passed through the incision and into the
puffed-up abdominal cavity. The area outside of the tubes, the ovaries,
and the uterus can now be examined, allowing scar tissue and adhesions to be seen. While the laparoscope is still in place, your doctor
will inject liquid blue dye through the cervix into the uterus. After a
short time, it should spill out of the fallopian tubes; this will prove
that they are clear and open. Because laparoscopy can tell a physician
so much about the health of the reproductive organs, it is extremely
valuable in an infertility investigation. But it is surgery, and it does
usually require anesthesia. So, as small as the risks involved may be—
and they are small—a physician will not usually opt for a laparoscopy
unless easier, quicker, noninvasive tests have proved inconclusive.

The hormone factors that can foul up the process of ovulation
also need to be evaluated. A lump of immobile scar tissue blocking a
tube is a clear, concrete obstacle to fertility. But the tiny invisible
drops of hormones coursing through the blood at the right times and
in the right amounts are just as important to the process. For it is
these hormones that prompt the body to prepare and release the egg
in the first place. Ovulation, as detailed in the chapter on the menstrual cycle, requires the efficient production of hormones from the
pituitary gland, the thyroid gland, and the ovaries themselves. Sometimes these hormones, and others related to the menstrual cycle, can
be measured in the blood itself. Measuring FSH, LH, prolactin, thyroid hormone, estrogen, and progesterone levels can confirm that the
glands are functioning correctly.

Charting your own temperature over a period of one or several
months is an indirect way for you to confirm that ovulation is taking
place. A basal body temperature chart is made by taking your temperature every morning as soon as you wake up, before you get out of bed,
and drawing a dot on the chart each day at the corresponding temperature. In a normal menstrual cycle, the BBT will show an average low

temperature before ovulation, with a jump after ovulation. The rise, usually to over 98°F, is maintained until menstruation starts. If you become pregnant, your temperature will remain elevated over 98°F (and, of course, you will not menstruate). Basal body temperature charting is very useful in confirming ovulation, the existence of a healthy postovulation or luteal phase, and an early pregnancy. BBT is easy, self-administered, and inexpensive but can be affected by many factors, leading to inaccurate results. A 2001 study found its accuracy to be only around 80 percent. Other methods for detecting ovulation are now available, with various results. One popular method is by studying the urine. The first morning urine can be tested with kits that look like pregnancy tests. These kits look for evidence of a chemical hormone that is detectable first in the blood and then in the urine. This chemical is called luteinizing hormone, or LH. This hormone is produced in high quantity, called the LH surge, immediately prior to ovulation. Once this chemical is first seen in the urine, ovulation is likely to occur in twelve to twenty-four hours. Detection of the LH surge in the urine is an accurate method of determining ovulation at home.

Endometrial biopsy, discussed earlier, can also be used to evaluate the functioning of your hormones. The procedure will show whether or not the uterus is responding in synchronization with the menstrual cycle.

Almost all of the tests we've discussed in this chapter are part of a standard complete fertility workup. Although it may seem unnecessary to do hormone studies—if, for example, another test has already shown blocked tubes—it is, in fact, critical that no single aspect of a fertility problem be the only focus; often more than one factor is at work, and the second, or even third, might be overlooked if a complete series of tests is not performed. It is usually necessary to complete the full workup and the evaluation before embarking on therapy, because the therapy chosen will depend on exactly what's wrong. The same problem may be treated differently, or not at all, if either partner has another condition demanding treatment. On average, once a couple has been completely evaluated, it turns out that 40 percent of the time the problems are with the man, 40 percent are with the woman, and 20 percent involve both.

THE TREATMENT OF INFERTILITY

Once your doctor has the diagnosis of infertility in hand, he or she can begin treatment. As we've said before, it is possible that in any given couple, more than one cause for infertility may be present, and treatment may vary if there are different combinations of causes. No one wants to plunge into an expensive, complicated treatment regimen only to discover, six months later, that something else entirely was preventing conception. And, always, the bottom line of successful treatment is having a baby. Obtaining a normal sperm count, opening blocked fallopian tubes, and making the uterus ready to nourish and support a fertilized egg are all critical parts of the whole, but none of them matters if correcting them doesn't achieve pregnancy.

Treating Male Infertility

The two main approaches to the treatment of fertility problems in men are hormone therapy and surgery.

If studies reveal a hormone problem, treatment is usually directed toward replacing what's missing or correcting an imbalance. For example, a thyroid deficiency causing poor sperm production is treated with thyroid hormone to bring the level in the body closer to normal.

Sometimes a man will have a poor sperm count, but his physical and laboratory examinations will have turned up no reason for it. In these cases, testosterone, the male hormone, is sometimes administered, but it is generally not very successful. Clomiphene citrate—a chemical also used to stimulate ovulation in women—has been tried in some hormone imbalances but has not proved promising. Current research is attempting to develop new methods of hormone therapy in these cases.

Surgery can be used to repair a varicocele. Each enlarged vein must be tied off individually, in an operation similar to those for hemorrhoids (enlarged veins in the anal canal) and varicose veins (swollen leg veins). The vessels that remain can easily take over the job from the unhealthy ones that are closed off. Varicocele operations can be successful, but it's difficult to know exactly how much help, if any, they will be in any particular man. Varicocele size itself seems to make no difference in how successful the surgery will be. The operation is much less effective for men who have sperm counts of under 60 million per ejaculation. But it has been shown that this procedure is one of the more successful forms of therapy in male infertility; in fact, 60 percent of the time surgical repair of the varicocele will be a success.

Artificial insemination with the sperm of the male partner may be of some help in cases of low sperm count. This technique involves depositing a man's sperm at the woman's cervix without intercourse. (The sperm is collected by masturbation.) The sperm produced can also be washed in a special way to remove certain chemicals that exist within. Often, the washed specimen has a higher concentration of "stronger" sperm. This specially prepared product can then be directly inserted into the uterus. The procedure is called an *intrauterine insemination*. Here, the doctor uses a tiny plastic tube to deposit sperm through the cervix. This may improve the chances of pregnancy because not only is the washed sperm deposited closer to the released egg, but it may be a better quality of sperm than before the wash. Often, healthy *donor* sperm is used, instead of the male partner's poor-quality sperm, if both partners agree. (For more on artificial insemination, see later in this chapter.)

Treating Female Infertility

Failure to ovulate is the most common reproductive problem in women and is thus a frequent cause of infertility. A major development of modern gynecology has been the production of drugs that can stimulate ovulation. Two basic types of medication are available. One is a synthetic chemical, clomiphene citrate, perhaps better known by one of its brand names, Clomid. The other is an extract refined from the urine of postmenopausal women, called pituitary gonadotropin, or human menopausal gonadotropin (HMG). This contains high concentrations of hormones produced in an area of the brain called the hypothalamus. More recently, the one important hypothalamic hormone produced (called FSH) has been isolated by using recombinant technology. Another less common method of ovulation induction includes a technique called "ovarian drilling." In this procedure, laparoscopy is performed and a laser is used to punch holes into the ovaries. This can stimulate the ovaries to ovulate. This is especially true when the woman has the diagnosis of PCOS.

Clomiphene Citrate

The "fertility pill," clomiphene citrate, is used when a woman's ovaries produce estrogen during the first half of the menstrual cycle but then fail to release an egg or produce progesterone during the second half of the cycle. In about 20 percent of infertile couples, this is the main problem to be overcome. Clomiphene can't help women who do not produce estrogen, but it can help women who ovulate regularly but don't produce enough progesterone, and women with luteal phase defects.

It's not known exactly how clomiphene works. Somehow, it apparently nudges the brain and the pituitary gland, so that the pituitary-released gonadotropins stimulate ovulation.

The drug is given in a start-up dose of 50 milligrams a day for five days, starting on the fifth day of the menstrual cycle. Ovulation usually occurs within three days after the drug is stopped. If it doesn't, treatment is repeated the next month—and the next, if necessary—with a slightly higher dose each time. Each month a careful pelvic examination must be done to see if any cysts have formed on the ovaries or to rule out pregnancy, before the next course of treatment is given. Treatment is discontinued for one cycle if ovarian cysts form.

Usually, if the drug is going to work, it does so fairly quickly: Most pregnancies occur within the first three cycles. In properly selected patients, 60 percent can be expected to ovulate following clomiphene therapy, and about 40 percent of these become pregnant. In any one cycle, there is a fifty-fifty chance the patient will become pregnant.

If the drug usually works well, occasionally it works *too* well: About 8 out of 100 pregnancies will be multiple—mostly twins, with a few cases of triplets or more. Ultrasound can usually reveal the number of eggs that have ripened, and, if a couple wishes to avoid a multiple birth, the partners may simply wait until the next cycle to attempt pregnancy. Except for the increased chances of a multiple pregnancy and its attendant risks, there are no bad effects for either mother or child when clomiphene is given. There is no increased risk of the baby having a birth defect, and infant survival and performance are normal.

Pituitary Gonadotropin

The fertility shot, which is now available under many names, is expensive. Some brand names are given as an intramuscular injection (a deeper shot that goes into the muscle), and some are given as a subcuticular injection (right under the skin). Treatment, which involves daily injections for approximately nine days, may cost more than $500 per cycle. Fortunately, it is also effective. Almost 90 percent of women with ovaries capable of responding will ovulate after the following treatment schedule. Most patients will be ready to ovulate after being given two ampules of medication per day for seven to twelve days. Unlike clomiphene, which stimulates the ovaries via the brain, gonadotropin works directly on the ovaries. The amount of estrogen the ovaries are producing with gonadotropin is carefully monitored with frequent blood tests. Then, when critical levels are achieved, a sonogram shows that the follicle of the ovary has matured, and a second drug, human chorionic gonadotropin or HCG, is injected to prompt actual release of the egg, or ovulation.

The pregnancy rate with this method is approximately 50 to 75 percent. There is no evidence of an increased risk of birth defects in babies born to mothers who have undergone this treatment regimen; but here again, there is a risk of multiple pregnancy—as high as one in five (20 percent): 15 percent of the pregnancies that result are with twins and 5 percent are with three or more fetuses. (Of course, since such multiple pregnancies are due to multiple eggs in ovulation, the siblings are not identical.) In multiple pregnancies, there is a higher chance of both prematurity and miscarriage. The miscarriage rate is, in fact, approximately 20 percent.

Other medications may be used in conjunction with either Clomid or gonadotropin when they fail to produce ovulation. They include a type of sugar-reducing (oral hypoglycemic) pill known as metformin or an adrenal hormone known as dexamethasone.

Hyperprolactinemia

Hyperprolactinemia, a problem in which the brain's master gland, the pituitary, causes too much of the hormone prolactin to be produced, has recently been identified. It is believed that microscopic tumors in this area of the brain might be to blame. Normally, prolactin is involved with milk production after birth. At that time, it appears also to be involved with suppressing ovulation—possibly as a kind of built-in birth control that prevents, although not infallibly, a new pregnancy from starting too soon after the last has ended. If this excess hormonal secretion happens when a woman is not nursing, it again interferes with ovulation.

Treatment for hyperprolactinemia, which can be detected by a blood test, involves the use of the drug bromocriptine mesylate. This drug curbs the production of prolactin by the pituitary and shrinks the microtumors. The measurement of prolactin is one of the basic tests in the hormonal evaluation of infertility.

Treatment of Cervical and Uterine Problems

Abnormalities of the cervix can be treated with several procedures: special douches to help sperm migrate; small doses of estrogens to improve cervical mucus; or antibiotics (either in pills to take by mouth or suppositories to insert vaginally) to treat infections. Your treatment will depend on the nature of the problem. Although abnormal antibodies can be detected with special test techniques, a successful way to treat this problem has not yet been discovered.

Treating uterine problems also depends on the nature of the problem. If, for example, the endometrium does not become ready for implantation each month, the problem is generally a hormonal one and may be treated by ovulation-induction techniques such as clomiphene.

Myomectomy

Fibroids may require an operation called myomectomy. This involves surgically removing the tumors from within the muscle mass of the uterine walls. If the fibroids are actually responsible for infertility in a particular case (and this is difficult to determine for sure), this type of surgery can be quite successful. Some congenital abnormalities, such as a bicornuate uterus, can also be treated with surgery, if necessary. An abnormally shaped uterus isn't actually considered to be a common cause of female infertility, however. When it does cause problems, they will more often be repeated miscarriages or prematurity. But most often, a woman born with an unusually shaped uterus will have no problems bearing children.

Tubal Surgery

Treating tube problems may involve various surgical techniques that reopen blocked fallopian tubes or cut away scar tissue that's choking them from the outside. But the success rate is not great: Even in the most experienced hands, pregnancy is achieved only about half the time. The fallopian tubes are extremely delicate structures, and despite meticulous, extraordinarily precise microsurgical techniques, normal egg and sperm movement through them may not occur.

Tubal surgery may also increase the risk of ectopic pregnancy (a pregnancy occurring in the tube itself). This happens only once or twice for every 100 pregnancies in the general population, but it happens in an extremely high 15 to 20 per 100 pregnancies following tubal surgery. Any woman who has undergone tubal surgery and subsequently becomes pregnant must make sure to rule out an ectopic pregnancy as early as possible. If allowed to continue, such a pregnancy can rupture the tube, causing serious internal bleeding and even death. Fortunately, this situation can be discovered more quickly today than ever before by careful measurement of chorionic gonadotropin and with early use of ultrasound.

Before undergoing tubal surgery, everyone involved must understand the risks of the procedure, the likelihood of success, and any alternatives that may exist. Since the success rates of in vitro fertilization have improved, and since, in some cases, in vitro simply bypasses closed tubes and allows for pregnancy, many doctors and patients choose that option.

The Latest Approaches to Treating Infertility

In Vitro Fertilization

"Test tube babies" are the successful result of bypassing malfunctioning fallopian tubes. In vitro fertilization (IVF) is, basically, the attempt to solve the problem of blocked or damaged fallopian tubes by simply leapfrogging their role altogether. This process was first successful with the birth of Louise Brown in 1978, through the work of two Englishmen, Dr. Patrick Steptoe and Robert Edwards. The National Academy of Sciences estimated that between 1 in 200 and 1 in 100 of all American women who are otherwise unable to bear children might be able to do so through IVF. In 1999, doctors performed approximately 90,000 in vitro fertilization procedures in the United States.

The process consists of four basic steps. The egg must be removed from a woman's ovaries, fertilized, allowed to grow a determined amount in a "test tube" (actually a flat, round dish), and then put back into the woman's uterus to implant. From then on, the pregnancy is exactly like any other. The first two steps are relatively simple. Obtaining the ovum and fertilization are usually successful. The harder part comes later. Most unsuccessful attempts at IVF are due to the inability of the embryo to implant in the uterine lining. And in IVF, the general rule of successful infertility treatment remains the same: Half-measures don't count; success is measured by the number of births.

Gonadotropin (Pergonal) is used to stimulate the production of eggs, just as it is for women whose ovaries are not ovulating spontaneously. Very often, this drug causes many eggs to develop, which increases the chances of an IVF success. By obtaining multiple eggs, the chances of fertilizing one that will successfully "take" are increased. Usually, up to three fertilized eggs are replaced in the womb.

In a woman's body, there is only a short period—about three hours—when eggs are fully mature and ripe for fertilization. The woman's cycle, then, must be monitored very carefully, in order to remove the eggs at precisely the right time.

The procedure used in most IVF clinics is fairly standard. Typically, a woman receives gonadotropin three days after menstruation begins, in order to stimulate her ovaries to mature several eggs during the next cycle. Often, the infertility specialist will use a series of additional drugs to tailor the cycle to the individual patient's needs. The approach of ovulation must be monitored extremely closely so that the short hours of prime readiness are not missed. Blood tests check for rising estrogen levels; ultrasound scans of the ovary measure the size of the follicles, the tiny sacs in which the eggs mature. After two weeks, the follicles should be close to the right size, and the woman is given a shot of HCG, which will bring on ovulation within thirty-eight hours.

Just before ovulation occurs, the eggs are carefully removed. Ultrasound is used to guide a needle to the follicles by way of the vagina. This technique, if successful, eliminates the need for the older method: using a laparoscope and anesthesia for egg retrieval. The follicular fluid is then rushed to an adjoining laboratory and checked under a microscope to make sure that at least one egg has been retrieved.

The ova are carefully washed and placed in small, round petri dishes that contain a mixture of nutrients designed to help the eggs grow. These petri dishes are incubated for four to eight hours at body temperature. Meanwhile, sperm that have been spun out of their semen with a centrifuge are washed and incubated in their own dish. After incubation, 500,000 to 1.5 million sperm are transferred into each egg-bearing petri dish. Sometime during the next twenty-four hours, if all goes well, fertilization will occur. If certain male factors are related to the infertility, sometimes success rates can improve if the sperm is injected directly into the egg (microinjection). This is referred to as intracytoplasmic sperm injection, or ICSI.

Just a few hours after fertilization, the fertilized egg (or zygote) is put into a new solution—this one specially formulated to support cell division and the maturing of the embryo. This is a critical time if development is to proceed normally. A proper balance of nutrients, a carefully monitored temperature, and a good supply of oxygen are all essential. Even so, only a small percentage of embryos will develop through the stage at which the embryo has sixteen cells. And sixteen cells is IVF's magic number, for then the embryo is ready for implantation. The doctor who works in the lab and helps the embryo develop is called an embryologist. The embryologist will study the developing blastocyst to determine its quality. The fertilized egg will be rated, and this will determine how many embryos will be transferred. If the fertilized eggs are of high quality, usually one or two will be transferred into the uterus. If they are all poor-quality embryos, the doctors may decide to transfer more than two to improve the chances of success. In the United States in 1999, around 63 percent of births after IVF were singleton births (just one baby); the remainder had two or more.

Of course, these carefully nurtured embryos can't just be plunked back into the uterus at any time. Implantation must be timed exactly so that the endometrium is at the right stage to accept the embryo. Unfortunately, at the current stage of medical knowledge, there is no way to be sure that the test tube embryo has developed at precisely the same speed as it would have in the body. Most failed in vitro attempts are due to a discrepancy between the readiness of the uterus and that of the egg.

Actually depositing the tiny, growing embryo into the uterus requires no anesthetic, but it demands a skilled physician. The uterus does not like things being put into it and responds to such attempts by contracting to push them out. The embryos must be carefully drawn up into a narrow Teflon tube, then slid through the cervix and into the uterus with as little disturbance as possible.

Now the embryo or embryos are on their own. Although the woman takes progesterone to keep the lining of her uterus receptive, there is nothing more that science can do at this point to encourage the embryo to burrow into the endometrium and grow. All that can be done is to watch and wait. Periodic samples of the woman's blood will be taken to check whether HCG levels are going up—a sign of pregnancy.

Many factors that may influence the success rate of IVF. Probably the most important is the age of the woman. For women over forty, the success rate is very low, less than 10 percent. This rate is not much different than with other forms of ovarian stimulation, such as Clomid alone or gonadotropins alone. Another important factor is the fertility center's lab. Finally, success rates are determined by the reason the couple is having IVF. For example, a very young woman with blocked tubes whose husband has a normal sperm count will do very well with IVF, whereas a woman who has had multiple operations on her ovaries and has difficulty producing eggs will do very poorly with IVF. In general, IVF success rates have improved in the United States. Congress enacted the Fertility Clinic Success Rate and Certification Act of 1992, in order to reliably inform the public about specific success rates of various centers in the United States. Currently, the Centers for Disease Control and Prevention (CDC) collaborates with the Society for Assisted Reproductive Technology and others to produce these figures. Women undergoing IVF should check the CDC's Web site to see how their particular clinic measures up. According to 1996 statistics, the IVF success rates were estimated to be approximately 25.9 percent. Since then, most centers report improved numbers, some as high as 50 percent.

Once implantation occurs, as many as one-third of IVF pregnancies spontaneously miscarry in the first three months. But while this is clearly a much higher than normal rate, a few important points must be kept in mind. For one thing, many of the protective mechanisms of in vivo (in the body) fertilization do not exist in the glass dishes of a lab. Normally, cervical mucus and the area where the tubes meet the uterus act as filtering stations, to keep abnormal sperm from getting through. Also, since much greater numbers of sperm are exposed to an egg in the dishes, there is a higher chance of an abnormal fertilization by more than one sperm. Embryos such as these will be spontaneously aborted. It's the body's backup screening to eliminate—early and easily—embryos that could not possibly survive anyway. It is also possible that the various stages of the procedure, including drug treatment and laparoscopy, may damage the lining of the uterus, leading to some of the early miscarriages. As more experience is gained with in vitro fertilization, perhaps these numbers will go down. Today, many labs that do IVF employ the technique known as preimplantation genetics. Here the fertilized egg can be studied for genetic defects prior to implantation into the uterus. If the fertilized egg is defective, it is discarded; if it is normal, it can be transferred into the uterus for implantation.

In vitro fertilization has primarily focused on women with blocked fallopian tubes. Occasionally, though, it has been used to bypass a blockage of the vas deferens—the narrow tubes through which sperm travel from testicles to penis. If the sperm can be removed from the testes through a small incision before the block in the vas deferens, they may then be used to fertilize an egg by the IVF method. (IVF is more efficient in this case than artificial insemination, since there are fewer sperm.)

Artificial Insemination

Artificial insemination and embryo transfer comprise another science-engineered way to beat fertility problems. This method involves depositing semen, via a syringe, right at a woman's cervix. In this country, an estimated 10,000 conceptions a year occur through this very successful method. There are two types of artificial insemination (AI). When the semen is obtained from a woman's partner, it's called homologous artificial insemination (HAI). Heterologous is the term used when the semen is from a donor. To avoid confusion, the latter is usually dubbed AID, for artificial insemination by donor. All donors are screened for genetic defects, infections, acquired immune deficiency syndrome, and fertility potential before their semen is accepted.

The sperm must be frozen or cryopreserved (see further on) and stored for six months, and then the donors are retested. This is a mandate from the Department of Health in many states, to protect the recipients from any infectious diseases that may not be clearly evident at the first time of testing. The AIDS virus, for example, may be present in a donor's sperm during his donation but might not be detectable for several months. Retesting the donor six months later reduces the likelihood of this happening.

HAI may be done if physical or psychological problems prevent a couple from being able to achieve fertilization through intercourse. For example, the sperm from several ejaculates can be pooled and deposited near the cervix in a concentrated form to compensate for poor sperm production. Or the first part of the ejaculate, which tends to contain the most active and well-developed sperm, is separated from the less-potent second part, and the resulting "split ejaculate" is used for insemination.

Artificial insemination by donor may be indicated if the partner is sterile—that is, producing no sperm—or when there is a risk of passing along a hereditary disease in the partner's genes. Artificial insemination by donor is also used when there is severe Rh incompatibility (as explained in chapter 12) and in most cases of deficient sperm production. AID also allows women without partners to bear children.

The availability of a method known as cryopreservation has broadened the potential for artificial insemination. Cryopreservation is a technique of freezing and preserving sperm by immersing tubes of semen in liquid nitrogen that's kept at 320 degrees below zero. At these temperatures, the sperm may be stored for years. Cryobanks make it possible for a man to store his semen before undergoing a vasectomy—in case he should one day in the future wish to have a child.

Cryopreservation is also being tested for use with in vitro fertilization. Several embryos may be frozen in liquid nitrogen, so that they can be thawed and inserted if the initial embryo does not implant or miscarries. This would eliminate the need to repeat the process of egg retrieval and fertilization. Although 30 to 50 percent of embryos do not survive the deep freeze, those that do have a higher chance of implanting. This is because the woman has not been given extra hormones to stimulate ovulation (as is done to retrieve eggs). The result is not only a better chance of implantation, but also a more natural and normal cycle and a healthier endometrium.

Sperm isn't the only reproductive product that can be donated. Eggs may be donated as well. Fertilization of a donor egg by either a male donor's sperm or the partner's sperm may be done in a petri dish, as in standard in vitro techniques. The only difference is that the embryo is put into an infertile woman's uterus, rather than into the female donor's.

Fertilization of a donor egg may also occur in the donor's own body in a rarely done procedure known as embryo transfer. In this method, a fertile woman (the donor) is artificially inseminated with semen from an infertile woman's partner. Five days after fertilization, the embryo is flushed out of the donor's uterus with a nutrient solution and then implanted in the infertile woman's uterus. This painless procedure is called lavage, which means "washing."

There are advantages and disadvantages to embryo transfer. Embryo transfer theoretically enables doctors to extend the childbearing years of women past menopause. It may also allow women whose infertility is caused by both malfunctioning ovaries and blocked fallopian tubes to become pregnant. Women who might pass on a hereditary disease are able to bear children without that risk. (Egg donors, like sperm donors, are carefully screened.) However, there is a risk that flushing may not recover an embryo from the donor's uterus; she could be left with an unwanted pregnancy.

Surrogate Motherhood

In this controversial method of reproduction, a fertile woman may be hired by an infertile couple to bear the couple's child. A surrogate mother may be artificially inseminated with the partner's sperm. Or, in cases in which the woman's ovaries can produce a normal egg but her uterus is not able to carry the child, the surrogate mother may be the recipient of an embryo that has been fertilized either in the other woman's uterus or in a petri dish. The surrogate mother then carries the fetus to full term and, upon delivery, relinquishes the baby to the couple. In theory it is simple, but in fact many legal and emotional problems may arise.

Moral and ethical questions are inevitable with in vitro fertilization, artificial insemination, embryo transfer, and surrogate motherhood, stemming from the replacement of some of the natural steps in the process of reproduction with artificial methods. Artificial insemination bypasses sexual intercourse, while in vitro fertilization not only does that but replaces tubal fertilization with fertilization in a dish in a lab. Many of the arguments concerning these reproductive technologies are similar to the ethical arguments over other "unnatural" life-support aids, like the artificial heart. These are issues a couple should consider, together with their doctor and maybe their pastor, rabbi, or even lawyer before making a decision.

The possibilities for procreation with the use of in vitro fertilization and artificial insemination are vast. The methods themselves are often time-consuming, extremely costly, and psychologically challenging. The moral questions raised may be difficult to wrestle with. And in some cases, the legality of these possibilities has yet to be considered. But modern medicine is for the first time able to give children to some couples who would otherwise be childless. To an infertile couple yearning for a family, that possibility may make all the struggles worthwhile.

Epilogue

We have worked in the field of reproductive health for over a combined fifty years. During that time, we have seen almost every aspect of obstetrics benefit from the tremendous advances in medical knowledge. Many of the medical discoveries discussed in this book simply didn't exist four decades ago: the now widely available procedure of amniocentesis and chorionic villus sampling that lets us check on the health of the unborn fetus; the advanced fertility tests with which we can pinpoint many problems of conception; the still-developing techniques of in vitro fertilization that allow previously infertile couples to achieve pregnancy; and the sophisticated monitors that alert us to the early signs of distress in a baby before or during delivery. Countless couples have healthy babies today because of these and other technological wonders.

But it's not only high-tech machines and sophisticated procedures that have brought the miraculous process of having a baby out of the dark ages and into the forefront of science. We have learned so much more about the intricate functioning of the human body: subtle details of how the organs of reproduction work; how a fetus is first conceived and then develops; how the complex interrelationship between mother and fetus is maintained. And we have learned so much more about the tremendous impact seemingly minor things can have on a woman's overall health and fertility—eating correctly during pregnancy, for example, and avoiding cigarettes, alcohol, and all but doctor-approved drugs.

If a woman wants to conceive, knowledge of conception, fertility, and implantation is available.

If pregnancy is to be avoided, contraception and abortion techniques have been developed and are readily available. Once pregnancy is established, the science of neonatology can be a great help in guaranteeing a healthy, normal baby.

Obstetrical prenatal care has advanced to the point where maternal mortality is practically zero. Perinatal and pediatric care are lowering the infant perinatal mortality rates. Advances in obstetrical analgesia, anesthesia, and the Lamaze technique have made delivery a safe, often comfortable, and conscious experience.

What is also important and striking about these findings is that women have so much control over most of them. So while technology has given health professionals new tools that have improved each woman's odds of bearing a healthy baby, increased knowledge has given women, too, a new measure of responsibility for their pregnancies. Today, women and their doctors find themselves working as a team to ensure that a pregnancy proceeds as smoothly and healthily as possible.

Our goal is to achieve healthier pregnancies—during which a woman will feel happy and healthy and be able to handle most of the same activities she has always handled. And, finally, our goal is healthier babies who come into the world with the best possible chance for a long, productive life.

It's a great time to be an obstetrician!

It's a great time to have a baby!

Index